T0372041

NEUROPSYCHOLOGY OF SPACE

NEUROPSYCHOLOGY OF SPACE

Spatial Functions of the Human Brain

ALBERT POSTMA

Experimental Psychology, Helmholtz Institute, Utrecht University, Utrecht, The Netherlands

Department of Neurology, University Medical Center, Utrecht, The Netherlands

Korsakov Center Slingedael, Rotterdam, The Netherlands

INEKE J. M. VAN DER HAM

Experimental Psychology, Helmholtz Institute, Utrecht University, Utrecht, The Netherlands

Department of Health, Medical and Neuropsychology Leiden University, Leiden, The Netherlands

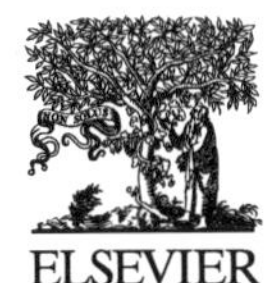

AMSTERDAM • BOSTON • HEIDELBERG • LONDON
NEW YORK • OXFORD • PARIS • SAN DIEGO
SAN FRANCISCO • SINGAPORE • SYDNEY • TOKYO
Academic Press is an imprint of Elsevier

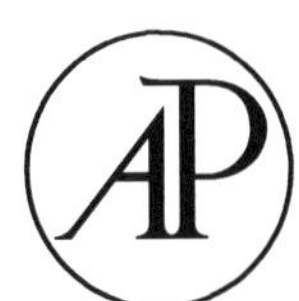

Academic Press is an imprint of Elsevier
125 London Wall, London EC2Y 5AS, United Kingdom
525 B Street, Suite 1800, San Diego, CA 92101-4495, United States
50 Hampshire Street, 5th Floor, Cambridge, MA 02139, United States
The Boulevard, Langford Lane, Kidlington, Oxford OX5 1GB, United Kingdom

Notices

Knowledge and best practice in this field are constantly changing. As new research and experience broaden our understanding, changes in research methods, professional practices, or medical treatment may become necessary.

Practitioners and researchers must always rely on their own experience and knowledge in evaluating and using any information, methods, compounds, or experiments described herein. In using such information or methods they should be mindful of their own safety and the safety of others, including parties for whom they have a professional responsibility.

To the fullest extent of the law, neither the Publisher nor the authors, contributors, or editors, assume any liability for any injury and/or damage to persons or property as a matter of products liability, negligence or otherwise, or from any use or operation of any methods, products, instructions, or ideas contained in the material herein.

British Library Cataloguing-in-Publication Data
A catalogue record for this book is available from the British Library

Library of Congress Cataloging-in-Publication Data
A catalog record for this book is available from the Library of Congress

ISBN: 978-0-12-801638-1

For Information on all Academic Press publications
visit our website at https://www.elsevier.com/

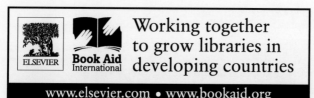

Publisher and Acquisition Editor: Nikki Levy
Editorial Project Manager: Barbara makinster
Production Project Manager: Susan Li
Designer: Greg Harris

CONTENTS

LIST OF CONTRIBUTORS

H. Chris Dijkerman
Experimental Psychology, Helmholtz Institute, Utrecht University, Utrecht, The Netherlands; Department of Neurology, University Medical Center, Utrecht, The Netherlands

Michiel H.G. Claessen
Experimental Psychology, Helmholtz Institute, Utrecht University, Utrecht, The Netherlands; Rudolf Magnus Institute of Neuroscience and Center of Excellence for Rehabilitation Medicine, University Medical Center Utrecht and Rehabilitation Center De Hoogstraat, Utrecht, The Netherlands

Annika Hellendoorn
Department of Education & Pedagogy, Utrecht University, Utrecht, The Netherlands

Marian J. Jongmans
Department of Education & Pedagogy, Utrecht University, Utrecht, The Netherlands

Jan J. Koenderink
Experimental Psychology, Helmholtz Institute, Utrecht University, Utrecht, The Netherlands; Laboratory of Experimental Psychology, University of Leuven, Leuven, Belgium

Hanna Mulder
Department of Education & Pedagogy, Utrecht University, Utrecht, The Netherlands

Tanja C.W. Nijboer
Experimental Psychology, Helmholtz Institute, Utrecht University, Utrecht, The Netherlands; Rudolf Magnus Institute of Neuroscience and Center of Excellence for Rehabilitation Medicine, University Medical Center Utrecht and Rehabilitation Center De Hoogstraat, Utrecht, The Netherlands; Department of Rehabilitation Medicine, University Medical Center, Utrecht, The Netherlands

Ora Oudgenoeg-Paz
Department of Education & Pedagogy, Utrecht University, Utrecht, The Netherlands

Albert Postma
Experimental Psychology, Helmholtz Institute, Utrecht University, Utrecht, The Netherlands; Department of Neurology, University Medical Center, Utrecht, The Netherlands; Korsakov Center Slingedael, Rotterdam, The Netherlands

Carla Ruis
Experimental Psychology, Helmholtz Institute, Utrecht University, Utrecht, The Netherlands; Department of Neurology, University Medical Center, Utrecht, The Netherlands

Francesco Ruotolo
Experimental Psychology, Helmholtz Institute, Utrecht University, Utrecht, The Netherlands; Laboratory of Cognitive Science and Immersive Virtual Reality, Second University of Naples, Naples, Italy

Marijn E. Struiksma
Utrecht Institute of Linguistics OTS, Utrecht University, Utrecht, The Netherlands

Esther van den Berg
Experimental Psychology, Helmholtz Institute, Utrecht University, Utrecht, The Netherlands; Department of Neurology, Erasmus MC University Medical Center, Rotterdam, The Netherlands

Ineke J.M. van der Ham
Experimental Psychology, Helmholtz Institute, Utrecht University, Utrecht, The Netherlands; Department of Health, Medical and Neuropsychology Leiden University, Leiden, The Netherlands

Stefan Van der Stigchel
Experimental Psychology, Helmholtz Institute, Utrecht University, Utrecht, The Netherlands

Nathan van der Stoep
Experimental Psychology, Helmholtz Institute, Utrecht University, Utrecht, The Netherlands

INTRODUCTION

Po says: you will find what you have lost but first you must remember where you have left it.

(Reading from a fortune cookie at a Chinese restaurant somewhere in the deep southwest)

SPACE IS SPECIAL

Our lives very much depend on our ability to perceive, remember, and act upon where things are in the world. From finding the things you want to buy in the supermarket, to packing them in your car; from recalling the way to your hotel during a weekend trip, to navigating the newest update of your computer's operating system; from combing your hair in the mirror, to solving a geometric problem during a university exam; each challenge requires some form of mental handling of spatial information.

Dealing with everyday life's spatial assignments may not always run very smoothly. One of us (Albert Postma) conducted a study some years ago in which he asked visitors to a shopping mall if they ever encountered problems in remembering where they parked their car (Postma, van Oers, Back, & Plukaard, 2012). Close to 50% of the interviewed participants reported occasional to regular difficulties. When tested more objectively on their efficiency to find their car back after the actual shopping mall visit, 15% of the participants made a considerable detour. Though annoying, these problems usually do not have a huge impact on our lives. We can typically find the desired object after some effort. In turn, we can collect additional cues such as road signs and names, in order to find the way when running the danger of getting lost. In contrast, various forms of brain damage do have a really profound effect on spatial orientation, memory, and reasoning. The central theme of this book is what happens to spatial cognitive functions after either global or local disturbances of the central nervous system. Importantly we intend not just to sketch the clinical profile for a given spatial disorder. We also try to give broader cognitive, neurocognitive, and applied perspectives. As such we use the described cases and groups of patients as models for further understanding of the (spatial) cognitive domain at stake. We will discuss how specific neuropsychological disorders inspire and can be used to modify relevant theoretical frameworks, and reversely, how theoretical frameworks can be used to better understand neuropsychological impairments. Both work with patient groups and exemplary cases will be featured. This can offer invaluable neurocognitive insights. Moreover, it will also illustrate methodological issues of neuropsychology at large (ie, the ins and outs of single case methodology, lesion overlap approaches in patient groups). Finally, we intend to also include an applied perspective: how does spatial cognition operate in the real world; what is the ecological validity of certain tasks; which daily life problems do neuropsychological patients encounter in certain domains; which rehabilitation possibilities for spatial functions exist; what is the potential of new techniques (virtual reality; GPS tracking) to support spatial cognition?

ON THE HISTORY OF SPACE (AT LEAST OF THE CURRENT BOOK ON SPACE)

The origins for this book go back to the first years of the 21st century when one of us (Albert Postma) started a research program on spatial cognition at Utrecht University, focusing on a variety of spatial functions, supported by a grant from the Dutch science foundation (NWO). He later was joined by Ineke van der Ham who completed her PhD thesis on the hemispheric lateralization of spatial functions within that program and stayed on as an assistant professor. From 1999 on we have been coordinating and giving lectures in the honours Bachelor course Spatial Cognition, University College Utrecht. A central idea in these lecture series as well as in the accompanying research program has been that spatial information processing is intrinsic to all cognitive domains: perception, attention, motor action, memory and representation, reasoning, and communication. This book intends to do justice to this idea and therefore entails a varied functional approach to the spatial cognition. We will trace space across the cognitive domains, and where possible try to highlight interconnections. Of course, throughout the chapters the special place of spatial cognition within neuropsychological research will be highlighted.

A MAP OF THE BOOK

In Chapter 1, A Sense of Space, Albert Postma and Jan Koenderink sketch an example from daily life that serves to set the floor for several conceptual questions that will be returned to later in that chapter. In particular it illustrates how different cognitive domains encompass a spatial element. A foremost question addressed in Chapter 1, A Sense of Space, concerns what is space and how do we measure it? This question has been at the center of many philosophical debates throughout the centuries. Some are briefly addressed here: is space absolute or relative; is it real or ideal; is the sense of space innate or does it have to be learned by an accumulation of experiences? This last debate returns in Chapter 9, How Children Learn to Discover Their Environment: An Embodied Dynamic Systems Perspective on the Development of Spatial Cognition, in which the development of spatial cognition is further addressed. Regarding the measurement of space the notion of reference frames is essential: we need to determine places, directions, and relations always with respect to some reference object or frame. Mentally we appear to be able to choose from a large repertoire of references frames, depending on the task at hand. Postma and Koenderink in Chapter 1, A Sense of Space, present a noninclusive overview of possible reference frames and related task domains.

One of the main channels through which we interact with space is our visual system. In Chapter 2, On Inter- and Intrahemispheric Differences in Visuospatial Perception, Ineke van der Ham and Francesco Ruotolo discuss the spatial features of visual perception. In the first part of this chapter they address a prominent dichotomy within visuospatial perception, that of categorical and coordinate spatial relations. We can perceive specific spatial situations in terms of categories (eg, "left of," "above") or metric properties (distances between elements), which are strongly linked to our left or right hemisphere, respectively. Reference frames also return in this chapter, as another important dichotomy within this domain. In particular, the distinction between egocentric and allocentric frames of reference is described. This distinction as well has a solid foundation in dissociated neural correlates.

Touch is particularly relevant to space very near to our bodies, peripersonal and/or body space, a topic thoroughly discussed in Chapter 3, On Feeling and Reaching: Touch, Action and Body Space. Chris Dijkerman shares his thoughts on peripersonal space, a prominent topic within neuropsychology. In addition to patient studies, also experiments are presented in which bodily illusions are induced in healthy participants. Peripersonal space is not just there for processing touch. It also constitutes a primary control center over spatiomotor actions. Many patient studies were consulted in the theoretical framing of the functions of the ventral and the dorsal stream and how they are involved in perception versus action.

In Chapter 4, Multisensory Perception and the Coding of Space, Nathan van der Stoep, Tanja Nijboer, and Albert Postma show that it is relevant to study spatial senses not only in isolation, such as within vision (see chapter: On Inter- and Intrahemispheric Differences in Visuospatial Perception) or touch (see chapter: On Feeling and Reaching: Touch, Action, and Body Space), but also in combination with one another. Apart from vision and touch, audition also provides us with vital spatial information, typically in combination with one of the other spatial senses. Special focus is given to the mechanisms of multisensory integration and how multisensory stimulation may help reduce or overcome some of the spatial impairments caused by cerebral brain damage. van der Stoep and colleagues also elaborate on what happens when one loses a sense completely. A closer look is taken at the effects of either visual or auditory deprivation on spatial cognition. The complexities of integrating different senses are all the more clear in the case of deafness or blindness.

Being able to perceive spatial information is only a first step, we also have to attend to it, in order to act on it. In Chapter 5, Spatial Attention and Eye Movements, Stefan Van der Stigchel and Tanja Nijboer therefore discuss the domain of spatial attention. In particular, eye movements allow for examination of spatial attention and are therefore the key variable in many spatial attention experiments. One of the landmark disorders of spatial cognition in the past century has been spatial neglect: patients who are completely unresponsive toward one side of space. This is typically explained in terms of spatial attentional failure. In Chapter 5, Spatial Attention and Eye Movements, the authors present a daring new theory on spatial neglect: a deficit in spatial remapping.

Once perceived and attended to, we can process spatial information in many different ways. One of the most prominent ways to do this is by spatial language. Marijn Struiksma and Albert Postma discuss this topic in Chapter 6, Tell Me Where to Go: On the Language of Space. We communicate about space, using spatial language at various scales: explaining a route to a tourist ("take a left turn here," "go north for three blocks"), and also telling your friend where to find the car keys ("on the kitchen table"). In this chapter the authors discuss how different sources of information are used to build representations of space, and what linguistic processes can tell us about these representations. Remarkably, reference frames appear to play a role not just in perception and memory but also in language understanding. Effective communication critically depends on choosing the appropriate reference frame.

A different way to process perceived and attended spatial input is to encode it into memory. Albert Postma and Ineke van der Ham elaborate on spatial memory in Chapter 7, Keeping Track of Where Things Are in Space: The Neuropsychology of Object Location Memory. A discussion of general memory theory highlights the importance of spatial information in working memory. Many of the spatial memory studies, some of which performed at Utrecht University, have focused on object location memory in particular. This memory has the distinct elements of memorizing object identities, object locations (which can be either categorical or coordinate, as discussed in chapter: On Inter- and Intrahemispheric Differences in Visuospatial Perception), and the connection between objects and their positions. Experimental studies in both healthy and brain-damaged patients have contributed to these findings.

In Chapter 8, Navigation Ability, Ineke van der Ham and Michiel Claessen go from more static spatial memory to dynamic spatial memory. Navigation includes interaction with space at a much larger scale: the process of finding your way around in the world. In the first part of this chapter they discuss the leading theoretical issues concerning navigation ability. Again, reference frames, or "perspective taking" are highly relevant here. The second part concerns the clinical perspective on navigation ability: a significant proportion of neuropsychological patients have specific complaints with regard to navigation. Yet, standardized diagnostic and treatment tools are currently lacking. The authors provide suggestions on how experimental and clinical findings can be used to work on the development of these much-needed tools.

The topics discussed in this book concern human cognition in general, but in Chapter 9, How Children Learn to Discover Their Environment: An Embodied Dynamic Systems Perspective on the Development of Spatial Cognition, Hanna Mulder, Ora Oudgenoeg-Paz, Annika Hellendoorn, and Marian Jongmans provide an overview of spatial cognition from a developmental perspective. In this chapter, embodiment, spatial memory, orientation, and navigation are discussed with a specific focus on children. In particular, the authors pay attention to experimental characteristics of task that are used to examine these domains for young children, and what methodological issues should be kept in mind. The overview offered in Chapter 9, How Children Learn to Discover Their Environment: An Embodied Dynamic Systems Perspective on the Development of Spatial Cognition, certainly also bears on the philosophical debate briefly addressed in Chapter 1, A Sense of Space, on the innateness of our spatial ability.

As this book is centered on neuropsychology, the final chapter concerns a discussion of how spatial cognition finds its place in clinical neuropsychology. In Chapter 10, Space in Neuropsychological Practice, Esther van den Berg and Carla Ruis, discuss case studies with specific spatial impairments and describe how such impairments are typically dealt with in clinical practice. A variety of standardized tests concerning spatial abilities is available, but technological advances such as virtual reality and other digital aids can be very helpful. The authors provide recommendations for both testing and treating spatial problems.

SPACE, THE FINAL FRONTIER: CONCLUDING THOUGHTS

There is a growing need to place the spatial functions of the brain within a broader context: philosophical, neuroscientific, comparative, geographical, cognitive psychological, and neuropsychological. We realize we have not done justice to all of these fields. We have chosen the clinical approach as a leading theme but always in combination with a cognitive and neurocognitive emphasis. We hope the book will be of interest to both researchers and clinicians with an interest in the human cognitive functioning in the spatial domain, from a broad range of backgrounds. We may finish here with a final thought on where exactly is spatial cognition in the human brain. This book shows that the human brain is capable of a wide repertoire of spatial mental operations and entails a large, dedicated neural circuitry underlying these operations. It is too simple to say that this circuitry is only found in the right side of the brain. Also the left hemisphere supports cognitive operations, which we could label as spatial in a broad sense. Given its versatility and relevance for everyday functioning as well as survival in general, the conclusion could be "spatial cognition is all over the brain." After finishing this book this only seems logical.

Albert Postma and Ineke J.M. van der Ham

Utrecht, April 1, 2016

REFERENCE

Postma, A., van Oers, M., Back, F., & Plukaard, S. (2012). Losing your car in the parking lot: Spatial memory in the real world. *Applied Cognitive Psychology, 26*(5), 680–686. Available from http://dx.doi.org/10.1002/acp.2844.

CHAPTER 1

A Sense of Space

Albert Postma[1,2,3] and Jan J. Koenderink[1,4]
[1]Experimental Psychology, Helmholtz Institute, Utrecht University, Utrecht, The Netherlands
[2]Department of Neurology, University Medical Center, Utrecht, The Netherlands
[3]Korsakov Center Slingedael, Rotterdam, The Netherlands
[4]Laboratory of Experimental Psychology, University of Leuven, Leuven, Belgium

We tend to perceive and understand the world in a spatial manner: distances, orientations, places, and sizes. These spatial features are integrated in a three-dimensional framework, and are extended to build internal notions of composite objects, layouts, and trajectories. In order to further appreciate the spatial activities of the human brain, let us start with a common example from daily life. Say your best friend has moved to a new place, a cute cottage on the edge of town. She invites you to come over next Sunday for a drink and gives you a detailed, though not necessarily comprehensive or accurate, route description. This first part of the example poses already a main decision to be made: do you keep the verbal instructions or do you somehow turn them in a more map-like representation? Choosing the first option will force you to translate the verbal commands in appropriate spatial behaviors along the way. Choosing the second raises another question: what exactly is the nature of a spatial representation. Which are its intrinsic qualities and how does it map to the outside world, that is, physical space?

Whatever your representational decision, you take the next step in reaching your friend's new place. Since the route is quite long, you choose to take the car. Finding your car keys becomes the next challenge, requiring spatial search (see chapter 4: Multisensory Perception and the Coding of Space). The difficulty here lies in scanning the visual world with a multitude of objects and locations trying to minimize the length and number of eye movements. Search efficiency clearly would benefit if you have some sort of spatial memory, either of where you placed them an hour ago or where you typically keep them (see chapter 7: Keeping Track of Where Things are in Space—The Neuropsychology of Object Location Memory). Keeping track of where we left things is a typical burden of daily life (Fig. 1.1).

Neuropsychology of Space.
DOI: http://dx.doi.org/10.1016/B978-0-12-801638-1.00001-X

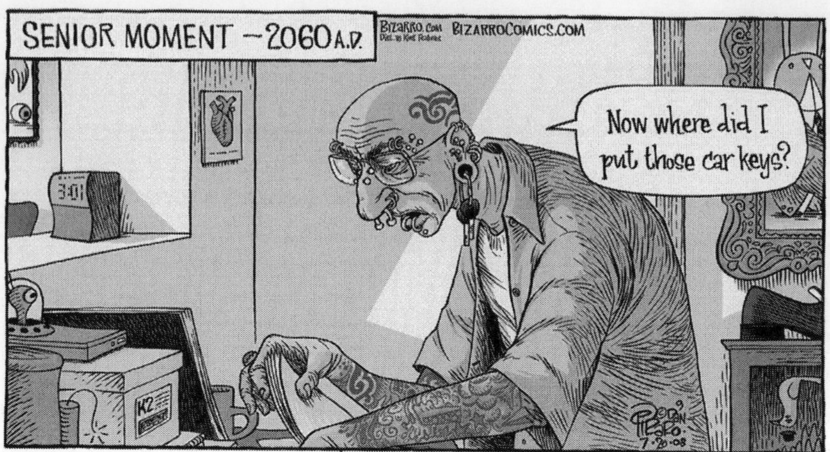
SENIOR MOMENT —2060 A.D.
BIZARROCOMICS.COM
Now where did I put those car keys?

Figure 1.1 Senior moment, from http://bizarro.com/, illustrating daily life difficulties in remembering where things are.

Assuming you have managed to find your keys you can get on your way. Negotiating traffic in a dynamic world requires a multitude of spatial abilities. We need to accurately perceive distances and orientations (see chapter 2: On inter and intra hemispheric differences in visuospatial perception), both in order to avoid collisions and to take the appropriate turns. The spatial world is dominated by the visual sense but our other sensory systems also offer marked sources of spatial information. When focusing eyes and attention straight ahead, a car horn from the left will force you to quickly reorient and integrate sound with the vision of a rapidly approaching vehicle. Multisensory integration is a special capacity of the brain's spatial system (see chapter 4: Multisensory perception and the coding of space). While seemingly effortless and inevitable, connecting one modality to another is quite a complex feat. In the given case auditory space is coded quite differently than visual space even in the early perceptual stages (ie, a tonotopic coding vs a retinotopic coding). Hence, the question may arise as to how we have learned to merge the spatial inputs from our senses (see Box 1.2; see also chapter 9: How Children Learn to Discover Their Environment: An Embodied Dynamic Systems Perspective on the Development of Spatial Cognition).

Finally, you have managed to arrive at your friend's new place. You spent the rest of the afternoon discussing work, holidays, other friends, news of the world, and maybe your efforts in reaching the place. After a pleasant afternoon you drive back home again. Did you retain anything from your earlier exposure to the route? In other words how does our navigation system learn and maintain route information (see chapter 8: Navigation Ability)? Notice, that on your way home the route has to be travelled in reverse order. Recognizing when to take a turn now might depend on your ability to change spatial perspective. A particular problem occurs when suddenly part of the way is blocked and you have to plan a detour. Much later than intended, and completely exhausted you arrive home. Without thinking you drop your keys in a rather unusual place—the fridge when grasping a can of beer. Hence the next day a strenuous spatial search will start again.

Our sense of space is critical for successful interaction with the outside world, whether we use it to estimate the distance towards an approaching car, program the grasping movement to pick up a can of beer, plan a route towards a new destination, or remember a route travelled many times. Spatial cognition is concerned with the acquisition, organization, utilization, and revision of knowledge about spatial environments. Spatial cognition involves the set of mental processes underlying spatial behaviors and thinking. In order to be labeled as "spatial," information or the behavior it supports needs to involve processing of features such as place/location, size/shape, direction/order, extent/continuity, relations/configurations, connectivity/sequence, and hierarchy/dimensionality (Montello & Raubal, 2012). Admittedly there is the danger of circularity here by defining spatial cognition using terms like "space" or "spatial." It is not our aim to give an encompassing, unequivocal definition, but rather to offer a more global notion of what the concept spatial cognition is about.

1.1 ON THE DEFINITION AND MEASUREMENT OF (PHYSICAL) SPACE

Of course a real understanding of spatial cognition and the human sense of space should begin with specifying what exactly space is and how we can measure it. A formal definition of "space" would be something like *structured simultaneous presence*. This is a very general definition that applies to formal (or mathematical), physical and mental spaces alike. When mentioning "physical space" one usually has the intuition that it is something that is infinitely and continuously extended. This feeling is perhaps best characterized by Newton's definition II in the *Scholium* (Newton, 1687). Notice that Newton obviously struggled to come up with a clear definition. So will you, just try! Space has seemingly mysterious properties both in the large and in the small. The Euclidean plane of high school geometry has no boundary and its area is "infinite." The surface of the earth is also unbounded—you can't fall off—but its area is only 510,072,000 km^2. An arbitrarily small patch of the Euclidean plane contains infinitely many points. One calls the plane "continuous" in contradistinction to the chessboard, a "discrete" space containing only 64 points ("fields"), a "point" being—in Euclid's definition—"that which has no parts." In the centuries following the various notions of boundedness, the infinite, and the nature of the continuum have been extensively studied by mathematicians (Bell, 2005; Rucker, 1995). These topics were already discussed by the Presocratics (Lloyd, 1970), but it is probably correct to say that they continue to be as mysterious as they ever were. When Bernhard Riemann delivered his famous habilitation lecture (Riemann, 1854), he mentioned that we know only two spaces by immediate intuition, namely "the space we move in," and the "space of colors." "The space we move in" is what people usually mean when they mention "physical space." It should not be confused with the concept of "space" used in modern physics, which is a formal, mathematical structure. "Physical space" is a naive, folk-science notion. Perhaps one should say "real life" instead of "physical," for that is usually implied, but we will use the conventional "physical" here. "Physical space" is a concept that covers a wide area of phenomenology.

Closely linked to the question of how we define space, there is the question of how to measure it. Throughout human history almost every culture has developed or adopted some system(s) of spatial measurement, both for economic, political, and cultural reasons. The most important are measurements of length, size, area, and volume. One often uses length and size interchangeably, but typically size relates to specific objects, whereas length can also be used to indicate a gap between different objects. Thus a sieve[1] is an instrument that applies to size, but not to length. In many cultures another important spatial property is the angle, although it is not necessarily quantified. This is because right angles tend

[1] A sieve (or "sifter") is a device that has numerous holes of some fixed size. It will pass objects that fit through the holes whereas it will stop larger ones from passing through. Thus it serves to separate smallish elements from large ones, say mustard seeds from peas. A template is a device that lets you check shape. A simple example it a taut wire—which is "straight"—commonly used by gardeners to ensure well-formed garden paths or lawns. Dividers (or "compasses") are used to compare or transfer distances from one place to another, for instance in drafting, or comparing distances on a map.

to be important, whereas others are merely considered "off." This does not apply to length, area, and volume, which range between very small (or even "nothing") to very large (or even "everything"), they denote "infinite" ranges, whereas angles live in a finite—although boundless—range.

The basis of measurement is *comparison*. There are many occasions where a mere comparison suffices, and a measurement proper is not even required. Common examples are the use of sieves, templates, straight-edges or taut wires, dividers, and so forth. The most basic comparison is that of *spatial coincidence*, that is, two objects are identical with respect to the spatial property central in the comparison.

Every measurement consists of a comparison with a conventional gauge, or reference object. A gauge object can take on many forms, but it is always used in essentially the same way. An observer notices a "fit," that is to say, the act of comparison yields a judgment of "equality," or "no difference." This is the basis of virtually every form of measurement, not just spatial ones. In physics one recognizes only two types of measurement, namely, the counting of discrete objects, and "pointer readings," for example, determining a distance value by reading out the corresponding mark on a ruler. Because pointer reading involves the judgment of "no difference," for example, the coincidence of a landmark with the mark on a scale, it involves no phenomenal qualities. Consequently, Sir Arthur Eddington famously argued (Eddington, 1927) that all physical quantities are completely meaningless. Physical quantities are not *qualia*. The physicist reasons formally from pointer reading to pointer reading, allowing for very precise quantitative predictions.

Consider a simple example of measurement in line with the foregoing. Because beer is perhaps the most efficient way to conserve grain, beer has been an important commodity in various cultures. Beer has value in all kinds of bartering, so one needs to be able to quantify it. The Egyptians used beer and bread as the currency to pay slaves, tradesmen, priests, and public officials. Their economy was based on grain. Different from bread, beer cannot be counted, so one needs a method of measurement. An obvious way to do this is to select a suitable jar and call it "unit beer measure." This jug is kept in an official place (eg, a temple), and is constantly guarded by absolutely trustworthy heavyweights. When the jug is used, an official is present to ensure that it is filled in the standard way. When the standard jug is emptied into another, larger, one, one may scratch a mark to indicate the "full measure." Thus all beer merchants can obtain a "secondary standard," which necessitates a special police to make sure that they keep it honest. No "theory of volume" is necessary to implement this technology. All that is needed is the judgment that the standard jug is full. Any fool is able to check that.

Notice that there are other ways to measure amounts of beer. For instance, it is not that hard to implement a method based on *weight*, choosing and guarding a standard stone. If you have both a standard volume and a standard weight, you might discover that the same full measure always has the same weight. It is these remarkable empirical facts between physical quantities that render such measurements *useful*. One should not fail to appreciate the fundamental importance of this point, however straightforward it might seem.

Consider the measurement of another spatial property: length. Here most cultures have used a conventional rod, or a rope with two knots. A rope can be used to measure length "around the corner," whereas the rod only applies to stretches that are fully exposed. You can try to find a rod that has exactly the same length as two copies of the standard rod placed in tandem. Or you can break a copy of the standard in two equal parts. Thus you can have rods of "two rods long" and rods of "half a rod long." In advanced cultures this leads to rods with a series of marks, so called "rulers," that make it easily possible to estimate arbitrary lengths. Notice that all that is ever needed to implement all this are judgments of spatial coincidences. No phenomenal qualities are involved. These are examples of Eddington's "pointer readings."

Why did length measurement with a rod become so useful? Well, mainly because *a rod is a rod*. This sounds trivial, but it is not. The point is that a rod does not change when you displace it over arbitrary distances, or when you put it in various spatial attitudes. Thus the rod allows you to compare the height of a building with its frontal width, or the size of a Celtic sword to a Roman one, even when these artifacts are a thousand miles apart. This is very remarkable if you come to think of it. And convenient too! (Fig. 1.2).

Length and volume fairly easily yield to the method of comparison. This is very different with *area*. Because areas come in many different shapes, it is not at all obvious what gauge object to use. There may be infinite possibilities! Historically one has employed various measures such as the "*Morgen*" (used in Germany, Poland, the Netherlands, and the Dutch colonies, including South Africa and Taiwan). A "morning"—the literal translation—is the amount of land tillable by one man behind an

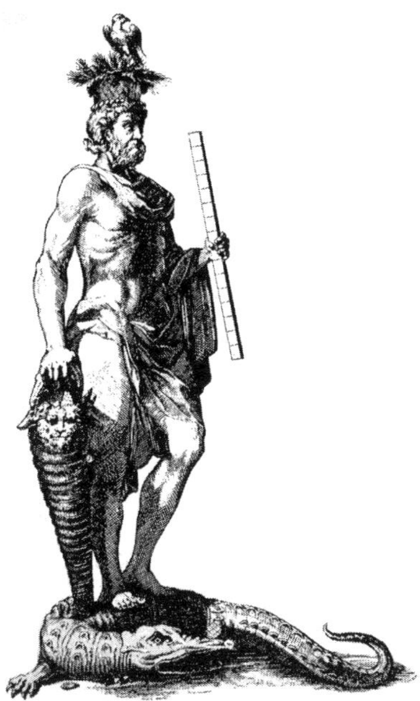

Figure 1.2 Graeco-Egyptian God Serapis with measuring rod. Notice the equal subdivisions. This rod allows one to define "length" (of anything) in terms of pointer readings.

ox in the morning hours of the day. Other measures include the number of olive trees a piece of land will accommodate. Early geometrical methods were often based on the *perimeter*. For instance, when Queen Dido was stranded on the coast of North Africa, she asked the Berber King Iardas for a bit of land as a temporary refuge, only as much as could be encompassed by an oxhide. She arrived at an agreement, and proceeded to cut the hide in thin strips, enough to encircle a nearby hill. This famously solved the isoperimetric problem—the circle has the shortest perimeter for a given area, and established the city of Carthage c. 814 BCE. A perimeter measure can be made to work for areas, but only if you use it only for a specific set of shapes, say squares or circles. A common instance is the forester measuring tree trunks with a tape measure. But perimeter-based area measures remain inconvenient. For instance, a square of twice the circumference of a unit square has four times the area of that unit square.

In agricultural societies area measurement was so important that the science of geometry (literally "land measurement") became established.

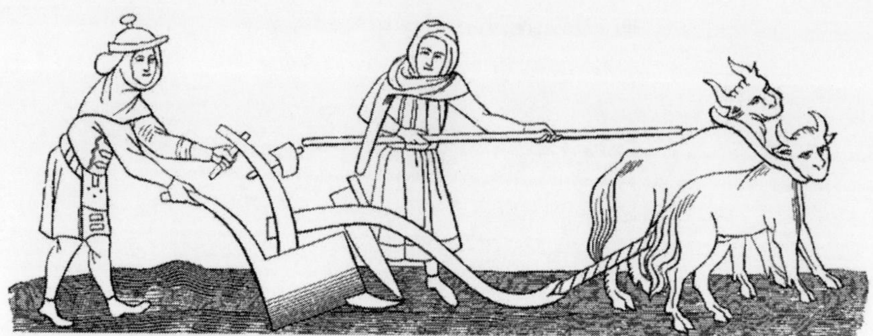

Figure 1.3 Anglo-Saxon plowmen using a rod.

This enabled areas of land to be measured by angle and length, albeit at the cost of nontrivial calculations. This can be considered the first step towards a formal description of space. A *geometry* is a set of rules with which we describe size, shape, position of figures, and the properties of space. Thus, although our current formal theories are remote from "land measurement," *geometry* remains an apt term (Fig. 1.3).

Although the official units for length, and so forth, are extremely important, it should not be forgotten that there are also convenient standards that are always literally "at hand." We mean such units as "a thumb," "a palm," or "an arm," "a step," "an hour's walk." These depend upon the fact that all humans are roughly of the same size. Even better, a mature human remains at fairly standard size for dozens of years. As Helmholtz remarked, "we use our legs as dividers." A "pint" was the volume—of beer—that was nourishing, but not too much. Aren't we all in sympathy with that?[2] Such "natural units" have been used for centuries in the Western world, and are still in frequent use in many cultures. Of course, the basic principle remains unchanged, it is only the "gauge objects" that are differently defined. The fundamental judgment is invariably that of equality, typically the spatial coincidence of two objects. No *qualia* are involved.

So where then did the meanings go? Well *they took refuge in the gauge objects*. The method of comparison manages to dodge matters of meaning

[2] Nowadays an "imperial pint" is 568.26 cm^3. Does that "make sense" to you? Of course, it isn't designed to do so. "568.26" is simply a meaningless number. "1" pint of beer is what many persons "understand." Here the meaningless number "1" stands for the gauge object "pint," which is "nourishing, but not too much."

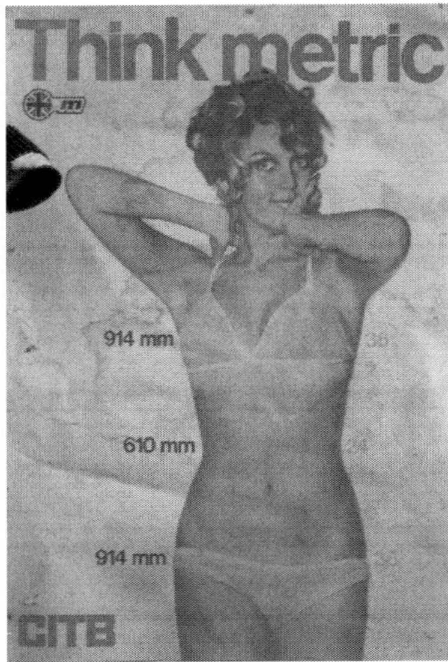

Figure 1.4 Poster by the British Metrication Board of the 1960s, converting 36–24–36 (the units—inches of course—not even indicated in the poster) to metric units (millimeters). "Lady Metric," a British C.I.T.B. (Construction Industry Training Board) poster of the late 1960s. "Miss Metric" Delia Freeman thought 914–610–914 made her look fat. Certainly, most people of that time intuitively understood "36–24–36." But numbers are just numbers, inches or millimeters are the corresponding qualities. Although conceptually equivalent, people apparently also "carry units in their heads."

and quality. The "mystery" is stored away with the gauge objects. Thus "a length of ten rods" is a formal statement that does not require one to understand "the nature of length" at all (Fig. 1.4). This is even more striking for cases like temperature, radiance, magnetic flux, and so forth.

So now we know how to measure spatial properties, do we understand any better what "physical space" is? Not really. Eddington (Eddington, 1927) was right in stating that physics is nothing but recording pointer readings, and formally reasoning from these to the prediction of possible pointer readings. This has nothing to do with an understanding of the objects being measured, in this case "physical space" or perhaps better the space you move in. If there is understanding somewhere, it is in the reasoning applied to the pointer readings. This can be regarding as a model of the area of interest. The theories of the physicist are of such nature. An understanding of this came rather late. Possibly Heinrich Herz (Herz, 1895) was the first one to offer a coherent exposition. The theories, or models, are usually not unique, and they are only provisionally, and almost certain only temporally, "true." They are best understood as our "user interface" (Hoffman, 2009). The interface allows one to interact efficiently with the world, but it should not be understood as being about some final or fundamental way "the world is" (Gibson, 1979). This insight certainly holds for "space" too. Thus "physical space" is perhaps best defined as your (that is to say, the academic society's) preferred interface. For many of our purposes that will be mainly Euclidean geometry, although for some purposes, like painting a landscape, projective geometry might be preferable, (ie, railway tracks, which are parallel lines in Euclidean space, meet at the horizon at a "vanishing point"; see also Box 1.1), and for aircraft transport Riemann geometry is advised (ie, airlines schedule New York–Singapore over the North pole using Riemannian geometry).

BOX 1.1 From 2D to 3D Space

One might argue that vision is the prime spatial sense. Intriguingly the initial visual input (ie, light falling on the retina) is two dimensional, whereas what we perceive is three dimensional (ie, depth). "From 2D to 3D space" suggests a well-defined progression in the processing of optical structure. Basically, and greatly simplified, first a "2D representation" is constructed on the basis of local "features" that have been extracted by such mechanisms as "edge finders," "corner detectors," and so forth. Then a "3D representation" is constructed on the basis of a variety of "cues" derived from the 2D representation. Such ideas have been acknowledged for ages, but might be said to have been canonized by David Marr in the 1970s (Marr, 1982). Alternatives (best known from the 1950s and 1960s) have particularly been advocated in the work of James Gibson (Gibson, 1950) that the observer directly picks up 3D information from the—partly self-generated through body movements—spatiotemporal optical structure. In that case there simply *is no* 2D stage. These notions are miles apart.

Conceptual complications are due to the fact that humans are able to obtain both 2D and 3D impressions from *pictures*, something animals are apparently unable to do (Deruelle, Barbet, Depy, & Fagot, 2000). Pictures are of particular interest here because they are doubtless 2D as physical structures. Pictures thus often stand for "retinal image" or "optical input" in scientific debates. The remarkable fact of 3D pictorial vision has not failed to puzzle many researchers, who consider the very notion of "monocular stereopsis" as paradoxical. The easiest way out of the dilemma is to simply ignore the phenomenon. Thus Gibson would understand a "picture" only as the illusion of a window opening up on an actual scene. Yet "pictorial space" is a striking

(*Continued*)

BOX 1.1 From 2D to 3D Space—cont'd

aspect of visual awareness (Ames Jr, 1925; Claparède, 1904; Schlosberg, 1941), to ignore this is hardly honest science. It is also important culturally. Artists rarely try to paint an illusory window; instead they rather tend to stress the existence of the physical picture plane. Pictures are aesthetically attractive *because* they are simultaneously 2D and 3D. From a Gibsonean perspective that is fully unpalatable.

In perceiving (interpreting) pictures as 3D scenes multiple cues are used. Cognitive processes are based on the interpretation of these "cues." Some cues are fully arbitrary, in the sense of being culturally determined. For instance, suppose you look a Caucasian person in the face and suddenly notice that the spectrum of scattered radiation skews towards the low energetic photons. This "reddening" will typically make you aware of "shame" in the face. Importantly though, there is no direct, necessary connection between the emotion of shame and turning red. This is a famous example by Bishop Berkeley (Berkeley, 1709) who may be said to have introduced the technical notion of "cue." Clearly "blushing" is not due to Gibson's "ecological physics," but is culturally determined.

In contradistinction, the blue tinge, which is often seen in landscapes and is a potent spatial cue for remoteness, can be interpreted in terms of the optics of the atmosphere. Clearly the latter and other cues depend on simple, direct physical causation. Another well-known example as such is the shading cue. A linear gradient of retinal illuminance is often experienced as the curvature of a surface in the scene in front of you. See for example Fig. 1.5. It is important to notice here that the 3D interpretation of 2D cues almost obligatorily invades our awareness. We would have great difficulties in deciding not to see any depth in Fig. 1.5.

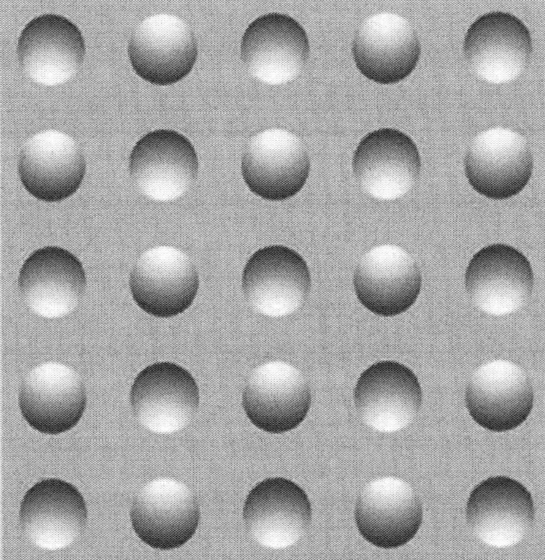

Figure 1.5 "Shape from shading." Most people see 3D "pictorial depth" here and cannot choose to not see it.

Given that there are multiple geometries to measure and describe (physical) space, we may wonder how our brain is tuned to appreciate space. Or in other words, what is the geometry of mental space. It is often said that Kant, one of the major philosophers of all time, displayed tunnel vision when he discussed space, perhaps because he never left Königsberg (present day Kaliningrad). However, another way to look at this is that Kant was not talking about "physical space"—whatever that may be, for Kant a mere "*Ding an sich*"—at all, but rather about *cognitive space*. Then he might well have been right, for most people intuit the Euclidean plane as "natural," whereas they experience a strong aversion against the notion of there being none, or infinitely many parallels to any given line.

1.2 SPATIAL REFERENCE FRAMES

In the foregoing, we saw there exist many mutually distinct formal geometries and there are various ways in which to operationalize spatial relations. But no matter what geometry we apply to understand the space surrounding us, we always have to decide on some appropriate frame of reference. Places and directions can only be determined relative to a chosen frame of reference (Mou & McNamara, 2002). A reference frame is a unit or an organization of units serving as a coordinate system with which spatial properties of objects in the world can be determined (Levinson, 2003). Reference frames typically include the notion of a "ground" object or unit with respect to which places are individuated. Klatzky and Wu (2008) point out that a reference frame gives a set of parameters that localize and orient an entity in space. A typical example of such parameters is the x,y,z that is used to define a point in Euclidean space. In a similar vein Wang (2012) distinguishes reference origin and reference direction or axes as basic elements making a reference frame system. Howard (1982) notes that a reference frame is an attribute of an object that does not normally vary and against which variations in the same attribute in other objects perceived at more or less the same time can be judged.

It has long been acknowledged that multiple spatial reference frames may exist and determine our perception, conception, and action in/of space at a given moment. We may employ these reference frames,

Table 1.1 Reference frames and their alleged functional properties

Subtype	Tasks/functions	Chapter
Egocentric frame of reference		
Retinotopic	Eye movements, attentional movements	5
Head	Attention movements	5
Shoulder	Reaching, grasping	3
Hand	Haptic object inspection and object handling	3, 4
Whole body	Linguistic communication (relative reference frame; Levinson, 2003) and sequential route learning and path integration	6
Allocentric frame of reference		
Single object	Object-based attention and linguistic communication (intrinsic reference frame; Levinson, 2003)	5, 6
Multiple objects	Object localization	7
Landmarks	Allocentric navigation; survey mapping	8
Environmental geometry	Object localization and allocentric navigation; survey mapping	8
Earth-bound features	Spatial thought and linguistic communication (absolute frame of reference; Levinson, 2003) and navigation in natural environments	6, 8

depending on the current perceptual conditions, task at hand, and personal preferences and skills (Table 1.1).

Reference frames have been described by a number of different terms and distinctions in the literature. A first main category includes so-called egocentric spatial reference frames: positions and objects in the outside world are coded relative to parts of the observer's body. Subclasses are retinotopic, head-centered, and body-centered. The latter in turn may include trunk/body midline, shoulder, and hand. Egocentric reference frames particularly play a role in direct motor actions such as grasping or pointing towards an object. In these situations it is vital to code the target object with respect to its spatial relation (distance, orientation) with a part of the body. In our example, picking up the car keys requires one to relate the keys both to the shoulder and the hand frame (see chapter 3: On feeling and reaching: Touch, Action, Body Space). Notably other cognitive activities may also engage egocentric (like) reference frames, such as navigation (see chapter 8: Navigation Ability) or communication (see chapter 6: Tell me Where to Go: On the Language of Space) (cf. Wang, 2012).

A second main category of reference frames is formed by the allocentric reference frames (sometimes also called exocentric reference frames). Here constellations of units outside the observer are used to offer an environment-based point of reference. Searching the car keys in our example could be facilitated by remembering where we left them in the room. Allocentric reference frames offer perspective independence, that is, the coding of positions is independent from your own current position or orientation. Different cues are used in allocentric reference frames: single objects, the relations between multiple external objects, landmarks (eg, salient, distal objects), and the geometry of an extended surface or boundary (cf. Chan, Baumann, Bellgrove, & Mattingley, 2012), for example, the shape of the room you search for your keys, or the contours of the landscape you drive through when visiting your friend. A special class of (allocentric) cues involves overarching features of the earth as a whole, such as perceived direction of gravity or the sun's azimuth, specifying cardinal directions (eg, North, South). Levinson (2003) uses the term absolute frame of reference whenever these more absolute place codings occur. Arguably repeated cross-checking with multiple environmental cues is needed to instantiate this frame of reference.

The reference frame chosen in turn determines the spatial representation employed in a given situation (see also below). Different reference frames may engage distinct neural networks in the brain. A popular division is that between the dorsal cortical route supporting egocentric spatial referencing and the ventral route involved in allocentric referencing (Milner & Goodale, 1995; Neggers, Van der Lubbe, Ramsey, & Postma, 2006; see also chapter 5: Spatial Attention and Eye Movements). An important consequence is that this makes it possible to observe qualitatively distinct disorders bound to selective impairments in a particular reference frame. The classical example is object-based spatial neglect (Driver, 1999) versus neglect for one side of egocentric space (see Committeri et al., 2004). We will address in more detail the underlying neural machinery of reference frames and representations when discussing particular spatial cognitive domains in the other chapters in this book.

1.3 THE NATURE OF SPATIAL REPRESENTATIONS

The reference frame chosen forms a main characteristic of the spatial representation employed in a given situation. But what exactly is the nature of this representation and the format of the information it contains? The example of the visit to your best friend's new home started with the question of whether to keep the route instructions in their original format or instead whether to use them to build a more map-like representation. The original instructions contain a verbal information format. Verbal information has certain notable characteristics: the representation is abstract, amodal, and relatively arbitrary, that is, words do not correspond in a natural, compulsory way to the objects, situations, or activities they refer to. Verbal elements are symbolic units, linked by overlearned, conventional associations (ie, the specific language adopted) to meaning and concrete referents in the world. Typically the information contained in verbal descriptions or instructions is thought to be based upon an underlying propositional network/representation.

Do we also possess information codes, which have a more direct spatial format? This question of course is reminiscent of the notorious imagery debate (Kosslyn, 1994; Pylyshyn, 1994). The central issue in this debate concerned whether knowledge representations are only propositional or instead may have a format more closely resembling the original perceptual inputs. Pylyshyn (2002) argued that the impression of possessing and inspecting (visual) mental images which are picture-like and intrinsically spatial of nature merely follows from us contemplating a nonspatial, propositional representation and deducing inferences from this representation on what the possible outside (physical and visuospatial) world could be. In contrast, proponents of a depictive knowledge representation theory claim that instead of single knowledge format (eg, propositional) we would also possess representations in the form of mental images. Mental images are presumed to have an analogue format. The analogue feature is typically interpreted by assuming that a representation is depictive and strongly comparable to the items in the physical world it represents. In consequence, analogue representations are presumed to be continuous (ie, properties of a representation may show a continuous variation rather than discrete steps) (Dretske, 1981).

In line with the foregoing, McCloskey (2001) differentiates between representations containing spatial information but in which the representation itself is not directly spatial and those which are intrinsically spatial to some extent. The instructions received from your friend could be an example of the former if you had kept them in purely verbal format in your memory. In contrast, in the latter case you would have converted the instructions into a more map-like format. Within this format one or more properties of the representation are isomorphic to the referent materials in the physical world (ie, distance of the streets you will pass through and orientations of the turns you need to take). Notice that the latter representations may differ in the extent of spatial correspondence or isomorphy. That is, you can construct either a more global, topological map, or a more metrically detailed topographic map. McCloskey (2001) further distinguishes mental representations in which the spatial properties of the representation are actually used to guide behavior and thinking from those in which they are contained in the mental representation but not used. Table 1.2 is a partial adaptation of Table 5.1 in McCloskey. We have chosen to ignore this last distinction but instead include a distinction between representations which contain limited isomorphy and those having isomorphy across multiple properties.

One of the concerns with depictive theories of mental images has been the question of who is doing the imagery. The metaphor often used is that of inspecting an image with one's mind's eye. The danger here is to assume some sort of homunculus who is interpreting the image. Related to this there is the question of whether images are necessarily conscious. A similar concern is linked to the three types of spatial representations described above. At the level of the neurons in the brain, none of the three representations is directly isomorphic to the outside world.[3] Hence we need a neurocomputational system to interpret and use the correlated patterns of neural activity to instantiate the functional characteristics associated with a particular type of spatial representation, either consciously or implicitly.

It goes beyond the scope of this chapter to address this interpretation stage here. Throughout this book we will entertain the idea that

[3] The one exception could be retinotopic maps in the visual cortex corresponding in a one-to-one fashion with the visual stimulus patterns reaching the observer's eyes.

Table 1.2 Distinguishing between spatial contents of a representation and the extent to which a representation has a "real" spatial format

Format of spatial representation	*Criteria*	Examples
Spatial1	*The represented information is spatial. The representation itself is not spatially organized*	Verbal description of a route; digital clock time
Spatial2	a. *Spatially defined parts of the representation correspond to (spatial or nonspatial) parts of the represented material* b. *At least one spatial property defined over the parts of the representation is isomorphic to a (spatial or nonspatial) property defined over the corresponding parts of the represented material*	Subway map; family tree (indicating generations but not exact age differences)
Spatial3	a. *Spatially defined parts of the representation correspond to (spatial or nonspatial) parts of the represented material* b. *Multiple spatial properties defined over the parts of the representation are isomorphic to a (spatial or nonspatial) properties defined over the corresponding parts of the represented material*	Topographical map; 3D model of landscape or building

Adapted from McCloskey, M. (2001). Spatial representation in mind and brain. In B. Rapp (Ed.), *What deficits reveal about the human mind/brain: A handbook of cognitive neuropsychology* (pp. 101–132). Philadelphia, PA: Psychology Press (Table 5.1).

multiple representations of spatial information can exist in the human mind and brain. They will differ in how far their properties are isomorphic to characteristics of the outside world. In turn this raises the question of their efficiency for guiding spatial behavior. We will return to this when discussing disorders in spatial cognition and techniques to remediate these (see also chapter: Space in Neuropsychological Practice). See also Box 1.2 for a discussion of the cognitive map concept in representing the spatial world.

BOX 1.2 On the Origins of the Cognitive Map

One of the first scientific papers on mental maps of space was published by Trowbridge in Science in 1913 (Trowbridge, 1913). As the paper states its purpose was to address the "reasons why civilized man is so apt to lose his bearings in unfamiliar surroundings." The author identifies two basic methods for spatial orientation: the domicentered strategy which would be employed by animals, children, and uncivilized individuals, with strong reliance on the home base as point of central orientation; and the egocentric strategy available only to educated, civilized citizens and critically rests on the ability to align oneself with compass directions.

We may take this paper as one of the first scientific essays in which the idea of a mental map was entertained. This notion later received more extended and empirically inspired attention in the monumental paper by Tolman on the cognitive map (Tolman, 1948).

Tolman started with discussing the concept of latent learning in rats in a maze. Fig. 1.6 shows the maze in which rats were trained to find food in a goal location, starting from another place in the maze. One group of animals was always rewarded by food and learned quickly given the same start and goal location every day. Two other groups of rats were also included in the experiment. One group was not rewarded in the goal location until day 3.

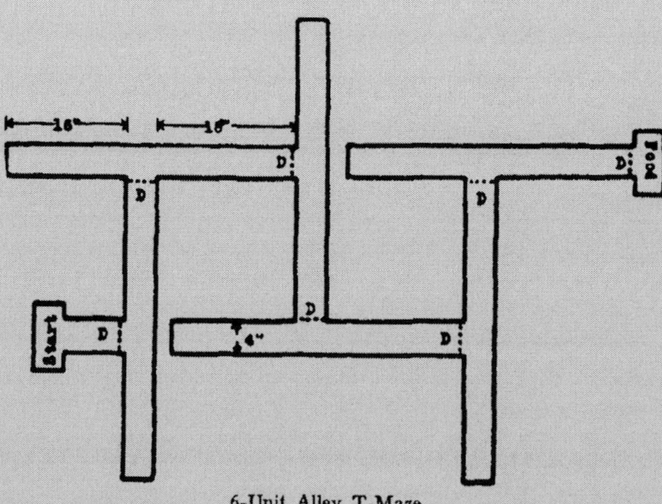

Figure 1.6 The maze discussed by Tolman in his paper on cognitive mapping in rats. *From Tolman, E. C. (1948). Cognitive maps in rats and men.* Psychological Review, *55(4), 189–208.*

(*Continued*)

BOX 1.2 On the Origins of the Cognitive Map—cont'd

The last group even had to wait until day 7 before they were rewarded in the goal location. As the (Figure 1.7) makes clear: the rate of learning was surprisingly high in the groups with delayed rewards in the goal location. Tolman took this as a sign that the rats engaged in some kind of spatial learning even when places in their environment did not contain any reward. Moreover, he argued that this spatial learning was not based on a chain of stimulus response associations, leading the animals from the start location to the goal location. Rather, he concluded that the rats gradually built up a field map or cognitive-like map of their environment. In a subsequent experiment Tolman showed that part of this map-like representation was a sense of direction.

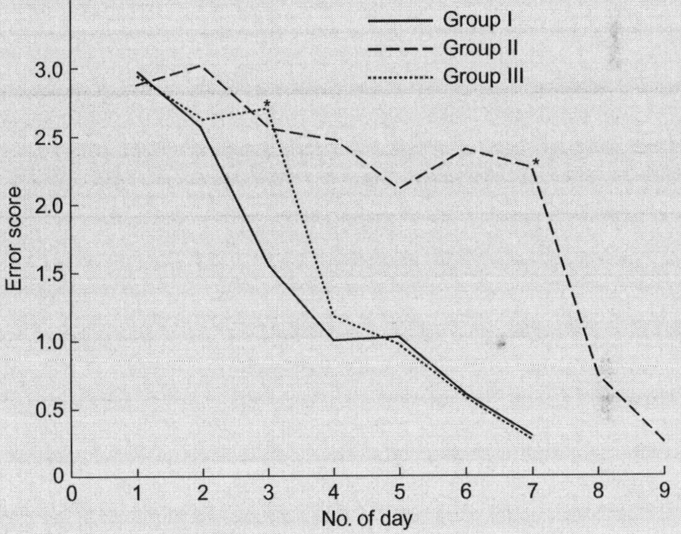

Figure 1.7 Maze performance by different groups of rats. *From Tolman, E. C. (1948). Cognitive maps in rats and men.* Psychological Review, *55(4), 189–208.*

Tolman's notion of a cognitive map did not exclude the possibility that the rats' mapping system was based on an egocentric spatial reference frame or an updated egocentric representation. Without doubt the move towards a more allocentric interpretation of the cognitive map has been inspired by the monumental book by O'Keefe and Nadel offering an ambitious neurocognitive model of the cognitive map (O'Keefe & Nadel, 1978). O'Keefe and Nadel defended the existence of a representational system for absolute space "... a non-centred stationary framework through which the organism and its egocentric spaces move" (O'Keefe & Nadel, 1978). Functionally the idea was that the cognitive

(*Continued*)

BOX 1.2 On the Origins of the Cognitive Map—cont'd

map provides a Euclidean description of the surroundings from an allocentric reference perspective (cf. Burgess & O'Keefe, 2002), informing on places in the environment, objects to be found in that places, and spatial relations, driving wayfinding, goal-directed behavior and exploration. Importantly the cognitive map system allows one to locate oneself in a familiar environment and to go from one place to another even through parts of the environment never visited before.

The neural building blocks of this cognitive map system are thought to involve several circuitries in the hippocampal formation. Various spatially specific types of cells have been found in these parts of the brain, including place cells, head direction cells, grid cells, and boundary vector cells, allowing for absolute sense of place, allocentric direction, Euclidean distance, and closeness of environmental borders, respectively (Spiers, 2012). Whereas the foregoing cellular print of the cognitive map within the hippocampal formation has mainly been based on animal work, it seems to make sense to suppose that the human hippocampus and related structures contain cells with similar properties. A further discussion of the cognitive map concept can be found in Kitchin (1994).

The importance of the discovery of the neural basis of the cognitive map has been widely acknowledged (http://www.nobelprize.org/nobel_prizes/medicine/laureates/2014/press.pdf). In the field of human cognitive neuroscience it has been argued that the cognitive map system might have been crucial for the evolution of episodic memory, in particular by storing in memory the spatiotemporal contexts of episodes (Bird & Burgess, 2008). Episodic memory records the personal events of one's life. Retrieving an episodic memory is thought to require connecting multiple different elements of an event: what happened, when it happened, and where it happened (Tulving, 2002; or as described by Hassabis, Kumaran, & Maguire, 2007) integrating a sense of time and self, with semantic and sensory details, and visuospatial imagination. We may speculate that the ideal way to bring these elements together and create an episodic memory trace is in the absolute place holders offered by the cognitive map. Within these location representations the activities of the stored event can cognitively unfold. Bird and Burgess (2008) point out that the allocentric spatial map allows viewpoint shifts across stored scenes, and as such is essential for mentally replaying what happened during the original event linked to that scene and for episodic recollection. The cognitive map thus engraves an *eventscape* in our memories. (See Eichenbaum, Dudchenko, Wood, Shapiro, & Tanila, 1999 for a nonspatial interpretation of the role of the hippocampus in memory.)

1.4 DIVISIONS IN MENTAL SPACE

Whereas the space we move in seems to be a property of the outside world, which expands in a unitary continuous fashion, mental space has long been argued to break down in a number of qualitatively distinct subregions. A classical distinction is that between space close to the body and more distal space. Brain (1941) already noted distinct effects of superior and inferior parietal lesions on perceptual motor performance in grasping distance versus in walking distance. Comparative monkey studies further support the notion of qualitative distinction between processing near and far regions of space (Mountcastle, 1976; Rizzolatti, Matelli, & Pavesi, 1983). Grusser (1983) was one of the first to sketch an extended model of the distinct spaces surrounding ourselves within the world. He distinguished personal space from extrapersonal space; the former including the ego sense with the body and depending on the interoceptors; the latter containing several further subdivisions and depending on exteroceptors and motor systems.

A most elaborate model of the division of (mental) space has been offered by Previc (1998), dividing extrapersonal space in peripersonal (0–2 m from the body center), extrapersonal focal (0,2 m to distant space), extrapersonal action (2 m to distant space), and ambient space (most distant). Interestingly the Previc model contends that these spaces serve separate functions (going from grasping/reaching, to visual search and object recognition, to scene recognition and navigation, to postural control during locomotion), depend on different sensory inputs, engage different motor systems and reference frames/coordinate systems. In turn, distinct neural circuitries may be involved. Table 1.3 gives our own adaptation of the Previc model. In the original scheme extrapersonal action space only involved a gaze-centered reference frame. As we have argued earlier, however, allocentric referencing is critically involved in navigation. Interestingly gravitation is the prime reference system used in ambient space. We speculate that ambient vision and cues such as the sun's azimuth and pattern of polarized light in the sky[4] also support ambient space and in particular help us to globally orient in space (knowing what is up and down, and perhaps also cardinal directions such as north south). Recent work by Cardinali, Brozzoli, and Farnè (2009) has further specified body and peripersonal space in terms of body schema,

[4] Polarized light in the sky is used by many insects for spatial orienting and apparently also by the ancient Vikings in the form of the so-called "sun-stones" (Ropars, Gorre, Le Floch, Enoch, & Lakshminarayanan, 2012).

Table 1.3 Spatial areas and their neurocognitive characteristics

	Spatial areas				
Characteristic:	**Body**	**Peripersonal**	**Extrapersonal focal**	**Extrapersonal action**	**Extrapersonal ambient**
Function	Posture; touch contact; pain; sense of agency; consumption	Multisensory space surrounding different body parts: hands, face, trunk, etc.; visually guided grasping; object manipulation	Visual search; object/face recognition	Navigation; scene memory; audiovisual target orientation	Spatial orientation; postural control; locomotion; long range navigation
Lateral extent	Front more than back; see Van der Stoep, Nijboer, Van der Stigchel, and Spence (2015)	Central 60°	Central 20–30°	Full 360°	Front 180°
Vertical bias	Depending on receptive fields body areas; see Longo, Mancini, and Haggard (2015)	Lower field	Upper field	Upper field	Lower field
Radial extent	0–0.5 m	0–2 m (reachable space depends on arm length); see Costantini, Ambrosini, Tieri, Sinigaglia, and Committeri (2010)	0.2 distance	2 m—distance	Very far
Primary coordinate/reference system	Body-centered	Body-centered (upper torso)	Retinotopic	Landmark-centered; environmental geometry	Gravitational; environmental geometry; stellar

					objects; polarized light
Sensory system	Somatosensory/ Proprioception; vestibular; gustatory; olfactory?	Visual (binocular); Somatosensory/ proprioception; vestibular	Visual (monocular)	Visual (monocular); auditory; olfactory; vestibular;	Visual (ambient motion, slant); vestibular; somatosensory/ proprioception
Motor system	Limbs and torso	Arm; smooth eye movements; head movements; saccades; leg kicks	Saccades	Head movements; saccades; upper-torso motion; leg movements	Leg movements; head movements
Neural correlates	Angular gyrus	Inferior parietal; dorsal stream; postarcuate frontal; cerebellum; globus pallidus; putamen; see also Aimola, Schindler, Simone, and Venneri (2012) for contrast with extrapersonal space	Inferior temporal; arcuate frontal; lateral intraparietal; Superior colliculus; caudate nucleus; lateral pulvinar	Superior + medial temporal; ventromedial frontal; posterior cingulate; hippocampal formation; auditory cortex; Superior colliculus; anterior thalamus	Parietal-occiptal; dorsal frontal; Ventroposterior thalamus; vestibular nuclei; cerebellum; putamen

Notice primary motor, sensory, and neural systems are given here, by no means intended to be a complete list.
Adapted from Previc, F. H. (1998). The neuropsychology of 3-D space. *Psychological Bulletin*, *124*(2), 123–164 (Table 1).

head- and hand-centered peripersonal space, and arm-centered reaching space. Chapter 5, Spatial Attention and Eye Movements, in the book deals mostly with personal and peripersonal space; Chapter 3, On Feeling and Reaching: Touch, Action, and Body Space, and Chapter 4, Multisensory Perception and the Coding of Space, are relevant for extrapersonal focal space; Chapter 8, Navigation Ability, addresses extrapersonal action and ambient space.

If the space we live in is mentally carved up in separate regions, and distinct modes of control at a perceptual, cognitive, motor and neural levels exist for different compartments of space, then it is likely that selective impairments can be detected after brain lesions. Indeed in particular for the disorder of spatial neglect double dissociations have frequently been reported between peripersonal and extrapersonal space (often labeled far space) (Berti & Frassinetti, 2000; Butler, Eskes, & Vandorpe, 2004; Keller, Schindler, Kerkhoff, von Rosen, & Golz, 2005; Van der Stoep et al., 2013). We will return to these selective disorders in Chapter 10, Space in Neuropsychological Practice. See also Box 1.3.

BOX 1.3 Historical Case of Spatial Disorder; Balint Syndrome

One of the first cases of a marked spatial disorder was recorded by Reszo Balint in 1909 (Balint, 1909). Balint (Figure 1.8) studied a patient suffering stroke followed by marked deficits in visual exploration. One particular symptom concerned the observation of neglect for stimuli in the left visual field. The anecdotal report describes that the patient was sitting on a bench looking straight ahead when the examiner approached him from the left but without evoking any reaction. In turn when the same procedure was repeated on the right side, the patient immediately detected the examiner (De Renzi, 1982, pp. 58–59).

Balint's patient suffered several additional symptoms of spatial impairments. An apparent inability to move his gaze once fixated on an object in the visual field to other elements in the visual world was most striking. Balint labeled this a psychic paralysis of gaze. Clearly this deficit had an impact on visual scanning behavior. A term coined somewhat later for this symptom is simultanagnosia: the inability to process multiple stimuli at the same time (see chapter: Multisensory Perception and the Coding of Space). A further symptom was disordered reaching and grasping. The patient could not produce adequate spatial actions upon target objects. For example, he lit a cigar in the middle and not at the end, and could not draw a simple (Figure 1.8) such as a triangle properly (De Renzi, 1982, pp. 59–60). This symptom was termed optic ataxia to denote severe impairment in visually guided motor action towards

(Continued)

BOX 1.3 Historical Case of Spatial Disorder; Balint Syndrome—cont'd

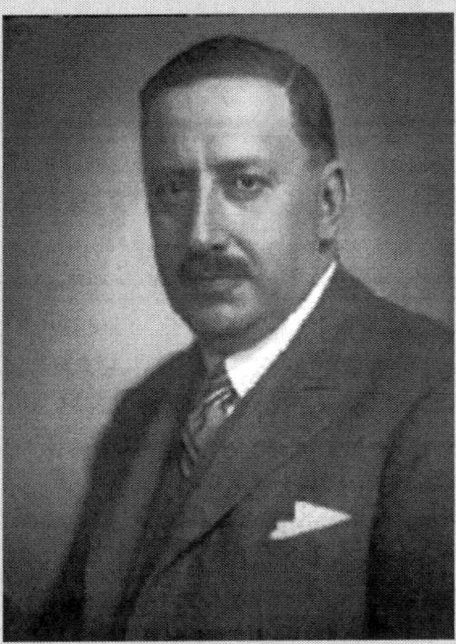

Figure 1.8 Reszo Balint.

objects (see chapter: Spatial Attention and Eye Movements). Postmortem neuroanatomical examinations revealed bilateral posterior parietal damage. The parietal circuitry since then became acknowledged as a particularly spatial circuitry, though its precise functionally has been open to discussion.

Why is the discovery of Balint syndrome so important for the neuropsychology of space? One reason lies in the fact that it has clear historical significance being one of the first documented cases with marked fall out in spatial domain whereas no clear degradation of cognition in other domains seems to exist. Throughout the following decades Balint syndrome has attracted scientific attention for various additional reasons. In particular there is the question of whether Balint syndrome should be regarded as a unitary syndrome or whether it is a complex of symptoms, which happen to vary over individual cases. Indeed symptoms often occur in isolation (Husain & Stein, 1988). If so there is the question of whether these symptoms are functionally linked and whether their co-occurrence is mediated by a single neurophysiological cause (see also Chechlacz & Humphreys, 2014). Clearly Balint's syndrome underscores the diversity of spatial cognition, composed of several more or less connected functional domains, similar to organization of this book.

See also:

http://www.frontiersin.org/Human_Neuroscience/researchtopics/The_enigma_of_B%C3%A1lint%E2%80%99s_syndrome:_complexity_of_neural_substrates_and_cognitive_deficits/1083

1.5 PHILOSOPHY OF SPACE

Given the historical importance of spatial concepts and the intrinsic complexities in both defining and measuring space, it will be no surprise that the concept of space has long dominated the philosophical debates. Actually several (sub)debates have been conducted about various, essential, spatial topics.

A most important topic concerns the question of whether space is absolute or relative. The absolute view states that space exists independently from the objects occupying it—space as such can be seen as a container. "Absolute space" would be like some substantial material of which any place is an "individual" because of some property. Objects occupy certain places because of the features of absolute space. The relative view in contrast holds that there are only objects and "space" is merely a name for the mutual relations between objects. Space as such can only be conceived because of the properties of the existing objects. "Relative space" in fact is literally nothing.

This particular debate became best known through the Leibniz–Clark correspondence (A Collection of Papers, which passed between the late Learned Mr. Leibniz, and Dr. Clarke, in the years 1715 and 1716; Collins, Clarke, Bulkeley, & Leibniz, 1717). Samuel Clarke strongly argued for Newton's notion of absolute space, whereas Leibniz considered this a nonobject. In his third letter Leibniz writes:

> As for my Own Opinion, I have said more than once, that I hold Space to be something merely relative, as Time is; that I hold it to be an Order of Coexistences, as Time is an Order of Successions. For Space denotes, in Terms of Possibility, an Order of Things which exist at the same time, considered as existing together; without enquiring into their Manner of Existing. And when many Things are seen together, one perceives That Order of Things among themselves.

Compare this with Newton's proposal of the absolute space concept in the *Principia* (Newton, 1687):

> Absolute, true and mathematical time, of itself, and from its own nature flows equably without regard to anything external, and by another name is called duration: relative, apparent and common time, is some sensible and external (whether accurate or unequable) measure of duration by the means of motion, which is commonly used instead of true time ... and Absolute space, in its own nature, without regard to anything external, remains always similar and immovable. Relative space is some movable dimension or

> measure of the absolute spaces; which our senses determine by its position to bodies: and which is vulgarly taken for immovable space...

And continuing, Newton argues:

> Absolute space, in its own nature, without relation to anything external, remains always similar and immovable. Relative space is some movable dimension or measure of the absolute spaces; which our senses determine by its position to bodies; and which is commonly taken for immovable space; such is the dimension of a subterraneous, an aerial, or celestial space, determined by its position in respect of the earth. Absolute and relative space are the same in figure and magnitude; but they do not remain always numerically the same. For if the earth, for instance, moves, a space of our air, which relatively and in respect of the earth remains always the same, will at one time be one part of the absolute space into which the air passes; at another time it will be another part of the same, and so, absolutely understood, it will be continually changed.

These are fully incompatible notions. Whereas modern physics might one day provide the ultimate solution, the present reader can easily appreciate the beauty contained in both views (see also Le Poidevin, 2003).

Linked to the question of whether space exists without objects and matter, another point of philosophical discussion is whether it is independent from the human observer, or in other words whether it is conceived as *ideal* or *real*. If *ideal*, it is subject-dependent, meaning depending on the (human) observer. If *real* it exists independently of the mind. Kant famously held that space is an a priori form of awareness, and is not real (Kant, 1781). In contrast modern mainstream science as well as analytical philosophy differentiate between "physical space" and "phenomenal space," and consider the latter a "representation" of the former. It is then suggested that biological fitness requires the representation to approach "veridicality," that is more or less fully matching with the former, "physical space." This renders physical space "real" but our mental representation possibly filled with gaps, or even distorted, but still having the possibility to support adaptive behavior in the world (cf. O'Keefe, 1993). In line with the latter, a major "constructivist" or "idealistic" undercurrent sides with Kant. It can be argued from ethology, especially Jakob von Uexküll's (Von Uexküll, 1909) work on the "Umwelt" of lower life forms, that an organism's "space" essentially equates with its "user interface." Since user interfaces shield the user from unnecessary complexity, they are typically not "veridical" at all. In that sense they are not fully "realistic," they are merely useful. O'Keefe argues that during evolution our brain has become tuned to order sensory inputs in an Euclidean interpretation of the physical world, even though the physical world is not organized in an Euclidean manner, because it offers direct survival value (O'Keefe, 1993).

Whether space is "real" and mentally represented in a more or less veridical manner or just a construct of the mind itself, the question remains how the mind's view on space is acquired. Are spatial concepts learned by sensory and behaviorally experiences or do we have an innate sense of space? The debate between nativists and empiricists has been going for ages with a peak in the 17th and 18th centuries. Kant argued that humans possess an innate, hardwired concept of space, which in turn would be one of the building blocks of human experience and knowledge. According to Kant: "*...Space is a necessary a priori representation, which underlies all outer intuitions. We can never represent to ourselves the absence of space, though we can quite well think it as empty of objects. It must therefore be regarded as the condition of the possibility of appearances, and not as a determination dependent on them*" (Kant, 1781; Wagner, 2006). In turn, empiricists argued that all our knowledge derives from our senses. In particular when mastering spatial concepts we would need to link motor actions (active touch) to sensory inputs (eg, visual perception). Box 1.4 addresses this last issue in more detail. Chapter 9, How Children Learn to Discover Their Environment: An Embodied Dynamic Systems Perspective on the Development of Spatial Cognition, explicitly deals with the development of spatial abilities and the way this can be disordered.

BOX 1.4 Molyneux' Question

In 1688 William Molyneux, philosopher, astronomer, and politician, wrote his colleague John Locke a letter in which he put forward the question of whether a person blind from birth could distinguish shapes by sight when by some intervention his sight was restored Fig. 1.9.

> Suppose Man born blind, and now adult, and thaught by his touch to distinguish between a Cube and a Sphere of the same metal, and nighly of the same bigness, so as to tell, when he felt one and t'other, which is the Cube, which the sphere. Suppose then the Cube and Sphere placed on a Table, and the Blind Man to be made to see: Quare, Whether by his sight, before he touch'd them, he could now distinguish, and tell, which is the Globe, which the Cube? (Molyneux's question)

(Continued)

BOX 1.4 Molyneux' Question—cont'd

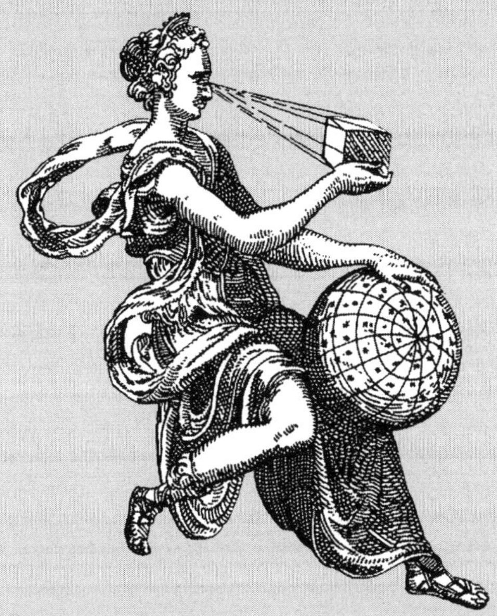

Figure 1.9 *Figure copied from: Degenaar, M. (1989). Het probleem van Molyneux: een psychologisch gedachtenexperiment.* Kennis en Methode *(13), 131–146.*

Intriguingly this question directly addresses the ontology of knowledge and the nature of conceptual reasoning. Do we automatically appreciate and interpret incoming external information or do we have to learn it in a slow, incremental manner? The version of this question which has become publicly known limits itself to the apprehension of shapes and forms. While shape and form perception also includes a spatial dimension, it is of particular relevance for our discussion on the origins of spatial thought that originally Molyneux did include a further formulation:

> . . . A Man, being born blind, ...suppose his Sight Restored to Him, ...Or Whether he Could know by his sight, before he stretched out his Hand, whether he Could not Reach them, tho they were Removed 20 or 1000 feet from him?
>
> ***(Degenaar, 1996; Jacomuzzi, Kobau, & Bruno, 2003)***

Interestingly, Molyneux' problem has not only initiated substantial philosophical discussion, but it has also inspired several empirical investigations (see also Wade & Gregory, 2006). Most of them have focused on the scarce cases of successful sight restoration in the ages following the formulation of the problem, typically after cataract operations. Due to

(*Continued*)

BOX 1.4 Molyneux' Question—cont'd

methodological limitations none of them has succeeded thus far in fully proving or discarding either the nativist or empiricist point of view. Still the question remains very intriguing as to whether we possess some innate ability to organize incoming sensory information in a truly spatial way or whether either a rapid or slow experience-based learning process is required. Modern neuroimaging research might provide a new line of discovery into this old question regarding the ontology of (visuo)spatial knowledge. Levin, Dumoulin, Winawer, Dougherty, and Wandell (2010) showed that in a man who had regained sight after 43 years of darkness structural changes in the visual cortex persisted even after 7 years of sight recovery, including enlarged population receptive field sizes and reduced longitudinal diffusivity in the optic track. Behaviorally this was accompanied by poor spatial resolution, monocular depth perception, and perception of illusory contours, against excellent motion processing (Fine et al., 2003). Together these results may indicate a critical period in life during which neural plasticity is high and several perceptual skills including spatial information processing have to be acquired, while at the same time some perceptual qualities (eg, motion) appear robust and hardwired, both neutrally and cognitively. A mixed yes/no to the question raised by Molyneux?

The quest to solve the nature of space (and time alongside it) has been of utmost significance for the progress of philosophy and science as well. The foregoing pages have only addressed a selection of central philosophical debates underlying this quest in a very cursory manner. For our exploration of psychological space (and the neuropsychological ailments that torture it) we are inclined to follow a pragmatic approach. Is space absolute or relative? Cognitively we can easily think about empty spaces or distances and space as a sort of container. Our memory for a certain place might improve over multiple learning episodes even though each day it is occupied by a different object. In contrast moving objects to new places might cause interference (see chapter 7: Keeping Track of Where Things are in Space—The Neuropsychology of Object Location Memory). On the other hand, the importance we have placed on the notion of reference frames, if anything, sides with a more relative view of space. Is space real or ideal? While acknowledging the complex relation between physical and mental/psychological space, for our daily functioning and survival in the world it would best to attribute some sort of reality to (physical) space. Is our sense of space innate or depending on critical learning periods and experiences? For the neuropsychological purposes of this book we intend to shed light on both innate constraints to process spatial information and on discovering which types of training programs might be best for development, education, and rehabilitation. A closing thought might be that one day training in special VR environments might help us to conceive of more than just three spatial dimensions.

REFERENCES

Aimola, L., Schindler, I., Simone, A. M., & Venneri, A. (2012). Near and far space neglect: task sensitivity and anatomical substrates. *Neuropsychologia, 50*(6), 1115–1123. Available from http://dx.doi.org/10.1016/j.neuropsychologia.2012.01.022.

Ames, A., Jr (1925). The illusion of depth from single pictures. *Journal of the Optical Society of America, 10*, 137–148.

Balint, R. (1909). Paralysis of the soul "blindness", optic Ataxia, spatial disorder of Attention. *Monatsschrift Fur Psychiatrie Und Neurologie, 25*(1), 51–81, Retrieved from <Go to ISI>://WOS:000206222700005.

Bell, J. L. (2005). *The continuous and the infinitesimal in mathematics and philosophy.* Monza: Polimetrica International Scientific Publisher.

Berkeley, G. (1709). *An essay towards a new theory of vision.* Dublin: A. Rhames.

Berti, A., & Frassinetti, F. (2000). When far becomes near: remapping of space by tool use. *Journal of Cognitive Neuroscience, 12*(3), 415–420. Retrieved from http://www.ncbi.nlm.nih.gov/pubmed/10931768.

Bird, C. M., & Burgess, N. (2008). The hippocampus and memory: insights from spatial processing. *Nature Reviews Neuroscience, 9*(3), 182–194. Available from http://dx.doi.org/10.1038/nrn2335.

Brain, W. R. (1941). Visual disorientation with special reference to lesions of the right cerebral hemisphere. *Brain, 64*(4), 244–272.

Burgess, N., & O'Keefe, J. (2002). Spatial models of the hippocampus. In M. A. Arbib (Ed.), *The Handbook of Brain Theory and Neural Networks* (2nd ed.). Cambridge MA: MIT Press.

Butler, B. C., Eskes, G. A., & Vandorpe, R. A. (2004). Gradients of detection in neglect: comparison of peripersonal and extrapersonal space. *Neuropsychologia, 42*(3), 346–358. Retrieved from http://www.ncbi.nlm.nih.gov/pubmed/14670573.

Cardinali, L., Brozzoli, C., & Farnè, A. (2009). Peripersonal space and body schema. In G. F. Koob, M. Le Moal, & R. R. Thompson (Eds.), *Encyclopedia of behavioral neuroscience* (pp. 40–46). Elsevier Science Ltd.

Chan, E., Baumann, O., Bellgrove, M. A., & Mattingley, J. B. (2012). From objects to landmarks: the function of visual location information in spatial navigation. *Frontiers in Psychology, 3*, 304. Available from http://dx.doi.org/10.3389/fpsyg.2012.00304.

Chechlacz, M., & Humphreys, G. W. (2014). The enigma of Balint's syndrome: neural substrates and cognitive deficits. *Frontiers in Human Neuroscience, 8*, 123. Available from http://dx.doi.org/10.3389/fnhum.2014.00123.

Claparède, E. (1904). Stéréoscopie monoculaire paradoxale. *Annales d'Oculistique, 132*, 465–466.

Collins, A., Clarke, S., Bulkeley, R., & Leibniz; G. W. (1717). *A collection of papers, which passed between the late learned Mr. Leibnitz, and Dr. Clarke, in the years 1715 and 1716: relating to the principles of natural philosophy and religion. With an appendix. To which are added, Letters to Dr. Clarke concerning liberty and necessity; from a gentleman of the University of Cambridge: with the Doctor's answers to them. Also remarks upon a book, entituled, A philosophical enquiry concerning human liberty.* Printed for James Knapton.

Committeri, G., Galati, G., Paradis, A. L., Pizzamiglio, L., Berthoz, A., & LeBihan, D. (2004). Reference frames for spatial cognition: different brain areas are involved in viewer-, object-, and landmark-centered judgments about object location. *Journal of Cognitive Neuroscience, 16*(9), 1517–1535. Available from http://dx.doi.org/10.1162/0898929042568550.

Costantini, M., Ambrosini, E., Tieri, G., Sinigaglia, C., & Committeri, G. (2010). Where does an object trigger an action? An investigation about affordances in space. *Experimental Brain Research, 207*(1–2), 95–103. Available from http://dx.doi.org/10.1007/s00221-010-2435-8.

De Renzi, E. (1982). *Disorders of space exploration and cognition.* Chichester: Wiley.

Degenaar, M. (1989). Het probleem van Molyneux: een psychologisch gedachtenexperiment. *Kennis en Methode, 13*, 131–146.

Degenaar, M. (1996). *Molyneux's problem: three centuries of discussion on the perception of forms.* London: Kluwer Academic Publishers.

Deruelle, C., Barbet, I., Depy, D., & Fagot, J. (2000). Perception of partly occluded figures by baboons (Papio papio). *Perception, 29*(12), 1483–1497. Retrieved from http://www.ncbi.nlm.nih.gov/pubmed/11257971.

Dretske, F. (1981). *Knowledge and the flow of information.* Cambridge, MA: The MIT Press.

Driver, J. (1999). Egocentric and object-based visual neglect. In N. Burgess, K. J. Jeffrey, & J. O'Keefe (Eds.), *The hippocampal and parietal foundations of spatial cognition.* Oxford: Oxford University Press.

Eddington, A. (1927). *).* The nature of the physical world: Gifford lectures. Cambridge University Press.

Eichenbaum, H., Dudchenko, P., Wood, E., Shapiro, M., & Tanila, H. (1999). The hippocampus, memory, and place cells: is it spatial memory or a memory space? *Neuron, 23*(2), 209–226. Retrieved from http://www.ncbi.nlm.nih.gov/pubmed/10399928.

Fine, I., Wade, A. R., Brewer, A. A., May, M. G., Goodman, D. F., Boynton, G. M., & MacLeod, D. I. (2003). Long-term deprivation affects visual perception and cortex. *Nature Neuroscience, 6*(9), 915–916. Available from http://dx.doi.org/10.1038/nn1102.

Gibson, J. J. (1950). *The perception of the visual world.* Oxford: Houghton Mifflin.

Gibson, J. J. (1979). *The ecological approach to visual perception.* Psychology Press.

Grusser, O.-J. (1983). Multimodal structure of the extrapersonal space. In A. Hein, & M. Jeannerod (Eds.), *Spatially oriented behavior* (pp. 327–352). New York, NY: Springer-Verlag.

Hassabis, D., Kumaran, D., & Maguire, E. A. (2007). Using imagination to understand the neural basis of episodic memory. *Journal of Neuroscience, 27*(52), 14365–14374. Available from http://dx.doi.org/10.1523/JNEUROSCI.4549-07.2007.

Herz, H. (1895). Die Prinzipien der Mechanik in neuen Zusammenhange dargestellt.

Hoffman, D. (2009). The interface theory of perception: Natural selection drives true perception to swift extinction. In S. Dickinson, M. Tarr, A. Leonardis, & B. Schiele (Eds.), *Object categorization: Computer and human vision perspectives* (pp. 148–165). Cambridge: Cambridge University Press.

Howard, I. P. (1982). *Human visual orientation.* Chichester: Wiley.

Husain, M., & Stein, J. (1988). Rezso Balint and his most celebrated case. *Archives of Neurology, 45*(1), 89–93. Retrieved from http://www.ncbi.nlm.nih.gov/pubmed/3276300.

Jacomuzzi, A., Kobau, P., & Bruno, N. (2003). Molyneux's question redux. *Phenomenology and the Cognitive Sciences, 2*, 255–280.

Kant, I. (1781). *Critique of pure reason*. Konigsberg: Riga.

Keller, I., Schindler, I., Kerkhoff, G., von Rosen, F., & Golz, D. (2005). Visuospatial neglect in near and far space: Dissociation between line bisection and letter cancellation. *Neuropsychologia*, *43*(5), 724–731. Available from http://dx.doi.org/10.1016/j.neuropsychologia.2004.08.003.

Kitchin, R. M. (1994). Cognitive maps: What are they and why study them? *Journal of Environmental Psychology*, *14*, 1–19.

Klatzky, R. L., & Wu, B. (2008). The embodied actor in multiple frames of reference. In R. Klatzky, M. Behrmann, & B. MacWhinney (Eds.), Embodiment, ego-space and action (pp. 145–177). New York, NY: Psychology Press.

Kosslyn, S. M. (1994). *Image and Brain: The Resolution of the Imagery Debate*. Cambridge, MA: MIT Press.

Le Poidevin, R. (2003). *Travels in four dimensions: The enigmas of space and time*. Oxford: Oxford University Press.

Levin, N., Dumoulin, S. O., Winawer, J., Dougherty, R. F., & Wandell, B. A. (2010). Cortical maps and white matter tracts following long period of visual deprivation and retinal image restoration. *Neuron*, *65*(1), 21–31, Retrieved from <Go to ISI>://WOS:000273791200005.

Levinson, S. C. (2003). *Space in language and cognition: Explorations in cognitive diversity*. Cambridge: Cambridge University Press.

Lloyd, G. E. R. (1970).). *Early Greek science: Thales to Aristotle*. New York, NY: Norton.

Longo, M. R., Mancini, F., & Haggard, P. (2015). Implicit body representations and tactile spatial remapping. *Acta Psychologica (Amst)*, *160*, 77–87. Available from http://dx.doi.org/10.1016/j.actpsy.2015.07.002.

Marr, D. (1982). *Vision: A computational investigation into the human representation and processing of visual information*. San Francisco, CA: : Freeman and Company.

McCloskey, M. (2001). Spatial representation in mind and brain. In B. Rapp (Ed.), *What deficits reveal about the human mind/brain: A handbook of cognitive neuropsychology* (pp. 101–132). Philadelphia, PA: Psychology Press.

Milner, A. D., & Goodale, M. A. (1995). *The visual brain in action*. Oxford: Oxford University Press.

Montello, D. R., & Raubal, M. (2012). Functions and applications of spatial cognition. In D. Waller, & L. Nadel (Eds.), *The APA handbook of spatial cognition* (pp. 249–264). Washington, DC: American Psychological Association.

Mou, W., & McNamara, T. P. (2002). Intrinsic frames of reference in spatial memory. *Journal of Experimental Psychology. Learning, Memory, and Cognition*, *28*(1), 162–170. Retrieved from http://www.ncbi.nlm.nih.gov/pubmed/11827078.

Mountcastle, V. B. (1976). The world around us: Neural command function for selective attention. *Neurosciences Research Program Bulletin*, *14*(Suppl), 1–47. Retrieved from http://www.ncbi.nlm.nih.gov/pubmed/818575.

Neggers, S. F., Van der Lubbe, R. H., Ramsey, N. F., & Postma, A. (2006). Interactions between ego- and allocentric neuronal representations of space. *Neuroimage*, *31*(1), 320–331. Available from http://dx.doi.org/10.1016/j.neuroimage.2005.12.028.

Newton, I. (1687). *The principia: Mathematical principles of natural philosophy*. University of California Press, (1999).

O'Keefe, J. (1993). Kant and the sea-horse: An essay in the neurophilosophy of space. In N. Eilan, R. McCarthy, & B. Brewer (Eds.), *Spatial representation*. Cambridge: Blackwell.

O'Keefe, J., & Nadel, L. (1978). *The hippocampus as a cognitive map*. Oxford: Oxford University Press.

Previc, F. H. (1998). The neuropsychology of 3-D space. *Psychological Bulletin*, *124*(2), 123–164. Retrieved from http://www.ncbi.nlm.nih.gov/pubmed/9747184.

Pylyshyn, Z. W. (1994). Mental images on the brain. [Review of the book Image and brain: The resolution of the imagery debate, by Stephen M. Kosslyn]. *Nature, 372*, 289–290.

Pylyshyn, Z. W. (2002). Mental imagery: in search of a theory. *Behavioral and Brain Sciences, 25*(2), 157–182. discussion 182–237. Retrieved from http://www.ncbi.nlm.nih.gov/pubmed/12744144.

Riemann, B. (1854). *Über die Hypothesen welche der Geometrie zugrunde liegen*. Göttingen.

Rizzolatti, G., Matelli, M., & Pavesi, G. (1983). Deficits in attention and movement following the removal of postarcuate (area 6) and prearcuate (area 8) cortex in macaque monkeys. *Brain, 106*(Pt 3), 655–673. Retrieved from http://www.ncbi.nlm.nih.gov/pubmed/6640275.

Ropars, G., Gorre, G., Le Floch, A., Enoch, J., & Lakshminarayanan, V. (2012). A depolarizer as a possible precise sunstone for Viking navigation by polarized skylight. *Proceedings of the Royal Society of London A: Mathematical, Physical and Engineering Sciences, 468*(2139), 671–684. Retrieved from http://rspa.royalsocietypublishing.org/content/468/2139/671.abstract.

Rucker, R. (1995).). *Infinity and the mind: The science and philosophy of the infinite*. Princeton, NJ: Princeton University Press.

Schlosberg, H. (1941). Stereoscopic depth from single pictures. *The American Journal of Psychology*, 601–605.

Spiers, H. J. (2012). Hippocampal formationIn V. S. Ramachandran (Ed.), *The encyclopedia of human behavior* (vol. 2, pp. 297–304). Academic Press.

Tolman, E. C. (1948). Cognitive maps in rats and men. *Psychological Review, 55*(4), 189–208. Retrieved from http://www.ncbi.nlm.nih.gov/pubmed/18870876.

Trowbridge, C. C. (1913). On fundamental methods of orientation and "imaginary maps". *Science, 38*(990), 888–897. Available from http://dx.doi.org/10.1126/science.38.990.888.

Tulving, E. (2002). Episodic memory: From mind to brain. *Annual Review of Psychology, 53*, 1–25. Available from http://dx.doi.org/10.1146/annurev.psych.53.100901.135114.

Van der Stoep, N., Nijboer, T. C., Van der Stigchel, S., & Spence, C. (2015). Multisensory interactions in the depth plane in front and rear space: a review. *Neuropsychologia, 70*, 335–349. Available from http://dx.doi.org/10.1016/j.neuropsychologia.2014.12.007.

Van der Stoep, N., Visser-Meily, J. M., Kappelle, L. J., de Kort, P. L., Huisman, K. D., Eijsackers, A. L., & Nijboer, T. C. (2013). Exploring near and far regions of space: distance-specific visuospatial neglect after stroke. *Journal of Clinical and Experimental Neuropsychology, 35*(8), 799–811. Available from http://dx.doi.org/10.1080/13803395.2013.824555.

Von Uexküll, J. (1909). *Umwelt und innenwelt der tiere*. Berlin: Springer-Verlag.

Wade, N. J., & Gregory, R. L. (2006). Editorial essay: Molyneux's answer I. *Perception, 35*(11), 1437–1440. Retrieved from http://www.ncbi.nlm.nih.gov/pubmed/17286115.

Wagner, M. S. (2006). *The geometries of visual space*. Routledge.

Wang, R. F. (2012). Theories of spatial representations and reference frames: what can configuration errors tell us? *Psychonomic Bulletin & Review, 19*(4), 575–587. Available from http://dx.doi.org/10.3758/s13423-012-0258-2.

CHAPTER 2

On Inter- and Intrahemispheric Differences in Visuospatial Perception

Ineke J.M. van der Ham[1,2] and Francesco Ruotolo[1,3]
[1]Experimental Psychology, Helmholtz Institute, Utrecht University, Utrecht, The Netherlands
[2]Department of Health, Medical and Neuropsychology Leiden University, Leiden, The Netherlands
[3]Laboratory of Cognitive Science and Immersive Virtual Reality, Second University of Naples, Naples, Italy

In this chapter we will cover the basics of human visuospatial perception and we will address the topic of dissociations within spatial perception, in particular the typical patterns of lateralization associated with spatial relation processing. We discuss various issues concerning the importance of studying spatial relation processing and the cognitive nature of this type of processing. Also, spatial relation processing appears to be linked to the use of spatial reference frames, which will be thoroughly discussed in the third part of this chapter.

PART 1: VISUOSPATIAL PERCEPTION

To understand what the term "Visuospatial perception" refers to, it is important to start with the difference between sensation and perception. Sensation refers to the process of sensing the environment through touch, taste, sight, sound, and smell. This information is sent to the brain where perception comes into play. Perception is the way humans select, organize, and interpret these sensations and therefore make sense of everything around them. The ability to interpret the surrounding environment by processing the information that is contained in visible light has been called "Visual Perception." As a consequence, "Visuospatial perception" refers to the ability to process and interpret visual information about "where" objects are in space.

Visuospatial processing encompasses a wide variety of neurocognitive operations ranging from the basic ability to analyze how parts or features of an object combine to form an organized whole, to the dynamic and interactive spatial processes required to track moving objects, to visualize

Neuropsychology of Space.
DOI: http://dx.doi.org/10.1016/B978-0-12-801638-1.00002-1

displacement, and to localize, attend, or reach for objects or visual targets in a spatial array (Stiles, Akshoomoff, & Haist, 2013).

Below, a general frame of how visuospatial perception works is given.

2.1 SEEING 3D FROM 2D IMAGES

The act of seeing starts when the cornea and then the lens of the eye focuses an image onto a light-sensitive membrane in the back of the eye, the retina. The retina is actually a part of the brain that is isolated to serve as a transducer for the conversion of patterns of light into neuronal signals (see also chapter: Multisensory Perception and the Coding of Space). These patterns of light are two-dimensional projection surfaces and represent the optical images of the external world. However, humans perceive the world in three dimensions and to do so they use a series of "depth cues." The depth cues can be monocular, based on the input of one eye (eg, an object that occludes another is closer; the larger object is closer; linear perspective), and binocular, based on cues that reflect the images from both eyes (eg, binocular disparity, ie, the difference between the images from the two eyes converted to depth information) (for further information about this topic, see Goldstein, 2014). Depth perception allows the perception of the distance between elements in an environment and a conception of the length, width, and height of an object.

Recent perceptual work has demonstrated that human observers make judgments about object size, shape, and orientation by integrating visual cues in close to a statistically optimal way (Hillis, Watt, Landy, & Banks, 2004; Jacobs, 1999; Knill & Saunders, 2003; Saunders & Knill, 2001). They rely more heavily on whatever cues are most reliable in a given stimulus. For example, under some conditions, monocular cues for 3D surface orientation (eg, surface texture and the outline shape of a figure) are more reliable than binocular cues; observers correspondingly give more weight to those cues when making surface orientation judgments (Knill & Saunders, 2003).

2.2 THE VISUAL PATHWAY FROM RETINA TO CORTEX

All sensory information must reach the cerebral cortex to be perceived and, with one exception, passes through the thalamus on its way to the cortex. In the case of the visual system, the thalamic nucleus is the lateral geniculate nucleus (LGN) and the cortex is the striate cortex of the

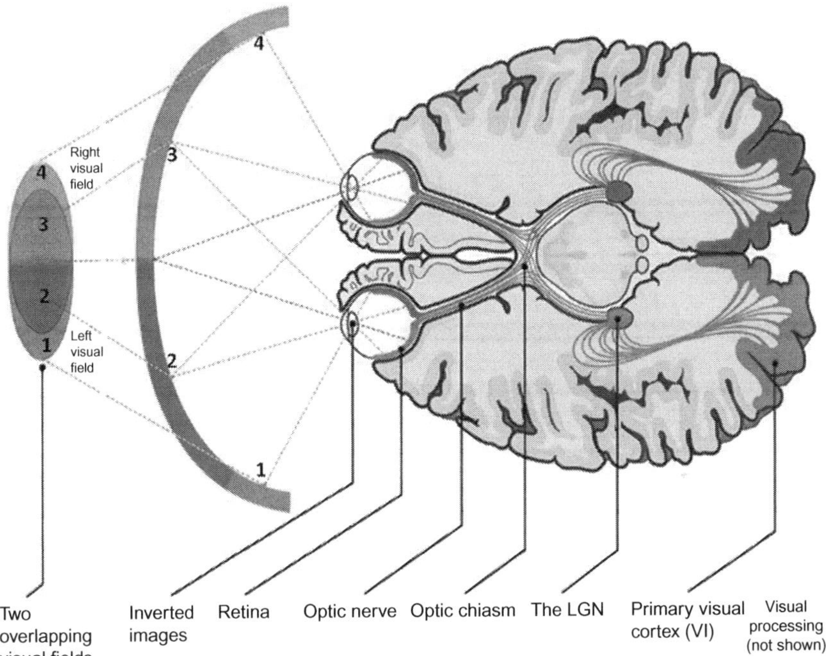

Figure 2.1 Pathway of optical processing from the stimulus to the visual cortex. *Taken from https://cdn-assets.answersingenesis.org/img/articles/am/v8/n3/eye-diagram.gif.*

occipital lobe. The vast majority of optic tract fibers terminate on neurons in the LGN. The optic tract fibers from each eye synapse in different layers of the LGN. Consequently, each LGN neuron responds to stimulation of one eye only. The axons of different types of LGN neurons terminate in different layers or sublayers of the primary visual cortex. The primary visual cortical receiving area is in the occipital lobe. The primary visual cortex is characterized by a unique layered appearance in Nissl stained tissue.[1] Consequently, it is called the striate cortex. It includes the calcarine cortex and extends around the occipital pole to include the lateral aspect of the caudal occipital lobe. The striate cortex is considered to be the primary visual cortex or V1 since it is involved in the initial cortical processing of all visual information necessary for visual perception (eg, information responsible for basic shapes such as horizontal lines) (see Fig. 2.1).

[1] Nissl-staining is a widely used method to study morphology and pathology of neural tissue. It is based on the interaction of basic dyes such as cresyl violet, thionine, toluidine blue, methylene blue, or aniline with the nucleic acid content of cells.

The primary visual cortex sends input to extrastriate cortex, to prestriate cortex, and to visual association cortex. The prestriate cortex (V2) is the second major area in the visual cortex. It receives strong feedforward connections from V1 and sends strong connections to the extrastriate cortex. The extrastriate cortex includes all of the occipital lobe areas surrounding the primary visual cortex (areas V3, V4, V5/MT). Instead, the visual association cortex extends anteriorly from the extrastriate cortex to encompass adjacent areas of the posterior parietal lobe and much of the posterior temporal lobe (Brodmann areas 7, 20, 37, and 39). In most cases, these areas receive visual input via the extrastriate cortex, which sends color, shape/form, location, and motion information to different areas of the visual association cortex.

Despite the complexity of the interconnections between these different areas, two broad "streams" of visual projections from area V1 and other early visual areas were identified in the primate brain: a ventral stream and a dorsal stream (Ungerleider & Mishkin, 1982).

The ventral stream begins at the retina and projects via the LGN of the thalamus to the primary visual cortex, area V1. From there, the pathway proceeds to prestriate and extrastriate visual areas V2 and V4, and then projects ventrally to the posterior (PIT) and anterior (AIT) regions of the inferior temporal lobe. Input to the ventral pathway is derived principally, though not exclusively, from the parvocellular layers of the LGN. Parvocellular input to V1 organizes into distinct areas called the blob and interblob regions (Kaas & Collins, 2004; Livingstone & Hubel, 1984; Wong-Riley, 1979). Cells in the blob regions are maximally sensitive to form, while cells in the interblob regions respond principally to color. Therefore, at a functional level the ventral stream processes information about visual properties of objects and patterns. In the original division between the two streams no spatial functions were attributed to the ventral stream (Ungerleider & Mishkin, 1982), instead later research has suggested that it would be involved in "spatial construction tasks" such as drawing or block assembly that provide insight into an individual's conceptualization of the organization of spatial arrays (eg, how people construe both the parts of an array and the relations among parts that combine to form the overall configuration) (for further details, see Stiles et al., 2013).

The dorsal visual pathway also begins at the retina and projects via the LGN to area V1. From there, the pathway proceeds to extrastriate areas V2 and V3, then projects dorsally to the medial (MT/V5) and medial superior (MST) regions of the temporal lobe, and then to the ventral inferior parietal (IP) lobe. Input to the dorsal pathway is derived principally, though not exclusively, from the magnocellular layers of LGN and then to layer 4C alpha of V1. Cells in this pathway are maximally sensitive to movement and direction and are less responsive to color or form. At a functional level, the dorsal stream is essentially involved in spatial localization tasks (ie, directly perceive), spatial attention (ie, ability to shift attention to different spatial locations), and mental rotation (ie, ability to mentally transpose the orientation of an object in space). Furthermore, the pathway is also involved in the integration of visual and motor functions (eg, Andersen, Snyder, Bradley, & Xing, 1997; Goodale, 2011; Goodale & Milner, 1992; Rizzolatti & Matelli, 2003).

According to Kravitz, Saleem, Baker, and Mishkin (2011), three principal projection pathways from the parietal lobe can be described (see Fig. 2.2): a parietal–prefrontal pathway (formed by the subregions LIP, VIP, MT, and MST; strongly involved in the initiation and control of eye movements and crucial for spatial working memory); a parietal premotor pathway (V6A, MIP, and VIP; maintain the continuously aligned representations of visual coordinates relative to the location of body parts that are necessary for visually guided action in peripersonal space); and a parietal medial temporal pathway (formed by a subregion of cIPL, area PG; involved in the processing of distant space, in the encoding of space in world or object-centered reference frames). All three pathways are served by an occipito–parietal circuit. It integrates information equally from central and peripheral visual fields and represents space largely in egocentric frames of reference, that is, according to the body parts and their orientation (see Part 3 of this chapter). The egocentric maps of space formed in the occipito–parietal circuit are the functional antecedents of the three proposed pathways. In the monkey, parietal neurons provide information about many egocentric aspects of vision, including optic flow and stimulus depth.

Regarding the ventral pathways, Kravitz and colleagues (2011) explain that the retinotopic organization, based on visual maps originated from the visual fields, can be found even in high levels of object representations (Arcaro, McMains, Singer, & Kastner, 2009).

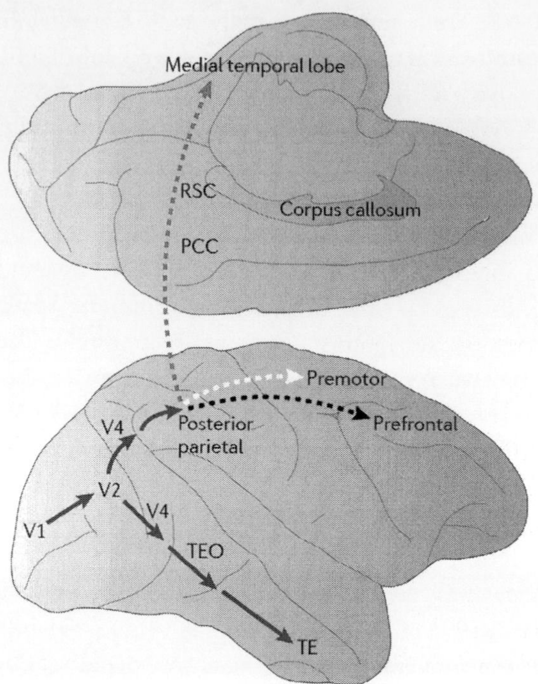

Figure 2.2 According to Kravitz et al. (2011) at least three distinct pathways emanate from the posterior parietal cortex. One pathway targets the prefrontal cortex (shown by a dashed green (black in print versions) arrow) and supports spatial working memory (the parieto–prefrontal pathway); a second pathway targets the premotor cortex (shown by a dashed red (white in print versions) arrow) and supports visually-guided actions (the parieto–premotor pathway); and the third targets the medial temporal lobe, both directly and through the posterior cingulate and retrosplenial areas (shown by a dashed blue (gray in print versions) arrow), and supports navigation (the parieto–medial temporal pathway). *PCC*, posterior cingulate cortex; *RSC*, retrosplenial cortex; *TE*, rostral inferior temporal cortex; *TEO*, posterior inferior temporal cortex; *V1*, visual area 1 (also known as primary visual cortex). *Taken from Kravitz, D. J., Saleem, K. S., Baker, C. I., & Mishkin, M. et al. (2011). A new neural framework for visuospatial processing.* Nature Reviews Neuroscience, 12*(4), 217–230 (April 2011). doi:10.1038/nrn3008.*

Therefore, following on from Milner and Goodale's suggestion (2008) about the interaction between the dorsal and the ventral stream, Kravitz and colleagues (2011) conceptualize the notion that spatial dimensions can contribute to ventral pathway representations and some aspects of object shape are necessary in the dorsal pathway to effectively guide action (Chao & Martin, 2000; Peeters, Simone, & Nelissen, 2009; see also van Polanen & Davare, 2015) Box 2.1.

BOX 2.1 Impaired Spatial Perception: Visual Agnosia and Optic Ataxia

Relevant understanding about the functions of the visual system comes from the examination of patients with brain lesions. An important case was that of D. F., a patient with a visual form of agnosia (VA) due to a bilateral lesion of the occipito–temporal cortex. D.F. was able to perform accurate visually-guided actions toward objects—that is, orient the hand or to size the finger grip in a way that is appropriate to the object—but she was not able to recognize them (Goodale, Milner, Jakobson, & Carey, 1991) (see also chapter: On Feeling and Reaching: Touch, Action and Body Space). This revealed that a close-to-normal visuomotor performance can be observed in spite of the complete deficit for object recognition. Evidence from patients with VA supports the idea that the ventral stream of the brain is responsible for recognition tasks ("What"), whereas the dorsal stream is responsible for guiding the hand toward visual objects ("How") (Goodale & Milner, 1992; Jeannerod & Rossetti, 1993; Milner & Goodale, 1995). Instead, according to Schenk (2006) the main problem of D.F. was that she was no longer able to perform tasks that required an allocentric encoding of spatial information, such as report verbally which of two targets was closer to a visual fixation point, whereas she did as well as normal subjects on egocentric both visuoperceptual and visuomotor tasks.

A second discovery comes from the cases of optic ataxia (OA), a neurological condition where patients have difficulties to reach toward visual objects presented in their peripheral visual field while they can accurately recognize them (eg, Garcin, Rondot, & deRecondo, 1967; Perenin & Vighetto, 1983). In this case, patients fail to code the spatial information of the object with respect to the effector requested to reach for and grasp the object. The most studied OA patient has been I.G., who had a bilateral parieto–occipital infarct following an ischemic stroke (Pisella et al., 2000). Therefore, OA is considered as a deficit in visuomotor functions with other visual functions preserved (including object recognition). Patients with VA and OA deficits have been considered as cases of "double-dissociation," for which an impairment of action is emphasized in OA and a deficit of visual recognition in VA as consecutive to dorsal and ventral damage, respectively. However, according to Pisella and colleagues (2006) this double dissociation becomes questionable when one introduces the visual eccentricity parameter. They indicate that in OA patients reaching and grasping are impaired in peripheral vision whereas they remain largely preserved in central vision, besides actions to peripheral targets remain undocumented in VA. Instead of a simple double-dissociation between perception and action, they argue for a far more complex organization with multiple parallel visual-to-motor connections in which at least three streams can be distinguished: (a) a dorso–dorsal pathway (involving the most

(*Continued*)

BOX 2.1 Impaired Spatial Perception: Visual Agnosia and Optic Ataxia—cont'd

dorsal part of the parietal and premotor cortices) necessary for immediate visuomotor control. Since the latest research about OA shows how these patients exhibit deficits restricted to the most direct and fast visuomotor transformations, a lesion to this pathway would result in OA; (b) a ventral stream—-prefrontal pathway with VA as typical disturbance. Indeed, preserved visuomanual guidance in patients with VA is restricted to immediate goal-directed guidance, whereas they exhibit deficits for delayed or pantomimed actions; (c) a ventro–dorsal pathway (involving the more ventral part of the parietal lobe and the premotor and prefrontal areas) responsible for complex planning and programming based on high representational. Lesions of this pathway would results in with mirror apraxia (ie, deficits in reaching to objects presented through a mirror), limb apraxia (ie, difficulty making precise movements with an arm or leg) and spatial neglect (ie, inability to process and perceive stimuli on one side of the body or environment).

PART 2: DICHOTOMIES IN SPATIAL PERCEPTION

We can interact with the spatial characteristics of our surroundings in different ways. When we ask someone for directions to a specific location, we often get a response that includes expressions similar to "take a left at the roundabout, then take the road between city hall and the library until you are in front of the supermarket." In contrast, in other situations, we are particularly aware of the geometric layout of a spatial situation. We know how we can walk through a building without bumping into anything, as we continuously update our own position and keep track of the location of the walls and other objects in the environment.

2.3 CATEGORICAL AND COORDINATE SPATIAL RELATIONS

These two examples illustrate the two parts of a dichotomy in how we process spatial relations. On the one hand we can describe spatial relations between objects in an abstract, propositional manner, using terms like "left at the roundabout" and "between city hall and the library." These relations are considered *categorical* and often used when we describe spatial situations or memorize locations of objects. The alternative way to describe spatial relations is in terms of metric properties, as happens when exact distances between objects are considered. Such *coordinate* relations

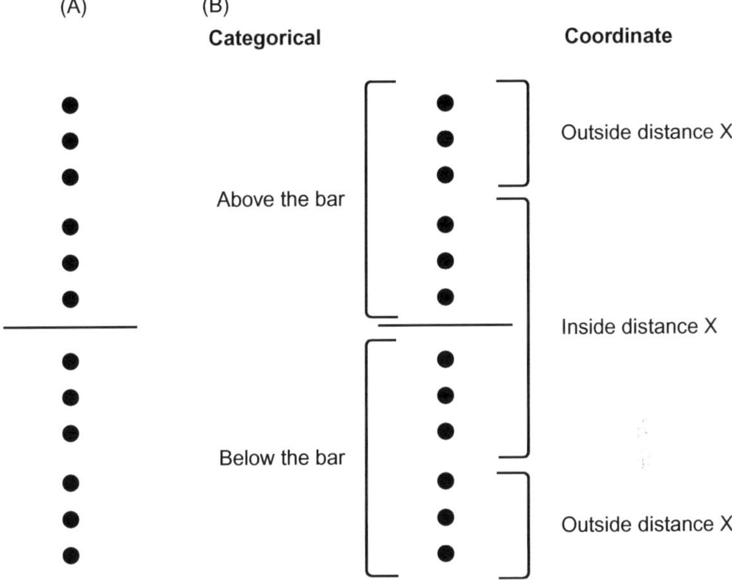

Figure 2.3 (A) The dot-bar stimulus and (B) all possible dot positions. The categorical decision is that a dot is either above or below the bar, the coordinate decision concerns the distance between the dot and the bar, which is either within or not within a specific distance. Note that for a single stimulus, only one dot position would be visible. *Taken from Van der Ham, I. J. M., Postma, A., & Laeng, B. (2014). Lateralized perception: The role of attention in spatial processing.* Neuroscience and Biobehavioral Reviews, 45, *142–148.*

are highly relevant for motor actions, for instance. Kosslyn (1987) was the first to report on a clear distinction between categorical and coordinate spatial relations, and many experimental reports soon followed (eg, Banich & Federmeier, 1999; Bruyer, Scailquin, & Coibion, 1997; Hellige & Michimata, 1989; Koenig, Reiss, & Kosslyn, 1990; Kosslyn et al., 1989; Wilkinson & Donnelly, 1999). The core finding of these studies was that the processing of categorical and coordinate spatial relations is dissociated based on the cerebral hemisphere that is involved; categorical relations are correlated with left hemisphere activity, whereas coordinate relation processing shows a right hemisphere bias. Initially, this was shown in behavioral paradigms, making use of dot-bar stimuli, as illustrated in Fig. 2.3. In such a stimulus, a single dot is presented along with a horizontal bar, the categorical instruction is to focus on the side of the bar the dot is at, regardless of distance (either above or below), and the coordinate instruction is to decide on the distance between the dot and the bar regardless of side (either within or not within a specific distance).

Such a perceptual task, in which a decision is made after a stimulus is shown, can reveal lateralization effects even when performance is only measured behaviorally. By showing a stimulus very briefly (<200 ms) to one side of the visual field (2–3 degrees of visual angle away from the center of the visual field), accuracy and response times reflect potential hemispheric biases for the decisions made (see, eg, Bourne, 2006).

Behavioral visual half field studies with the dot bar stimuli were followed by other reports making use of the same or similar stimuli in various neuroimaging and neuropsychological patient studies (eg, Baciu et al., 1999; Kosslyn, Thompson, Gitelman, & Alpert, 1998; Laeng, 1994; Trojano et al., 2002; van der Ham, Duijndam, et al., 2012; van der Ham, Raemaekers, van Wezel, Oleksiak, & Postma, 2009). Taken together, these studies have highlighted the importance of the left and right parietal cortex in processing spatial relations, further substantiating the dissociation between categorical and coordinate processing, respectively.

The dichotomy between categorical and coordinate relation processing has not only been shown with different methods. It has also been found in different task designs. The first studies on this topic were all perceptual: direct responses to single stimuli were measured. Later on, also designs were applied including the comparison of two separate stimuli in working memory task designs (eg, Laeng, 1994). In such a task design, a participant is asked to interpret and memorize the spatial relation depicted in a single stimulus, and then to compare it to the spatial relation in another stimulus, presented later. Van der Ham and colleagues (2007, 2009) have shown that differential lateralization mainly appears during stimulus retrieval and comparison and for intervals of 500 and 2000 ms. The same pattern of lateralization has also been found for mental imagery (Michimata, 1997; Palermo et al., 2008), in tasks where participants imagined clock faces for certain times presented digitally and answered spatial questions concerning the angle between the short and the long arm in that clock face. Experimental approaches like these make clear that the dissociation between categorical and coordinate relation processing is not restricted to visual perception but can be generalized to cognitively more complex processes like working memory and even mental imagery.

2.4 THEORETICAL FRAMING OF SPATIAL RELATION PROCESSING

One could wonder whether it is really meaningful to study this spatial distinction: what are its implications? It is important to realize that the lateralization effects itself can be considered instrumental; not the fact that a specific type of relation is linked to one of two hemispheres is crucial, but the fact that the two hemispheres are differentially involved. The evidence points out that at least to a certain extent categorical and coordinate spatial representations are processed by different underlying mechanisms. Those mechanisms have been shown to be differentially located in the two hemispheres of the brain. Lateralization can be considered a "divide-and-conquer" method of the brain to increase efficiency of information processing. By having just one hemisphere process a specific type of information, there is no need for intensive interhemispheric communication (see, eg, Cook, 1986; Hugdahl, 2000). Moreover, research on this distinction may contribute to other scientific domains as well. Recently, the distinction between categorical and coordinate processing has also raised interest outside the cognitive sciences. Hamami and Mumma (2013) discuss how this distinction can be considered the cognitive expression of Euclidean diagrammatic reasoning. From a philosophical point of view, the concepts "co-exact" and "exact" as used in Euclidean diagrammatic reasoning (Manders, 2008) can be aligned with categorical and coordinate spatial relations, respectively. The definition given by Hamami and Mumma (2013) illustrates this: "*Exact relations obtain between objects instantiating the same kind of magnitude: for any two line segments, angles or areas, the magnitude of one will be greater than the magnitude of the other, or they will be equal. Co-exact relations between objects are positional. A point can realize one of three co-exact relations to the region defined by a line segment or circle: it can lie inside the region, outside it, or on its boundary.*" In other words, exact relations concern metric, or coordinate, spatial properties and co-exact relations are categorical as they are linked to propositional categories of space like "inside" and "outside."

2.5 ALTERNATIVE VIEWPOINTS

Despite the large body of evidence supporting at least a partial functional and neurological distinction between categorical and coordinate processing, some have presented alternative explanations. Roughly, these explanations can be divided into two groups, those concerning language and those concerning task difficulty.

As categorical spatial processing is often defined as "propositional" and verbal processing which is evidently a left hemispheric process, it is not surprising to consider language as a potential determinant in the lateralization patterns discussed here (see chapter 6). In most experimental designs verbal labels like "above," "below," "inside," and "outside" suffice to correctly perform categorical tasks. Kemmerer and Tranel (2000) for instance, argue for a triad of spatial relations, as opposed to a dichotomy. They suggest splitting up categorical relations into verbal categories and spatial categories. However, the majority of studies specifically looking into this, report that the left hemisphere is involved in categorical processing, regardless of whether the task is explicitly verbal or perceptual (Franklin, Catherwood, Alvarez, & Axelsson, 2010; Holmes & Wolff, 2012; Suegami & Laeng, 2013; van der Ham & Postma, 2010).

Variation in difficulty has also been considered as an alternative explanation for the lateralization patterns found. In the vast majority of experiments, the categorical decisions were easier to make than the coordinate decision. Some have argued that not the spatial characteristics of the tasks, but the difference in difficulty level determined the hemispheric advantages (Martin, Houssemand, Schiltz, Burnod, & Alexandre, 2008; Sergent, 1991a, 1991b; van der Lubbe, Schölvinck, Kenemans, & Postma, 2006). Yet, in multiple experimental studies difficulty level has been specifically addressed and found to be unrelated to the lateralization pattern found (Franciotti, D'Ascenzo, Di Domenico, Tommasi, & Laeng, 2013; Kosslyn, Chabris, Marsolek, & Koenig, 1992; Slotnick, Moo, Tesoro, & Hart, 2001; van der Ham, Dijkerman, et al., 2012; van der Ham, Duijndam, et al., 2012).

2.6 THE ROLE OF ATTENTION IN SPATIAL RELATION PROCESSING

Although language and difficulty cannot satisfactorily explain all of the typical lateralization patterns found, another factor might be able to do this: spatial attention. As reviewed by van der Ham et al. (2014), the size of attentional scope during a task may substantially affect hemispheric lateralization. In Fig. 2.4, the resulting model presented by van der Ham and colleagues is shown. Not only the instruction to pay attention to either the categorical or coordinate features of a certain stimulus determines the lateralization patterns associated with a given task. Stimulus size and the resulting size of attention scope also play a part. Several researchers performed experiments in which the size of the attended area was manipulated (Borst & Kosslyn, 2010; Franciotti et al., 2013; Franconeri, Scimeca, Roth, Helseth, & Kahn, 2012; Laeng, Okubo, Saneyoshi, & Michimata, 2011; Michimata, Saneyoshi, Okubo, & Laeng, 2011; Okubo, Laeng, Saneyoshi, & Michimata, 2010). These manipulations may consist of priming the size of

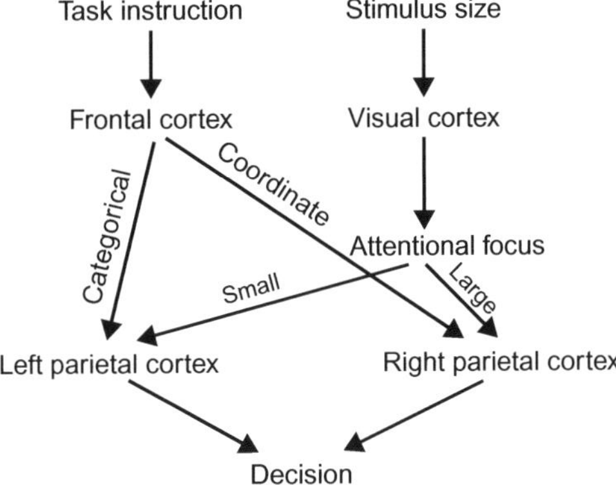

Figure 2.4 A decision about a spatial relation is based on both the task instruction, which can be categorical or coordinate, and stimulus size, which results in an attentional focus of a certain size. Categorical task instruction with a small attentional focus results in a left hemispheric bias, whereas a coordinate instruction and a large attentional focus leads to a right hemispheric bias (van der Ham, Postma, & Laeng, 2014) Box 2.2.

BOX 2.2 Spatial Relations in Objects and Faces

All of the studies concerning spatial relation processing in this chapter concern inanimate objects or geometric shapes. However, as mentioned at the end of Part 2 of this chapter, it is highly relevant to consider the impact of problems with spatial relation processing in daily life. One class of visual stimuli might be of particular interest here: faces. Most of the visuospatial processing of objects also applies to faces. Yet, there are some distinct differences showing that faces are more than just complex objects. For instance, functional neuroimaging has repeatedly indicated that activity in the fusiform face area, a structure in the fusiform gyrus (BA 37), is selectively related to the perception of faces. Moreover, face processing is highly sensitive to orientation: inverted faces are more difficult to recognize than inverted objects. Cooper & Wojan, (2000) have addressed this effect by looking at the impact of changes in spatial relations. In a recognition task with upright and inverted faces, they moved either one eye (categorically different) or two eyes (coordinate change, categorically intact), according to the categorical and coordinate properties defined in Fig. 2.10.

These manipulations allowed for a dissociation of the effect of categorical change in addition to coordinate change (moving either one or two of the eyes). Performance patterns showed that faces are processed both categorically and coordinately, but that the type of instruction determines which type of relation is processed more easily. When participants were asked to identify the face of a famous person, performance relied more on coordinate properties, whereas

(*Continued*)

BOX 2.2 Spatial Relations in Objects and Faces—cont'd

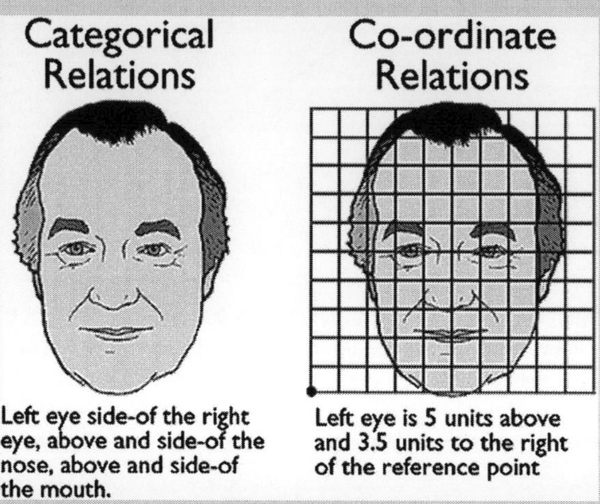

Figure 2.10 Categorical and coordinate relations in faces, as defined by Cooper & Wojan (2000).

the question was asked if the image displayed a face or not, categorical properties were more important. This finding can also be extrapolated to lateralization patterns; coordinate relations are linked to the right hemisphere and a right hemisphere advantage is typically found for face identification as well. This example shows that findings in traditional spatial relations experiments can be valuable for other domains within visual perception as well.

attentional focus by first performing a task relying on either a small or large field of focus, or by using visual indications of a to be attended area during spatial relation task performance. All these studies found that a small attentional focus was linked to a left hemisphere bias and a large attentional focus was related to right hemisphere processing. These findings are further substantiated by observations in patient N.C., who due to her condition showed a significantly larger scope of attention than healthy controls. So, the case study of N.C. offered the opportunity to assess the consequences of a large attentional scope in the absence of manipulation (van der Ham, Dijkerman, et al., 2012). She suffers specific problems with coordinate tasks, but performed at control level in various categorical tasks.

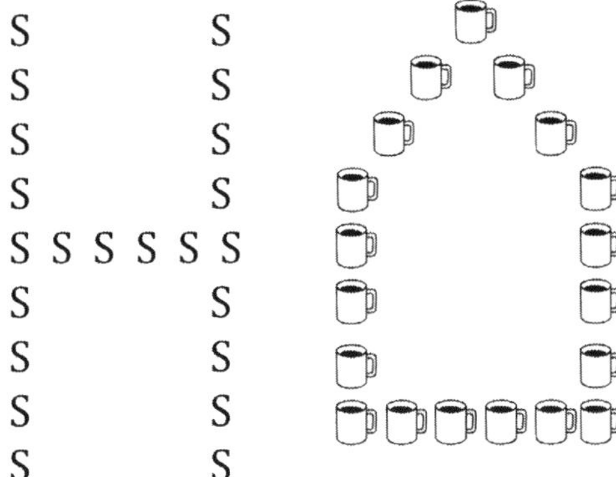

Figure 2.5 Two examples of embedded figures, consisting of local and global letters or objects.

2.7 OTHER DICHOTOMIES IN VISUOSPATIAL PERCEPTION

Categorical versus coordinate spatial relation processing is not the only clear dichotomy within visuospatial perception characterized by differential hemispheric preferences. Local versus global processing research has led to similar findings (Martin, 1979; Navon, 1977). The definition of local and global is inherently different, as it concerns an indication of relative size, and is therefore continuous; "smaller" versus "larger." A very popular method to assess local and global processing is to use hierarchical figures and ask participants to detect a specific letter or object in such a figure as shown in Fig. 2.5. In multiple studies this distinction has been shown to be left and right lateralized, respectively (for a review, see Van Kleeck, 1989). The dissociation often described for spatial frequency processing is closely linked to the classical local/global distinction. Similarly, it has been found that the left hemisphere is more proficient in processing high frequency input, whereas the right hemisphere is better equipped to process low frequency input (eg, Mecacci, 1993; Proverbio et al., 1997). Yet, very little empirical work is available on the potential overlap or interaction between these three different dichotomies. The model proposed by van der Ham et al. (2014) might provide a solution here, as attentional focus is now introduced to better understand the lateralization patterns for categorical and coordinate processing. In turn, attentional focus could well be a key factor for local versus global and high versus low spatial frequencies, as they all refer to spatial size of visual input. More experimental work on examining the potential overlap of these distinctions would surely benefit theoretical advances in this field.

2.8 SPATIAL RELATION PROCESSING IN CLINICAL NEUROPSYCHOLOGY

Laeng (1994) was the first to address spatial relation processing in clinical patients. He found support for the typical lateralization pattern in patients with brain lesion in either the left or the right hemisphere. For these experiments he needed to adjust the existing stimulus materials. Instead of using dots and lines, he resorted to nameable figures, like animals. Also, he adjusted the task design, as very brief presentation times were not suitable for this type of patients. He used two different approaches, both based on working memory: one that required accurate recollection of an image, and one in which the question was asked which pictures were most alike. In his stimuli, he manipulated either the categorical or coordinate relationship. For instance in Fig. 2.6, either the racket and the bat can be switched in position (categorical change) or the distance between them can be altered (coordinate change). The data showed that patients with left hemisphere damage were less likely to answer correctly when a categorically different distractor was used and thought that a categorically different picture was more similar than a coordinately different picture. The opposite patterns were found for patients suffering from right hemisphere damage, to them coordinately different distractors were harder to identify, and coordinately different stimuli looked more similar than categorically different stimuli.

This study has inspired a later study, in which participants were presented with search tasks in visual scenes. A specific scene in two pictures simultaneously, in one picture one object has moved. This displacement was either within the same spatial category with regard to the nearest object or not. For instance a chair could be on a rug and moved to a different location on the rug (categorically same), or moved to a different location off the rug (categorically different). Healthy participants show that categorical changes are easier to detect, even when the metric (or coordinate) properties of the displacement are identical; a change in category helps participants to find the change (see also Rosielle & Cooper, 2001). This task was also administered in clinical patients with either left or right hemisphere damage. The results again confirmed the typical lateralization pattern.

Importantly, these studies show that also with more natural stimuli and task instructions, the lateralization pattern emerges. In line with this a number of other studies have also focused on realistic stimuli like objects (Saneyoshi et al., 2006; Saneyoshi & Michimata, 2009), faces (Cooper & Wojan, 2000), and even navigation (Baumann et al., 2012), and found

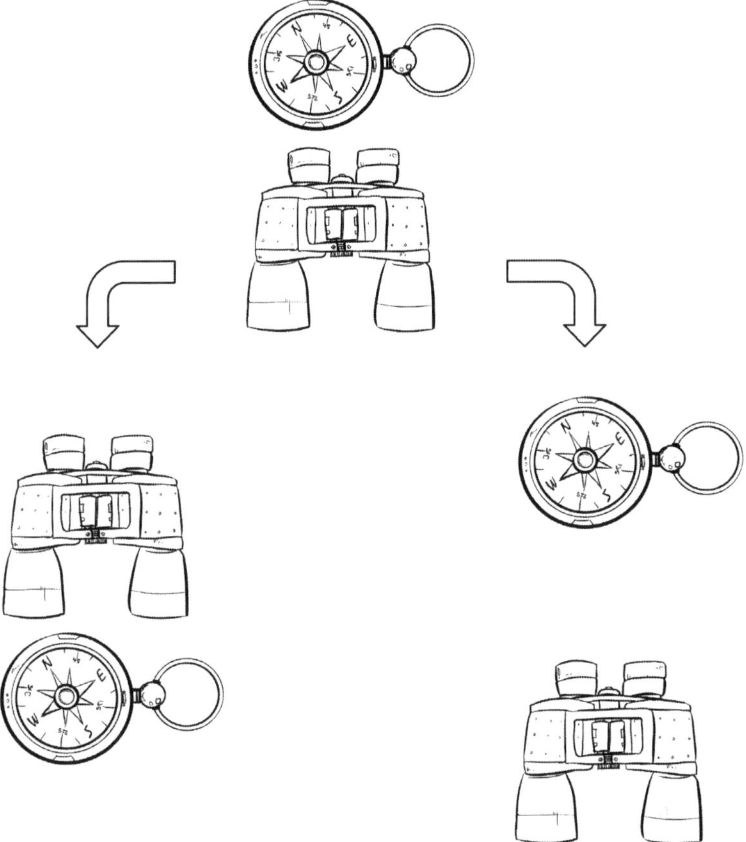

Figure 2.6 Examples of stimuli similar to those used by Laeng (1994). The top figure can be altered in a categorical way; in the bottom left figure the compass has moved to "below" the binoculars, or in a coordinate way; in the bottom right figure, the distance between the compass and the binoculars has changed.

highly similar lateralization outcomes. Therefore it is important to be aware of the potential spatial problems that are expected during everyday activities in patients with unilateral brain damage, in particular in the parietal cortex. For example, patient N.C., with very specific impairment in coordinate processing, described to have problems in daily life with tasks that demand correct processing of coordinate spatial relations. She would experience problems with filling out forms for instance, as they required writing in predefined spatial areas for instance. Later testing on her writing skills showed, that she had no problem in writing, or even very small writing, but she did have problems with fitting her writing between lines.

PART 3: SPATIAL REFERENCE FRAMES

The distinction between categorical and coordinate spatial relations is intrinsically linked to another important dichotomy in the field of spatial cognition: egocentric and allocentric frames of reference. Human beings cannot specify any kind of abstract or metric spatial relation without the use of one of these reference frames (eg, an object will be always on the right or on the left, or at some centimeters or meters with respect to something, be it your own body or an external element in the environment).

In this part of the chapter, we will report evidence supporting the distinction between egocentric and allocentric frames of reference and discuss their relationship with categorical and coordinate spatial relations.

2.9 EGOCENTRIC AND ALLOCENTRIC SPATIAL FRAMES OF REFERENCE

One of the aims of spatial cognition is to study how humans and animals acquire spatial information but also how they organize this knowledge in order to deal with a variety of daily tasks; from the recognition of a scene or a place to the guide of a movement into the environment. Coding spatial information means to determine an element's position with respect to another that is used as point of anchorage. Humans use frames of reference to code spatial relations between elements in the environment, by means of either a categorical or coordinate representation (see Fig. 2.7).

The notion of "frames of reference" is crucial to the study of spatial cognition. The Gestalt theories of perception in the 1920s defined the "frame of reference" as "a unit or organization of units that collectively serve to identify *a coordinate system* with respect to which certain properties of objects, including the phenomenal self, are gauged" (Levinson, 1996; Rock, 1992). This construct has been presented by various disciplines and each discipline has proposed a different distinction between the frames of reference (see Levinson, 1996). In this chapter we adopt the distinction proposed by developmental and behavioral psychology and brain sciences that identifies "egocentric" and "allocentric" frames of reference. In synthesis, it can be said that for egocentric representations retinotopic coordinates, head-centered, and body-centered reference systems are used to organize spatial information (Franklin & Tversky, 1990; Kosslyn, 1994; Levinson, 1996; O'Keefe & Nadel, 1978; Paillard, 1991). These representations are dependent on the egocentric perspective and therefore, the access to spatial

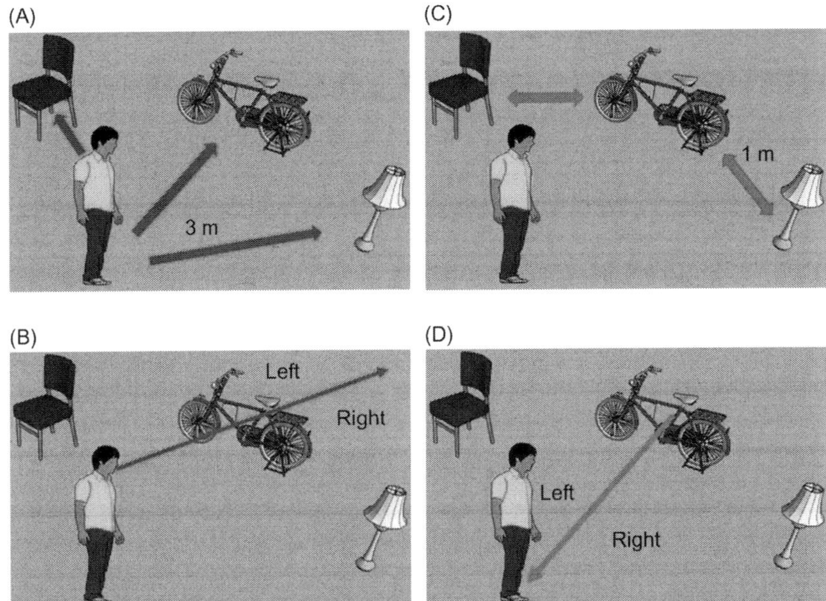

Figure 2.7 (A) Egocentric and (C) allocentric frames of reference combined with metric distances (coordinate spatial relations); (B) egocentric and (D) allocentric frames of reference combined with abstract spatial relations (ie, right/left: categorical spatial relations).

locations is not equally easy but depends on the relation between the required location and the observer. Instead, the allocentric frames of reference specify spatial information independently of the observer's position. Some theories specify that external objects are chosen like anchor-points: objects or part of objects (Humphreys & Riddoch, 1984; Kosslyn, 1994), salient landmarks, local features like walls and global features like mountains (McNamara, 2003; McNamara, Rump, & Werner, 2003), intrinsic axes defined by interobject relations (Mou & McNamara, 2002), the Sun's azimuth, and the direction of gravity (Paillard, 1991). This implies that all spatial positions in the environment are equally available and derived spatial representations are "orientation-free" (Rieser, 1989; Roskos-Ewoldsen, McNamara, Shelton, & Carr, 1998; Waller, Montello, Richardson, & Hegarty, 2002) (see also Chapter 1 and 7).

There is extensive literature concerning frames of reference revealing a general acceptance (Paillard, 1991) of the need for a distinction (O'Keefe & Nadel, 1978; Tolman 1948) between egocentric and allocentric systems. For example, this distinction is useful to distinguish the egocentric measurements of distance and direction toward a set of landmarks from the resulting "mental map" of that environment (eg, O'Keefe, 1993), or to explain the human conceptual development. Acredolo (1988) showed that infants, during their first 6 months, only use egocentric frames of reference with which to encode spatial information. Thenceforth, they acquire the ability to compensate for their own rotation, so that by 16 months they can identify a window in one wall as the relevant stimulus even when entering the room (with two identical windows) from the other side. This can be thought of as the acquisition of a nonegocentric, "absolute," or "geographic" orientation or frame of reference.

2.10 DISSOCIATION BETWEEN EGOCENTRIC AND ALLOCENTRIC FRAMES OF REFERENCE: EVIDENCE FROM NEUROSCIENCE

Best and White (1998), in their commentary about the spatial functions of the hippocampus, indicate that the first experimental evidence that spatial information can be encoded according to an allocentric reference frames was presented in 1971 by O'Keefe and Dostrovsky (1971). The discovery of place-cells (ie, cells firing maximally when the rats were in a rather small, well-defined region of the environment) led O'Keefe and Nadel (1978) to propose that the hippocampus serves as a cognitive map. According to the theory, an environment is represented by a collection of place-cells, each of which represents a specific region of space.

Other studies made use of a variety of topographical tasks, such as landmark knowledge, orientation in large-scale space and navigation, and have detected activation in the posterior parahippocampal cortex (Aguirre & D'Esposito, 1997; Aguirre, Detre, Alsop, & D'Esposito, 1996; Ghaëm et al., 1997; Grön, Wunderlich, Spitzer, Tomczak, & Riepe, 2000; Maguire, Frackowiak, & Frith, 1997; Maguire, Frith, Burgess, Donnett, & O'Keefe, 1998; Mellet et al., 2000), the hippocampus (Ghaëm et al., 1997; Grön et al., 2000; Maguire, Frackowiak, & Frith, 1996; Maguire et al., 1997), and the retrosplenial cortex (Maguire, 2001), as well as the posterior parietal cortex (Aguirre et al., 1996; Grön et al., 2000; Mellet et al., 2000). Since the tasks used in these studies were too complex and entailed spatial operations referring to both the viewer and to external references, it was difficult to disentangle between brain areas involved in egocentric or allocentric representations. Instead, in the following sections, a brief overview of neuropsychological and neurophysiological studies, showing anatomically and functionally separate neuronal circuits for allocentric and egocentric spatial coding, will be presented.

2.10.1 Disorders in Reference Frames Use

Neuropsychological investigations on unilateral spatial neglect have provided indications for distinct spatial frames of reference. Patients with spatial neglect fail to explore the side of space contralateral to the lesion and to report stimuli presented in that portion of space. Neuropsychological investigations of brain-damaged patients suffering from spatial unilateral neglect (Vallar, 1998), have generally revealed an egocentric disorder, where the affected sector of space is defined according to coordinate frames such as the midsagittal plane of the body (Vallar, Guariglia, & Rusconi, 1997), that is, a fundamental egocentric spatial principle (Jeannerod & Biguer, 1989). Spatial neglect may also concern the contralesional side of individual objects, independent of their position relative to the egocentric frame ("object-based" neglect: Bisiach, 1997; Driver, 1999). According to Hillis and colleagues (Hillis et al., 2005) egocentric neglect can be associated with frontal and dorsal hypofusion in right posterior inferior frontal gyrus, angular gyrus, supramarginal gyrus, and the visual association cortex. Object-based neglect can be associated with more ventral hypofusion, including right superior temporal gyrus and posterior inferior temporal gyrus.

Reports on topographical disorientation have also provided evidence that supports the hypothesis of separate and specific egocentric and allocentric frames of reference. Topographically, disorientation is a disorder in which patients have selectively lost the ability to find their way within their locomotor environment. Within this class of patients, there is a disorder caused by loss of the egocentric representation (egocentric disorientation) distinct from "heading disorientation" that is due to impairment in the allocentric domain (Aguirre & D'Esposito, 1999). In the words of Aguirre and D'Esposito (1999): "*These egocentrically disoriented patients are uniformly impaired in way-finding tasks in both familiar and novel environments. Most remain confined to the hospital or home, willing to venture out only with a companion* (Kase, Troncoso, Court, Tapia, & Mohr, 1977; Levine, Warach, & Farah, 1985). *Route descriptions are impoverished and inaccurate* (Levine et al., 1985) *and sketch-map production is disordered* (Hanley & Davies, 1995). *In contrast to these impairments, visual—object recognition has been informally noted to be intact.*" All egocentrically disoriented patients above mentioned had either bilateral or unilateral right lesions of the posterior parietal lobe, commonly involving the superior parietal lobule.

A second group of brain damaged patients appeared to be affected by a *Heading Disorientation*, with selective damage of the allocentric spatial representations. These patients are able to recognize salient landmarks but are unable to derive directional information from them. The lesion reported by these patients mainly involves the right retrosplenial (ie, posterior cingulate) region.

2.10.2 Neuroimaging Studies

Among the first neuroimaging evidence showing the involvement of a posterior parietal–frontal premotor network, bilateral but more extensive on the right, when stimuli are localized with respect to the body's midsagittal plane was that by Vallar and colleagues (Vallar et al., 1999). Successively, a similar activation was found by Galati and colleagues (2000) but much larger in the egocentric than in the allocentric judgments (Galati et al., 2000), for both visual and tactile stimuli (Galati, Committeri, Sanes, & Pizzamiglio, 2001). In addition, activation of the lingual gyrus and the region around the tail of the hippocampus, including the parahippocampal gyrus, was found when the allocentric task was directly compared with the egocentric one. Similar results were also reported by Committeri and colleagues (Committeri et al., 2004) in an fMRI study. In their research, participants saw 3D images of an environment and they had to estimate distances between objects in the environment (object-centered condition), between objects and a salient landmark in the environment (landmark-centered condition), and between objects and the observer (viewer-centered condition). Results revealed an activation of the posterior parietal and frontal premotor network during the viewer-centered condition more extensive in the right hemisphere, and the center of activity was quite superior and medial. Further, the bilateral ventromedial occipito–temporal cortex and retrosplenial cortex were exclusively activated in the landmark-centered condition, where the geometrical structure of the environment had to be taken as a reference. Instead, the ventrolateral occipito-temporal cortex was more activated by the object-centered judgment. Another study comparing the neural bases of egocentric and allocentric frames of reference (Zaehle et al., 2007) found that the processing of egocentric verbal descriptions of spatial relations are mediated by medial superior-posterior areas with an important role of the precuneus, whereas allocentric spatial reasoning requires an additional involvement of right parietal cortex, the ventral visual stream and the hippocampal formation. They interpreted their data as evidence of a hierarchically organized processing system in which the egocentric spatial coding requires only a subsystem of the processing resources of the allocentric condition. Finally, Chen and colleagues (Chen et al., 2014) have shown that the egocentric encoding of spatial locations for guiding a reaching movement activates the parietofrontal cortex more than the allocentric encoding of the same locations.

In synthesis, data from neuroimaging studies reveal that distinct but also partially overlapping brain areas support egocentric and allocentric encoding of spatial information. Overall a fronto–parietal network subtends egocentric spatial processing, whereas a subset of these regions associated with some ventral areas and hippocampal formation subtends allocentric spatial processing. Importantly, other studies (Hartley, Maguire, Spiers, & Burgess, 2003; Iaria, Petrides, Dagher, Pike, & Bohbot, 2003) demonstrated that the hippocampus is tied to the destiny of allocentric representation of spatial information and, even if there is still a debate on the status of long-term spatial memory, the involvement of the hippocampus in allocentric spatial memory is commonly accepted (Feigenbaum & Morris, 2004; Kesner, 2000; Nadel & Hardt, 2004; Save & Poucet, 2000).

2.11 DISSOCIATION AND INTERACTION BETWEEN EGOCENTRIC AND ALLOCENTRIC FRAMES OF REFERENCE: EVIDENCE FROM BEHAVIORAL STUDIES

Interesting evidence about how human beings encode and represent spatial information comes from behavioral studies about "visuospatial information in perceptual- and action-oriented tasks" and "visuospatial memory." Both these lines of studies seem to support the idea that even though egocentric and allocentric frames of reference are distinct components of human visuospatial system they seem to strictly cooperate during the encoding phase of spatial information in healthy people and the representation and the storing of spatial properties of the environments (Burgess, 2006).

2.11.1 Visuospatial Information in Perceptual- and Action-Oriented Tasks

Although the neuroscientific studies suggest a relative neural specialization for egocentric and allocentric processing, it is not clear to what extent or for what tasks such a specialization is necessary or, instead, a close interaction would be more efficient. This raises the question as to whether egocentric and allocentric processing of spatial information may interact.

Some studies about the effect of visual illusions on spatial judgments demonstrated that participants were more accurate when they performed spatial tasks by using motor actions (eg, pointing) than verbal judgments (Bridgeman, Peery, & Anand, 1997; Gentilucci Chieffi, Daprati, Saetti, & Toni, 1996). Such dissociations of accurate sensorimotor and inaccurate nonmotor localization are accounted for by modeling two separate spatial "maps," one, more egocentric, used in motor tasks and one, more allocentric, in cognitive/perceptual tasks (Bridgeman, 1991; Milner & Goodale, 1995; Sterken, Postma, de Haan, & Dingemans, 1999). However, there is evidence that in motor tasks allocentric information is also used. For instance, in Bridgeman's (1991) study, participants had to judge by pointing the position of a stimulus target whose reference background (a rectangle) was laterally displaced. They had to respond immediately after stimulus offset or after 8 seconds of delay. Results revealed that the visual illusion induced by the displacement of the reference background (Roelofs effect) influenced the pointing judgment when participants had to give the response after 8 seconds and not when the response was immediate. The author argued that when the motor representation was no longer available, participants had to utilize the cognitive representation in order to give a response. Further, Heat and colleagues (Heath, Rival, Neely, & Krigolson, 2006) studied the performance of participants that had to regulate their grip aperture (GA) with respect to a visual object embedded within fins-in and fins-out Müller–Lyer figures (ML). In the first part of the task, participants formulated a premovement GA based on the size of a neutral preview object. Preview objects were smaller, veridical, or larger than the size of the to-be-grasped target object. As a result, premovement GA associated with the small and large preview objects required significant online reorganization to appropriately grasp the target object. It was found that the online reorganization of GA was reliably influenced by the ML figures, regardless of the size of the preview object, albeit the small and large preview objects elicited more robust illusory effects than the veridical preview object. These results counter the view that online grasping control is mediated by absolute visual information computed with respect to the observer (Milner & Goodale, 1995). Instead, the impact of the ML figures suggests a level of interaction between egocentric and allocentric visual cues in online action control. Whether or not action is subject to visual illusions is still a matter of debate (Bruno, Bernardis, & Gentilucci, 2008; Franz, 2001; Smeets & Brenner,

2006). According to Smeets and colleagues (2002) "whether an illusion influences the execution of a task will depend on which spatial attributes are used rather than on whether the task is perceptual or motor." As a consequence, the two-visual-systems hypothesis should be based not on a dissociation between perception and action but on the kind of spatial representation used to accomplish the task, that is, egocentric or allocentric (Schenk, 2006; Smeets & Brenner, 2006). However, besides this issue what several authors agree upon is the fact that a strict interconnection between both egocentric and allocentric spatial information is used to deal with a huge number of everyday tasks (eg, Byrne & Crawford, 2010).

Neggers and colleagues (2005) studied the interaction between egocentric and allocentric frames of reference just in the cognitive domain. In the "egocentric judgment task" participants judged the position of a vertical target bar (at one out of five different fixed positions) relative to themselves, where the task-irrelevant horizontal bars were located at five different positions relative to each of the target bars. In the "allocentric judgment" task, the position of the vertical target bar relative to the center of the background bar had to be judged, for different egocentric position of the object-background ensemble. Neggers and colleagues (2005) observed that the judgments of the target's position with respect to the body were systematically biased by the irrelevant positions of the horizontal background. Since there was no effect from egocentric target location on position judgments with respect to the background, it was concluded that a unidirectional influence from allocentric to egocentric space representations existed. This influence appeared to be limited to occipito–temporal areas, subserving the biased cognitive reports of location, and was not found in parietal areas, subserving unbiased goal-directed action (Neggers, Van der Lubbe, Ramsey, & Postma, 2006).

However, another study indicates that the reverse, that is, the influence of egocentric spatial changes on allocentric spatial judgments, could also be possible. Sterken and colleagues (Sterken et al., 1999) showed that the perceived displacement (jump) of an object with respect to a surrounding frame (allocentric coordinate) of a dot can be influenced by the displacement of that dot with respect to the body. The reverse was also true; jumps in egocentric position were also influenced by the jump in the position of the background frame, an interaction similar to the induced Roelofs effect. Furthermore, the detection of displacements involves a comparison of current frame position with previously perceived frame position, indicating that some memory processes might be involved in the interactions observed by Sterken and colleagues (1999).

Although detection of a displacement is different from determining the exact location of a stimulus, similar perceptual processes might underlie position judgments, indicating that the interaction between egocentric and allocentric coordinate representations could be bidirectional. The relevance of egocentric spatial processing within the cognitive domain was also highlighted by Neggers and colleagues (2006). In their fMRI study activation of the parietal cortex during the egocentric cognitive judgments of the participants appeared. More recently, Bridgeman and Hoover (2008) pointed out that also a task that does not require motor control can be critically dependent on body posture and distortion of bodily coordinates.

2.11.2 Visuospatial Memory

Wang and Spelke (2002) suggested a simple model of spatial memory that combines: a viewpoint-dependent scene recognition process; a spatial updating of egocentric locations by self-motion information; and a geometric module that represents the surface geometry of the surrounding environment. This model is endorsed by several studies. Shelton and McNamara (1997) demonstrated that when people are asked to point to an object from an imagined viewpoint, they are faster and more accurate when the imagined viewpoint has the same direction as the studied viewpoint. This *alignment effect* indicates storage of a viewpoint-dependent representation of the visual scene. The absence of a stable allocentric representation is also revealed by other researches in which the "spatial updating" paradigm is used. In the study by Wang and Spelke (2000), participants learned locations of objects scattered around a room. Afterward, they had to point to the objects with eyes either open or blindfolded or blindfolded after disorientation by rotating the chair where they seated. The results indicate that participants were able to capture the environmental geometry of the room but they used mainly egocentric spatial representation to solve the task at hand.

However, other studies have shown that the locations of objects might be stored in allocentric representations based on landmarks or intrinsic axes in the external environment. For example, in an experiment by McNamara and colleagues (2003), participants learned the locations of objects while following a route through a park, which encircled a large rectangular building, and after they had to point to the objects from several imagined viewpoints. Participants in this experiment were more accurate when pointing to objects from imagined viewpoints aligned with a salient landmark (eg, a large lake), even when this viewing direction was not experienced.

As suggested by Burgess (2006), the simple egocentric model for object–location memory proposed by Wang and Spelke (2002) is more consistent with a "two-system model" in which transient egocentric representations exist in parallel to (rather than instead of) more endurable allocentric ones (Waller & Hodgson, 2006; see also Mou, McNamara, Valiquette, & Rump, 2004; Sholl & Nolin, 1997). Importantly, the use of one or the other spatial representation can depend on the way of learning spatial information (Presson & Hazelrigg, 1984), size (Presson, DeLange, & Hazelrigg, 1989), geometric structure (McNamara et al., 2003), and degree of familiarity of the environment (Iachini, Ruggiero, Conson, & Trojano, 2009; Ruggiero & Iachini, 2006).

In conclusion, the literature reveals a broad acceptance of the functional distinction between egocentric and allocentric frames of reference. Egocentric frames of reference seem to have the role of primary interface between humans and the environment (Iachini & Logie, 2003); this role is revealed in primacy on learning new environments. Instead, increased familiarity with the environment provides an allocentric representation (Iachini, Ruotolo, & Ruggiero, 2009). However, several factors can influence the selection of the frames of reference more useful to solve the task at end. Several studies about spatial memory have shown that egocentric and allocentric information is combined to produce mental representation of the environment (Burgess, 2006) or to guide the movement toward a remembered position (Byrne & Crawford, 2010) and that this could be the product of an encoding phase in which egocentric and allocentric information influence each other (Neggers, Schölvinck, van der Lubbe, & Postma, 2005; Ruotolo, van der Ham, Iachini, & Postma, 2011; Sterken et al., 1999).

2.11.3 Relation between Frames of Reference and Categorical and Coordinate Spatial Information

In the first section of this part of the chapter we have presented a huge number of studies endorsing the functional and neurological distinction between egocentric and allocentric frames of reference as well as between categorical and coordinate spatial information. However, it is also important to put these elements in a more general theory of the functioning of the mind. We propose a theoretical analysis starting from Milner and Goodale's theory (1995) about the division of labor in the human visual pathway. The segregation is between a ventral channel (occipito–temporal pathway) that mediates processing of information useful for object recognition (what), while a dorsal channel (occipito–parietal pathway) subserves visually guided behavior (how). On the basis of this theoretical framework these processing streams may depend upon different classes of spatial information for performing their distinct roles. For example, motor responses like skilled reaching and grasping and the control of eye movements could not function without specific, precise coordinate computations that code the location of visual targets relative to the body or its parts such as the hand or the eye (ie, egocentrically). In contrast, the representations of spatial layouts or objects in the absence of perceptual stimuli require less fine-grained spatial information that can be built upon the relative positions of salient objects or parts of objects. Such cruder but more robust spatial coding based on allocentric spatial relationships would primarily require categorical rather than coordinate information (Kosslyn, 1987; Kosslyn et al., 1989; Kosslyn et al., 1992). Perceptually based categorical representations can last indefinitely, irrespective of the imagined viewpoint, whereas coordinate reporting from memory can be attempted, but it would be highly inaccurate (Carey, 2004).

Therefore, according to Milner and Goodale's theory (1995), if the encoding primarily subserves visuomotor action, dorsal stream circuits encode targets relative to the observer, and do so in egocentric effector-specific codes that are coordinate-based (such as degrees of visual angle, or absolute distance/direction vectors from the hand or shoulder). Recent functional fMRI evidence supports the idea that egocentric spatial coding is subserved by a posterior parietal and frontal premotor network (Committeri et al., 2004). Visual circuits associated with the occipito–temporal ventral stream encode spatial relationships in multipurpose codes which enjoy considerable flexibility, while losing the precision of the viewpoint-dependent, short-lasting, coordinates that characterize dorsal stream function (Goodale & Humphrey, 1998; Rossetti & Pisella, 2002).

From this theory derives an important issue. Indeed, the theory suggests a connection between egocentric and allocentric frames of reference and coordinate and categorical spatial information, respectively. Carey, Dijkerman, & Milner (1998) suggested that another relation between the two basic aspects of the spatial cognition could be theoretically possible. The second possibility is that the egocentric/allocentric and the categorical/coordinate distinctions form orthogonal dimensions, which can be fully combined (Murphy, Carey, & Goodale, 1998). That is, while the former defines the point of reference to anchor a location, the latter specifies the grain of the spatial relation. We would thus have four possible situations: (a) egocentric-categorical (the chair is on your left); (b) egocentric-coordinate (the chair is 50 cm from yourself);

(c) allocentric-categorical (the chair is on the left of the table); (d) allocentric-coordinate (the chair is 50 cm from the table) (Jager & Postma, 2003).

These two possible relationships between egocentric and allocentric frames and categorical and coordinate spatial relations have been formalized by Jager and Postma (2003). They proposed two opposing hypotheses concerning this question. The *interaction hypothesis* states that allocentric processing "more or less equates" categorical coding of spatial relations, whereas egocentric processing is closely linked to coordinate coding. Therefore, categorical spatial representations should be favored when an allocentric frame is used, whereas coordinate spatial relations processing should benefit from an egocentric anchoring. Instead, the *independence hypothesis* states that frames of reference and spatial relations are distinct spatial dimensions that can be fully combined without preference for a particular kind of association.

Iachini and colleagues (Iachini, Ruggiero, et al., 2009) compared left- and right-parietal brain damaged patients on egocentric and allocentric spatial memory tasks. The results strongly suggest that the right hemisphere is specialized in processing metric information according to egocentric frames of reference. These results seem to be in favor of an interaction between frames of reference and grain of spatial information. Instead, results from a study by Carey, Dijkerman, Murphy, Goodale, and Milner (2006) support the hypothesis of independence between egocentric-allocentric and categorical-coordinate distinctions. In this study, performance of DF, a patient with bilateral damage to the ventral stream (see Box 2.1), was compared with the performance of nondamaged subjects. They had to point to a set of spatially distributed stimuli either by direct pointing or by copying or "pantomiming" the response in an adjacent homologous workspace. The three conditions required either categorical or coordinate processing of spatial information that relied on an allocentric frame of reference. The results showed that even when DF performed quite poorly with respect to the control group when copying target arrays on the pantomimed pointing task, her performance was more accurate with categorical than coordinate relations between the elements in the array. It is possible that DF's degraded performance reflected a relative preservation of allocentric categorical coding, despite a loss of allocentric coordinate coding. Instead, nondamaged subjects did perform the allocentric coordinate and allocentric categorical tasks at the same level. Moreover, results indicated accurate sensorimotor localization when DF pointed directly to single targets or to

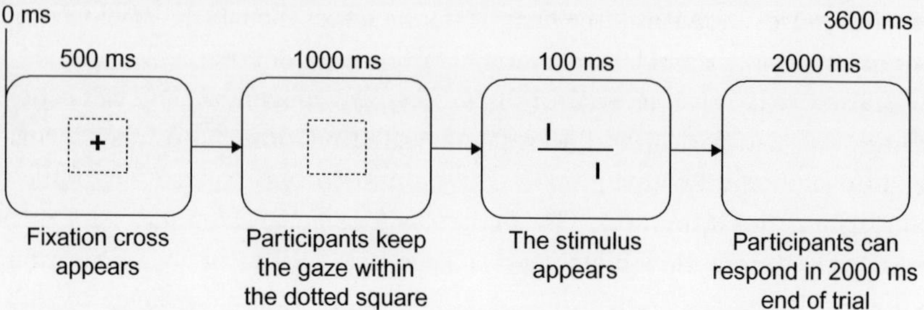

Figure 2.8 The figure shows a schematic overview of one trial. At $t = 0$, the fixation cross is displayed for 500 ms; then the cross disappears, and only the dotted square remains for 1000 ms. When the square disappears, the to-be-judged stimulus is displayed for 100 ms, after which the participants have 2000 ms to give their response. After this, a new trial starts. *Taken from Ruotolo, F., van der Ham, I. J. M, Iachini, T., & Postma, A. (2011). The relationship between allocentric and egocentric frames of reference and categorical and coordinate spatial information processing.* The Quarterly Journal of Experimental Psychology, *64(6), 1138–1156. doi:10.1080/17470218.2010.539700.*

sequences of targets, presumably as she could use egocentric visual coding. According to the authors these results are consistent with the idea that the egocentric–allocentric and coordinate–categorical are not interacting processes but rather form orthogonal dimensions (Jager & Postma, 2003; Murphy et al., 1998).

In order to spread light on this pattern of results, Ruotolo and colleagues (Ruotolo, Iachini, et al., 2011; Ruotolo, van der Ham, et al., 2011; Ruotolo, van der Ham, Postma, Ruggiero, & Iachini, 2015) studied in a complementary way the use of the frames of reference and of the categorical and coordinate information. In their first study (Ruotolo, van der Ham, et al., 2011), participants were presented, via a computer screen, with stimuli comprising two vertical bars, one above and the other below a horizontal bar. Afterward, they were requested to visually judge coordinate and categorical spatial relations of the two vertical bars with respect to their body-midline (egocentric frame) or with respect to the center of the horizontal bar (allocentric frame) (see Fig. 2.8).

Specifically, the spatial judgments that had to be given included: (a) were the two vertical bars at the same distance with respect to you? (egocentric coordinate judgment); (b) were the two vertical bars at the same distance with respect to the center of the horizontal bar? (allocentric coordinate judgment); (c) were the two vertical bars on the same side with respect to you? (egocentric categorical judgment); (d) were the two

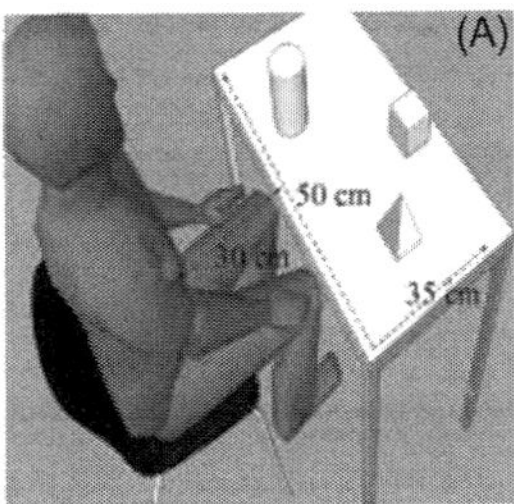

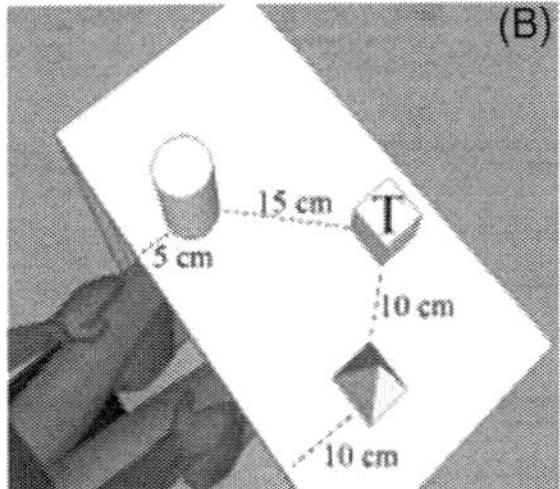

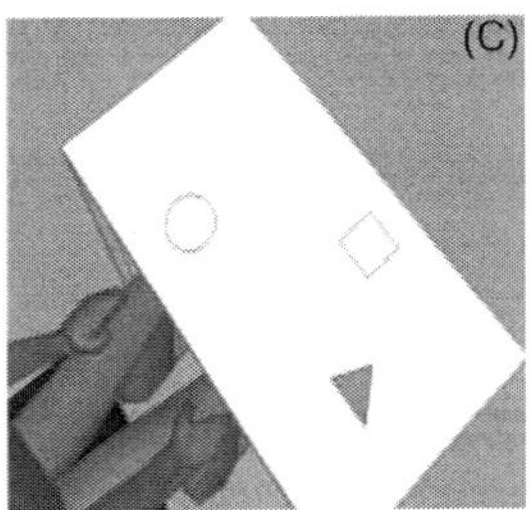

Figure 2.9 (A) Participants seated at a distance of 30 cm from a desk on which 3D manipulable objects (B) or 2D images (C) could be presented. *Taken from Ruotolo, F., van der Ham, I., Postma, A., Ruggiero, G., & Iachini, T. (2015). How coordinate and categorical spatial relations combine with egocentric and allocentric reference frames in a motor task: Effects of delay and stimuli characteristics.* Behavioural Brain Research, 284, *167–178. doi:10.1016/j.bbr.2015.02.021.*

vertical bars on the same side with respect to the center of the horizontal bar? (allocentric categorical judgment). Results revealed an advantage of allocentric categorical judgments over all the other judgments, whereas egocentric coordinate judgments were less accurate than all others. However, when the luminance of the horizontal bar was reduced, this specifically improved egocentric coordinate judgments. These data were taken as an evidence partially supporting the independence hypothesis. Indeed, they showed that frames of reference and spatial relations are distinct dimensions, but the use of the four kinds of spatial representation deriving from their combination can be modulated by the characteristics of the task at hand. Indeed, according to Milner and Goodale's theory (1995), the visuoperceptual task used by Ruotolo and colleagues could have favored the encoding of allocentric categorical spatial relations to the detriment of an egocentric encoding of coordinate spatial relations. To verify this hypothesis, recently Ruotolo and colleagues (2015) used an experimental paradigm in which participants were requested to perform a motor action (ie, pointing) toward the locations of previously seen objects (3D, manipulable objects) or images (2D, nonmanipulable geometrical figures) (see Fig. 2.9).

Specifically, participants were presented with triads of objects or images (6 seconds). Afterward they were requested to indicate: (a) where was the object/image closest/farthest with respect to them (egocentric coordinate task); (b) where was the object/image closest/farthest with respect to another object (allocentric coordinate task); (c) where was the object/image X with respect to them (egocentric categorical task);

(d) where was the object/image X with respect to the object/image Y (allocentric categorical task). Pointing movements could be executed immediately after stimuli presentation or after 5 seconds they have been removed. Contrary to the results from the visuoperceptual task (Ruotolo, van der Ham, et al., 2011), results indicated that coordinate judgments were more precise and faster when made with respect to an egocentric rather than an allocentric frame of reference and this was independent from the kind of stimuli used and from the temporal parameters of the response. Instead, when the visuoperceptual characteristics of the task were stressed with the use of 2D images and when the action was memory-based, allocentric and categorical spatial representations improve.

A similar paradigm was also used by Ruggiero and colleagues to explore spatial memory in blind people (Ruggiero, Ruotolo, & Iachini, 2012) and the spatial abilities of a patient with "heading disorientation" (Ruggiero, Frassinetti, Iavarone, & Iachini, 2014). In the former study, congenitally blind, adventitiously blind, and sighted blindfolded participants had to memorize through haptic and haptic plus visual exploration (only the sighted) as accurately as possible the positions of three 3D geometrical objects. Afterward, they were asked to verbally provide four spatial judgments: "which object was closest/farthest to you?" (egocentric-coordinate); "which object was on your left/right?" (egocentric-categorical); "which object was closest/farthest to a target object (eg, cone)?" (allocentric-coordinate); "which object was on the left/right of the target object (eg, cone)?" (allocentric-categorical). Results revealed that congenitally blind participants were slower than all other groups in processing the coordinate—allocentric spatial relations, whereas adventitiously blind participants were slower in processing the categorical—egocentric combination. In the latter study, the same task was used with the exception that the patient and control participants provided the combined egocentric—allocentric and coordinate—categorical spatial judgments by means of verbal and visuomotor response modalities. The results indicated a selective deficit in the coordinate component in verbal (combined with both egocentric and allocentric frames) and visuomotor (only with the egocentric frame) spatial judgment tasks. In contrast, the categorical component looked always preserved in both frames of reference.

Finally, Ruotolo, Iachini, et al. (2011) showed that the relationship between frames of reference and spatial relations can be thought as hierarchically organized. Participants in this study were more accurate in judging categorical and coordinate spatial relations when they knew in advance the frame of reference (egocentric vs allocentric) than when they received information about frame of reference after the information about the kind of spatial relations to be judged. This was taken as an evidence of the fact that frames of reference have a primary role with respect to spatial relations in organizing spatial information.

In sum, these studies suggest that the four spatial representations deriving from the combination of frames of reference and spatial relations can be selectively damaged and influenced by the characteristics of the task at hand. This would suggest that they represent distinct and independent spatial dimensions. However, Baumann and Mattingley (2014) suggest that to answer the question whether and how reference frame processing and spatial relation coding interact, it will be necessary to determine the neural correlates of these cognitive processes in one common experiment. Based on current evidence, they hypothesize that spatial relation coding and reference frame processing are independent cognitive mechanisms that engage different subregions of the hippocampus and posterior parietal cortex. An allocentric–coordinate task should therefore be entirely hippocampal dependent, whereas an egocentric–categorical task would be solely dependent on the parietal cortex. On the other hand, allocentric–categorical and egocentric–coordinate navigation tasks should rely on both the hippocampus and the parietal cortex.

2.12 GENERAL CONCLUSION

Two main distinctions within visuospatial perception concern spatial relation processing and reference frames. Categorical and coordinate spatial relations have shown to be processed mainly by the left and right hemispheres, respectively. This lateralization pattern is found regardless of task characteristics or stimulus layout. However, recent evidence highlights the impact of stimulus size: a smaller attentional focus facilitates categorical processing, whereas a larger attentional focus is linked to coordinate processing.

Egocentric and allocentric frames of reference represent two distinct dimensions within the visuospatial domain and their relevance for action- or recognition-oriented tasks depends on the kind of spatial relation that is processed (ie, categorical vs coordinate), on the temporal parameters of the response (ie, online vs memory-based), and on the kind of elements we have to deal with (eg, manipulable vs nonmanipulable objects).

REFERENCES

Acredolo, L. (1988). Infant mobility and spatial development. In J. Stiles-Davis, M. Kritchevsky, & U. Bellugi (Eds.), *Spatial cognition: Brain bases and development* (pp. 157–166). Hillsdale, NJ: Lawrence Erlbaum.

Aguirre, G. K., & D'Esposito, M. (1997). Environmental knowledge is subserved by separable dorsal/ventral neural areas. *Journal of Neuroscience*, *17*, 2512–2518.

Aguirre, G. K., & D'Esposito, M. (1999). Topographical disorientation: A synthesis and taxonomy. *Brain*, *122*(9), 1613–1628.

Aguirre, G. K., Detre, J. A., Alsop, D. C., & D'Esposito, M. (1996). The parahippocampus subserves topographical learning in men. *Cerebral Cortex*, *6*, 823–829.

Andersen, R. A., Snyder, L. H., Bradley, D. C., & Xing, J. (1997). Multimodal representation of space in the posterior parietal cortex and its use in planning movements. *Annual Review of Neuroscience*, *20*, 303–330.

Arcaro, M. J., McMains, S., Singer, B., & Kastner, S. (2009). Retinotopic organization of human ventral visual cortex. *Journal of Neuroscience*, *29*, 10638–10652.

Baciu, M., Koenig, O., Vernier, M.-P., Bedoin, N., Rubin, C., & Segebarth, C. (1999). Categorical and coordinate spatial relations: fMRI evidence for hemispheric specialization. *Neuroreport*, *10*, 1373–1378.

Banich, M. T., & Federmeier, K. D. (1999). Categorical and metric spatial processes distinguished by task demands and practice. *Journal of Cognitive Neuroscience*, *11*, 153–166.

Baumann, O., Chan, E., & Mattingley, J. B. (2012). Distinct neural networks underlie encoding of categorical versus coordinate spatial relations during active navigation. *NeuroImage*, *60*(3), 1630–1637.

Baumann, O., & Mattingley, J. B. (2014). Dissociable roles of the hippocampus and parietal cortex in processing of coordinate and categorical spatial information. *Frontiers in Human Neuroscience*, *8*, 73. Available from http://dx.doi.org/10.3389/fnhum.2014.00073.

Best, P. J., & White, A. M. (1998). Hippocampal cellular activity: A brief history of space. *Proceedings of the National Academy of Sciences USA*, *95*(6), 2717–2719.

Bisiach, E. (1997). The spatial features of unilateral neglect. In P. Their, & H. O. Karnath (Eds.), *Parietal lobe contributions to orientation in 3D space* (pp. 465–495). Heidelberg: Springer-Verlag.

Borst, G., & Kosslyn, S. M. (2010). Varying the scope of attention alters the encoding of categorical and coordinate spatial relations. *Neuropsychologia*, *48*(9), 2769–2772.

Bourne, V. J. (2006). The divided visual field paradigm: Methodological considerations. Laterality: Asymmetries of body. *Brain and Cognition*, *11*(4), 373–393.

Bridgeman, B. (1991). Complementary cognitive and motor image processing. In G. Obrecht, & L. Stark (Eds.), *Presbyopia research: From molecular biology to visual adaptation* (pp. 189–198). New York, NY: Plenum Press.

Bridgeman, B., & Hoover, M. (2008). Processing spatial layout by perception and sensorimotor interaction. *The Quarterly Journal of Experimental Psychology*, *61*(6), 851–859.

Bridgeman, B., Peery, S., & Anand, S. (1997). Interaction of cognitive and sensorimotor maps of visual space. *Perception & Psychophysics*, *59*, 456–469.

Bruno, N., Bernardis, P., & Gentilucci, M. (2008). Visually guided pointing, the Müller-Lyer illusion, and the functional interpretation of the dorsal-ventral split: Conclusions from 33 independent studies. *Neuroscience and Biobehavioral Reviews*, *32*(3), 423–437. Available from http://dx.doi.org/10.1016/j.neubiorev.2007.08.006.

Bruyer, R., Scailquin, J.-C., & Coibion, P. (1997). Dissociation between categorical and coordinate spatial computations: Modulation by the cerebral hemispheres, task properties, mode of response, and age. *Brain and Cognition*, *33*, 245–277.

Burgess, N. (2006). Spatial memory: How egocentric and allocentric combine. *Trends in Cognitive Sciences*, *10*(12), 551–557. Available from http://dx.doi.org/10.1016/j.tics.2006.10.005.

Byrne, P. A., & Crawford, J. D. (2010). Cue reliability and a landmark stability heuristic determine relative weighting between egocentric and allocentric visual information in memory-guided reach. *Journal of Neurophysiology*, *103*(6), 3054–3069. Available from http://dx.doi.org/10.1152/jn.01008.2009.

Carey, D. P. (2004). The exploration of (neuropsychological) space. *Cortex*, *40*, 645–650.

Carey, D. P., Dijkerman, H. C., & Milner, A. D. (1998). Perception and action in depth. *Consciousness and Cognition*, 7(3), 438–453.

Carey, D. P., Dijkerman, H. C., Murphy, K. J., Goodale, M. A., & Milner, A. D. (2006). Pointing to places and spaces in a patient with visual form agnosia. *Neuropsychologia*, *44*, 1584–1594.

Chao, L. L., & Martin, A. (2000). Representation of manipulable man-made objects in the dorsal stream. *NeuroImage*, *12*, 478–484.

Chen, Y., Monaco, S., Byrne, P., Yan, X., Henriques, D. Y., & Crawford, J. D. (2014). Allocentric versus egocentric representation of remembered reach targets in human cortex. *Journal of Neuroscience*, *34*(37), 12515–12526. Available from http://dx.doi.org/10.1523/JNEUROSCI.1445-14.2014.

Committeri, G., Galati, G., Paradis, A., Pizzamiglio, L., Berthoz, A., & LeBihan, D. (2004). Reference frame for spatial cognition: Different brain areas are involved in viewer-, object-, and landmark-centered judgments about object location. *Journal of Cognitive Neuroscience*, *16*(9), 1517–1535.

Cook, N. D. (1986). *The brain code: Mechanisms of information transfer and the role of the corpus callosum*. London: Methuen.

Cooper, E. E., & Wojan, T. J. (2000). Differences in the coding of spatial relations in face identification and basic-level object recognition. *J Exp Psychol Learn*, *26*, 470–488.

Driver, J. (1999). Egocentric and object-based visual neglect. In N. Burgess, K. J. Jeffery, & J. O'Keefe (Eds.), *Spatial functions of the hippocampal formation and the parietal cortex* (pp. 67–89). Oxford: Oxford University Press.

Feigenbaum, J. D., & Morris, R. G. (2004). Allocentric versus egocentric spatial memory after unilateral temporal lobectomy in humans. *Neuropsychology*, *18*, 462–472.

Franciotti, R., D'Ascenzo, S., Di Domenico, A., Tommasi, L., & Laeng, B. (2013). Focusing narrowly or broadly attention when judging categorical and coordinate spatial relations: A MEG study. *PLoS One*, *8*(12), e83434.

Franconeri, S. L., Scimeca, J. M., Roth, J. C., Helseth, S. A., & Kahn, L. E. (2012). Flexible visual processing of spatial relationships. *Cognition*, *122*, 210–227.

Franklin, A., Catherwood, D., Alvarez, J., & Axelsson, E. (2010). Hemispheric asymmetries in categorical perception of orientation in infants and adults. *Neuropsychologia*, *48*, 2648–2657.

Franklin, N., & Tversky, B. (1990). Searching imagined environments. *Journal of Experimental Psychology: General*, *119*, 63–76.

Franz, V. H. (2001). Action does not resist visual illusions. *Trends in Cognitive Sciences*, *5* (11), 457–459.

Galati, G., Committeri, G., Sanes, J. N., & Pizzamiglio, L. (2001). Spatial coding of visual and somatic sensory information in body-centered coordinates. *European Journal of Neuroscience*, *14*, 737–746.

Galati, G., Lobel, E., Berthoz, A., Pizzamiglio, L., Le Bihan, D., & Vallar, G. (2000). The neural basis of egocentric and allocentric coding of space in humans: A functional magnetic resonance study. *Experimental Brain Research*, *133*, 156–164.

Garcin, R., Rondot, P., & de Recondo, J. (1967). Optic ataxia localized in 2 left homonymous visual hemifields (clinical study with film presentation). *Revue Neurologique (Paris)*, *116*, 707–714.

Gentilucci, M., Chieffi, S., Daprati, E., Saetti, M. C., & Toni, I. (1996). Visual illusion and action. *Neuropsychologia*, *34*, 369–376.

Ghaëm, O., Mellet, E., Crivello, F., Tzourio, N., Mezoyer, B., Berthoz, A., & Denis, M. (1997). Mental navigation along memorized routes activates the hippocampus, precuneus, and insula. *Neuroreport*, *8*, 739–744.

Goldstein, E. B. (2014). *Sensation and perception* (ninth ed.) Pacific Grove, CA: Wadsworth.

Goodale, M. A. (2011). Transforming vision into action. *Vision Research*, *51*(13), 1567–1587.

Goodale, M. A., & Humphrey, G. K. (1998). The objects of action and perception. *Cognition*, *67*(1–2), 181–207.

Goodale, M. A., & Milner, A. D. (1992). Separate visual pathways for perception and action. *Trends in Neurosciences*, *15*(1), 20–25.

Goodale, M. A., Milner, A. D., Jacobson, L. S., & Carey, D. P. (1991). A neurological dissociation between perceiving objects and grasping them. *Nature*, 154–156.

Grön, G., Wunderlich, A. P., Spitzer, M., Tomczak, R., & Riepe, M. W. (2000). Brain activation during human navigation: Gender-different networks as substrate of performance. *Nature Neuroscience*, *3*, 404–408.

Hamami, Y., & Mumma, J. (2013). Prolegomena to a cognitive investigation of Euclidean diagrammatic reasoning. *Journal of Logic, Language, and Information*, *22*, 421–448.

Hanley, J. R., & Davies, A. D. (1995). Lost in your own house. In R. Campbell, & M. A. Conway (Eds.), *Broken memories: Case studies in memory impairment* (pp. 195–208). Oxford: Blackwell.

Hartley, T., Maguire, E. A., Spiers, H. J., & Burgess, N. (2003). The well-worn route and the path less travelled: Distinct neural bases of route following and wayfinding in humans. *Neuron*, *37*, 877–888.

Heath, M., Rival, C., Neely, K., & Krigolson, O. (2006). Müller-Lyer figures influence the online reorganization of visually guided grasping movements. *Experimental Brain Research*, *169*(4), 473–481. Available from http://dx.doi.org/10.1007/s00221-005-0170-3.

Hellige, J. B., & Michimata, C. (1989). Categorization versus distance: Hemispheric differences for processing spatial information. *Memory and Cognition*, *17*, 770–776.

Hillis, A. E., Newhart, M., Heidler, J., Barker, P. B., Herskovits, E. H., & Degaonkar, M. (2005). Anatomy of spatial attention: Insights from perfusion imaging and hemispatial neglect in acute stroke. *Journal of Neuroscience*, *25*, 3161–3167.

Hillis, J. M., Watt, S. J., Landy, M. S., & Banks, M. S. (2004). Slant from texture and disparity cues: Optimal cue combination. *Journal of Vision*, *14*(12), 967–992.

Holmes, K. J., & Wolff, P. (2012). Does categorical perception in the left hemisphere depend on language. *Journal of Experimental Psychology*, *141*(3), 439–443.

Hugdahl, K. (2000). Lateralization of cognitive processes in the brain. *Acta Psychologica*, *105*, 211–235.

Humphreys, G. W., & Riddoch, M. J. (1984). Routes to object constancy: Implications from neurological impairments of object constancy. *The Quarterly Journal of Experimental Psychology*, *36*(A), 385–415.

Iachini, T., & Logie, R. H. (2003). The role of perspective in locating position in a real--world, unfamiliar environment. *Applied Cognitive Psychology*, *17*, 715–732.

Iachini, T., Ruggiero, G., Conson, M., & Trojano, L. (2009). Lateralization of egocentric and allocentric spatial processing after parietal brain lesions. *Brain and Cognition*, *69*(3), 514–520. Available from http://dx.doi.org/10.1016/j.bandc.2008.11.001.

Iachini, T., Ruotolo, F., & Ruggiero, G. (2009). The effects of familiarity and gender on spatial representation. *Journal of Environmental Psychology, 29*(2), 227–234.

Iaria, G., Petrides, M., Dagher, A., Pike, B., & Bohbot, V. (2003). Cognitive strategies dependent on hippocampus and caudate nucleus in human navigation: Variability and change with practice. *Journal of Neuroscience, 23*, 5945–5952.

Jacobs, R. A. (1999). Optimal integration of texture and motion cues to depth. *Vision Research, 39*(21), 3621–3629.

Jager, G., & Postma, A. (2003). On the hemispheric specialization for categorical and coordinate spatial relations: A review of the current evidence. *Neuropsychologia, 41*, 504–515.

Jeannerod, M., & Rossetti, Y. (1993). Visuomotor coordination as a dissociable visual function: experimental and clinical evidences. *Bailliere's clinical neurology, 2*, 439–460.

Jeannerod, M., & Biguer, B. (1989). Reference égocentrique et espace represente. *Revue Neurologique, 145*, 635–639.

Kaas, J. H., & Collins, C. E. (2004). *The Primate Visual System*. Boca Raton, FL: CRC Press.

Kase, C. S., Troncoso, J. F., Court, J. E., Tapia, J. F., & Mohr, J. P. (1977). Global spatial disorientation, clinico-pathologic correlation. *Journal of the Neurological Sciences, 34*, 267–278.

Kemmerer, D., & Tranel, D. (2000). A double dissociation between linguistic and perceptual representations of spatial relationships. *Cognitive Neuropsychology, 17*, 393–414.

Kesner, R. P. (2000). Behavioral analysis of the contribution of the hippocampus and parietal cortex to the processing of information: Interactions and dissociations. *Hippocampus, 10*, 483–490.

Knill, D. C., & Saunders, J. A. (2003). Do humans optimally integrate stereo and texture information for judgments of surface slant? *Vision Research, 43*(24), 2539–2558.

Koenig, O., Reiss, L. P., & Kosslyn, S. M. (1990). The development of spatial relation representations: Evidence from studies of cerebral lateralization. *Journal of Experimental Child Psychology, 50*, 119–130.

Kosslyn, S. M. (1987). Seeing and imagining in the cerebral hemispheres: A computational analysis. *Psychological Review, 94*, 148–175.

Kosslyn, S. M. (1994). *Image and brain: The resolution of the imagery debate*. Cambridge, MA: MIT Press.

Kosslyn, S. M., Chabris, C. F., Marsolek, C. J., & Koenig, O. (1992). Categorical versus coordinate spatial relations: Computational analyses and computer simulations. *Journal of Experimental Psychology: Human Perception and Performance, 181*, 562–577.

Kosslyn, S. M., Koenig, O., Barrett, A., Backer Cave, C., Tang, J., & Gabrieli, J. D. E. (1989). Evidence for two types of spatial representations: Hemispheric specialization for categorical and coordinate relations. *Journal of Experimental Psychology: Human Perception and Performance, 15*, 723–735.

Kosslyn, S. M., Thompson, W. L., Gitelman, D. R., & Alpert, N. M. (1998). Neural systems that encode categorical versus coordinate spatial relations: PET investigations. *Psychobiology, 26*, 333–347.

Kravitz, D. J., Saleem, K. S., Baker, C. I., & Mishkin, M. (2011). A new neural framework for visuospatial processing. *Nature Reviews Neuroscience, 12*(4), 217–230.

Laeng, B. (1994). Lateralization of categorical and coordinate spatial functions: A study of unilateral stroke patients. *Journal of Cognitive Neuroscience, 6*, 189–203.

Laeng, B., Okubo, M., Saneyoshi, A., & Michimata, C. (2011). Processing spatial relations with different apertures of attention. *Cognitive Science, 35*(2), 297–329.

Levine, D. N., Warach, J., & Farah, M. J. (1985). Two visual systems in mental imagery: Dissociation of "what" and "where" in imagery disorders due to bilateral posterior cerebral lesions. *Neurology, 35*, 1010–1018.

Levinson, S. C. (1996). Frames of reference and Molyneux's question. In P. Bloom, M. A. Peterson, L. Nadel, & M. F. Garrett (Eds.), *Language and space* (pp. 109–169). Cambridge, MA: MIT Press.

Livingstone, M. S., & Hubel, D. H. (1984). Anatomy and physiology of a color system in the primate visual cortex. *Journal of Neuroscience*, *4*(1), 309–356.

Martin, M. (1979). Hemispheric specialization for local and global processing. *Neuropsychologia*, *17*, 33–40.

Maguire, E. A. (2001). The retrosplenial contribution to human navigation: A review of lesion and neuroimaging findings. *Scandinavian Journal of Psychology*, *42*, 225–238.

Maguire, E. A., Frackowiak, R. S. J., & Frith, C. D. (1996). Learning to find your way: A role for the human hippocampal formation. *Proceedings of the Royal Society of London, Series B, Biological Sciences*, *263*, 1745–1750.

Maguire, E. A., Frackowiak, R. S. J., & Frith, C. D. (1997). Recalling routes around London: Activation of the right hippocampus in taxi drivers. *Journal of Neuroscience*, *17*, 7103–7110.

Maguire, E. A., Frith, C. D., Burgess, N., Donnett, J. G., & O'Keefe, J. (1998). Knowing where things are: Parahippocampal involvement in encoding object locations in virtual large-scale space. *Journal of Cognitive Neuroscience*, *10*, 61–76.

Manders, K. (2008). The Euclidean diagram. In P. Mancosu (Ed.), *The Philosophy of Mathematical Practice*. Oxford University Press.

Martin, R., Houssemand, C., Schiltz, C., Burnod, Y., & Alexandre, F. (2008). Is there continuity between categorical and coordinate spatial relations coding: Evidence from a grid/no-grid working memory paradigm. *Neuropsychologia*, *46*(2), 576–594.

McNamara, T. P. (2003). How are the locations of objects in the environment represented in memory? In C. Freksa, W. Brauer, C. Habel, & K. Wender (Eds.), *Spatial cognition III: Routes and navigation, human memory and learning, spatial representation and spatial reasoning* (pp. 174–191). Berlin: Springer-Verlag.

McNamara, T. P., Rump, B., & Werner, S. (2003). Egocentric and geocentric frames of reference in memory of large-scale space. *Psychonomic Bulletin & Review*, *10*, 589–595.

Mecacci, L. (1993). On spatial frequencies and cerebral hemispheres: Some remarks from the electrophysiological and neuropsychological points of view. *Brain Cognit*, *22*, 199–212.

Mellet, E., Kosslyn, S. M., Mazoyer, N., Bricogne, S., Denis, M., & Mazoyer, B. (2000). Functional anatomy of high resolution mental imagery. *Journal of Cognitive Neuroscience*, *12*, 98–109.

Michimata, C. (1997). Hemispheric processing of categorical and coordinate spatial relations in vision and visual imagery. *Brain Cognit*, *33*, 370–387.

Michimata, C., Saneyoshi, A., Okubo, M., & Laeng, B. (2011). Effects of the global and local attention on the processing of categorical and coordinate spatial relations. *Brain and Cognition*, 77(2), 292–297.

Milner, A. D., & Goodale, M. A. (Eds.). (1995). *The visual brain in action*. Oxford: Oxford University Press.

Milner, A. D., & Goodale, M. A. (2008). Two visual systems re-viewed. *Neuropsychologia*, *46*, 774–785.

Mou, W., & McNamara, T. P. (2002). Intrinsic frames of reference in spatial memory. *Journal of Experimental Psychology: Learning, Memory and Cognition*, *28*, 162–170.

Mou, W., McNamara, T. P., Valiquette, C. M., & Rump, B. (2004). Allocentric and egocentric updating of spatial memories. *Journal of Experimental Psychology: Learning, Memory, and Cognition*, *30*, 142–157.

Murphy, K. J., Carey, D. P., & Goodale, M. A. (1998). The perception of allocentric spatial relationships in a visual form agnostic. *Cognitive Neuropsychology*, *15*, 705–722.

Navon, D. (1977). Forest before trees: The precedence of global features in visual perception. *Cognit Psychol*, *9*, 353–383.

Nadel, L., & Hardt, O. (2004). The spatial brain. *Neuropsychology, 18*, 473–476.

Neggers, S. F. W., Schölvinck, M. L., van der Lubbe, R. H. J., & Postma, A. (2005). Quantifying the interactions between allocentric and egocentric representations of space. *Acta Psychologica, 118*, 25–45.

Neggers, S. F. W., van der Lubbe, R. H. J., Ramsey, N. F., & Postma, A. (2006). Interactions between ego- and allocentric neuronal representations of space. *Neuroimage, 31*, 320–331.

O'Keefe, J. (1993). Kant and the sea-horse: An essay in the neurophilosophy of space. In N. Eilan, R. McCarthy, & B. Brewer (Eds.), *Spatial representation: Problems in philosophy and psychology* (pp. 43–64). Oxford: Blackwell.

O'Keefe, J., & Dostrovsky, J. (1971). The hippocampus as a special map: Preliminary evidence from unit activity in the freely moving rat. *Brain Research, 34*, 171–175.

O'Keefe, J., & Nadel, L. (1978). *The hippocampus as a cognitive map*. Oxford: Clarendon Press.

Okubo, M., Laeng, B., Saneyoshi, A., & Michimata, C. (2010). Exogenous attention differentially modulates the processing of categorical and coordinate spatial relations. *Acta Psychologica, 135*(1), 1–11.

Paillard, J. (1991). *Brain and space*. Oxford: Oxford Science Publications.

Palermo, L., Bureca, I., Matano, A., & Guariglia (2008). Hemispheric contribution to categorical and coordinate representational processes: A study on brain-damaged patients. *Neuropsychologia, 46*(11), 2802–2807.

Peeters, R., Simone, L., Nelissen, K., et al. (2009). The representation of tool use in humans and monkeys: Common and uniquely human features. *Journal of Neuroscience, 29*, 11523–11539.

Perenin, M.-T., & Vighetto, A. (1983). Optic ataxia: A specific disorder in visuomotor coordination. In M. Hein, & M. Jeannerod (Eds.), *Spatially oriented behavior* (pp. 305–326). New York: Springer-Verlag.

Pisella, L., & Rossetti, Y. (2000). Interaction between conscious identification and non-conscious sensori-motor processing: temporal constraints. In Y. Rossetti, & A. Revonsuo (Eds.), *Beyond dissociation: interaction between dissociated implicit and explicit processing* (pp. 129–151). Amsterdam: Benjamins.

Pisella, L., Binkofski, F., Lasek, K., Toni, I., & Rossetti, Y. (2006). No double dissociation between optic ataxia and visual agnosia: Multiple sub-streams for multiple visuo-manual integrations. *Neuropsychologia, 44*, 2734–2748.

Presson, C. C., DeLange, N. Z., & Hazelrigg, M. D. (1989). Orientation specificity in spatial memory: What makes a path different from a map of the path? *Journal of Experimental Psychology: Learning, Memory and Cognition, 15*, 887–889.

Proverbio, A. M., Zani, A., & Avella, C. (1997). Hemispheric asymmetries for spatial frequency discrimination in a selective attention task. *Brain Cognit, 34*, 311–320.

Presson, C. C., & Hazelrigg, M. D. (1984). Building spatial representations through primary and secondary learning. *Journal of Experimental Psychology: Learning, Memory and Cognition, 10*, 716–722.

Rieser, J. J. (1989). Access to knowledge of spatial structure at novel points of observation. *Journal of Experimental Psychology: Learning, Memory and Cognition, 15*, 1157–1165.

Rizzolatti, G., & Matelli, M. (2003). Two different streams form the dorsal visual system: Anatomy and functions. *Experimental Brain Research, 153*(2), 146–157.

Rock, I. (1992). Comment on Asch & Witkin's "Studies in space orientation II." *Journal of Experimental Psychology, General, 121*(4), 404–406.

Roskos-Ewoldsen, B., McNamara, T. P., Shelton, A. L., & Carr, W. S. (1998). Mental representations of large and small spatial layouts are orientation dependent. *Journal of Experimental Psychology: Learning, Memory and Cognition, 24*, 215–226.

Rossielle, L. J., & Cooper, E. E. (2001). Categorical perception of relative orientation in visual object recognition. *Memory and Cognition, 29*(1), 68–82.

Rossetti, Y., & Pisella, L. (2002). Several "vision for action" systems: A guide to dissociating and integrating dorsal and ventral functions (Tutorial). In W. Prinz, & B. Hommel (Eds.), *Attention and performance XIX: Common mechanisms in perception and action* (pp. 62–119). Oxford: Oxford University Press.

Ruggiero, G., Frassinetti, F., Iavarone, A., & Iachini, T. (2014). The lost ability to find the way: Topographical disorientation after a left brain lesion. *Neuropsychology, 28*(1), 147–160. Available from http://dx.doi.org/10.1037/neu0000009.

Ruggiero, G., & Iachini, T. (2006). The effect of familiarity on egocentred and allocentred spatial representations of the environment. *Cognitive Processing*, 7(5), 88–89.

Ruggiero, G., Ruotolo, F., & Iachini, T. (2012). Egocentric/allocentric and coordinate/categorical haptic encoding in blind people. *Cognitive Processing, 13*(Suppl. 1), S313–S317. Available from http://dx.doi.org/10.1007/s10339-012-0504-6.

Ruotolo, F., Iachini, T., Postma, A., & van der Ham, I. J. M. (2011). Frames of reference and categorical and coordinate spatial relations: A hierarchical organisation. *Experimental Brain Research, 214*(4), 587–595. Available from http://dx.doi.org/10.1007/s00221-011-2857-y.

Ruotolo, F., van der Ham, I. J. M., Iachini, T., & Postma, A. (2011). The relationship between allocentric and egocentric frames of reference and categorical and coordinate spatial information processing. *Quarterly Journal of Experimental Psychology (2006), 64* (6), 1138–1156. Available from http://dx.doi.org/10.1080/17470218.2010.539700.

Ruotolo, F., van der Ham, I., Postma, A., Ruggiero, G., & Iachini, T. (2015). How coordinate and categorical spatial relations combine with egocentric and allocentric reference frames in a motor task: Effects of delay and stimuli characteristics. *Behavioural Brain Research, 284*, 167–178. Available from http://dx.doi.org/10.1016/j.bbr.2015.02.021.

Saneyoshi, A., & Michimata, C. (2009). Lateralized effects of categorical and coordinate spatial processing of component parts on the recognition of 3-D non-namable objects. *Brain Cognit, 71*, 181–186.

Saneyoshi, A., Kaminaga, T., & Michimata, C. (2006). Hemispheric processing of categorical/metric properties in object recognition. *NeuroReport, 17*, 517–521.

Saunders, J. A., & Knill, D. C. (2001). Perception of 3D surface orientation from skew symmetry. *Vision Research, 41*(24), 3163–3183.

Save, E., & Poucet, B. (2000). Involvement of the hippocampus and associative parietal cortex in the use of proximal and distal landmarks for navigation. *Behavioural Brain Research, 109*, 195–206.

Schenk, T. (2006). An allocentric rather than perceptual deficit in patient D.F. *Nature Neuroscience, 9*, 1369–1370.

Sergent, J. (1991a). Judgments of relative position and distance on representations of spatial relations. *Journal of Experimental Psychology: Human Perception and Performance, 91*, 762–780.

Sergent, J. (1991b). Processing of spatial relations within and between the disconnected cerebral hemispheres. *Brain, 114*, 1025–1043.

Shelton, A. L., & McNamara, T. P. (1997). Multiple views of spatial memory. *Psychonomic Bulletin & Review, 4*, 102–106.

Sholl, M. J., & Nolin, T. L. (1997). Orientation specificity in representations of place. *Journal of Experimental Psychology: Learning, Memory and Cognition, 23*, 1494–1507.

Slotnick, S. D., Moo, L. R., Tesoro, M. A., & Hart, J. (2001). Hemispheric asymmetry in categorical versus coordinate visuospatial processing revealed by temporary cortical activation. *Journal of Cognitive Neuroscience, 13*, 1088–1096.

Smeets, J. B. J., & Brenner, E. (2006). 10 Years of illusions. *Journal of Experimental Psychology: Human Perception and Performance, 32*(6), 1501–1504.

Smeets, J. B. J., Brenner, E., de Grave, D. D. J., & Cuijpers, R. H. (2002). Illusions in action: Consequences of inconsistent processing of spatial attributes. *Experimental Brain Research, 147*, 135–144.

Sterken, Y., Postma, A., de Haan, E. H. F., & Dingemans, A. (1999). Egocentric and exocentric spatial judgements of visual displacement. *The Quarterly Journal of Experimental Psychology, 52A*(4), 1047–1055.

Stiles, J., Akshoomoff, N., & Haist, F. (2013). The development of visuospatial processing. In J. L. R. Rubenstein, & P. Rakic (Eds.), *Comprehensive developmental neuroscience: Neural circuit development and function in the brain* (vol. 3, pp. 271–296). Amsterdam: Elsevier.

Suegami, T., & Laeng, B. (2013). A left cerebral hemisphere's superiority in processing spatial-categorical information in a non-verbal semantic format. *Brain and Cognition, 81*, 294–302.

Tolman, E. C. (1948). Cognitive maps in rats and men. *The Psychological Review, 55*(4), 189–208.

Trojano, L., Grossi, D., Linden, D. E. J., Formisano, E., Goebel, R., Cirillo, S., … Di Salle, F. (2002). Coordinate and categorical judgements in spatial imagery. An fMRI study. *Neuropsychologia, 40*, 1666–1674.

Ungerleider, L. G., & Mishkin, M. (1982). *Two cortical visual systems. Analysis of visual behavior*. MIT Press.

Van Kleeck, M. (1989). Hemispheric differences in global versus local processing of hierarchical visual stimuli by normal subjects: New data and a meta-analysis of previous studies. *Neuropsychologia, 27*, 1165–1178.

Vallar, G. (1998). Spatial hemineglect in humans. *Trends in Cognitive Sciences, 2*, 87–97.

Vallar, G., Guariglia, C., & Rusconi, M. L. (1997). Modulation of the neglect syndrome by sensory stimulation. In P. Their, & H. O. Karnath (Eds.), *Parietal lobe contributions to orientation in 3D space* (pp. 555–578). Heidelberg: Springer-Verlag.

Vallar, G., Lobel, E., Galati, G., Berthoz, A., Pizzamiglio, L., & Le Bihan, D. (1999). A fronto-parietal system for computing the egocentric spatial frame of reference in humans. *Experimental Brain Research, 124*, 281–286.

van der Ham, I. J. M., Dijkerman, H. C., & van den Berg, E. (2012). The effect of attentional scope on spatial relation processing: A case study. *Neurocase, 19*(5), 505–512.

van der Ham, I. J. M., Duijndam, M. J. A., Raemaekers, M., van Wezel, R. J. A., Oleksiak, A., & Postma, A. (2012). Retinotopic mapping of categorical and coordinate spatial relation processing. *PLoS One*, 7(6), e38644.

van der Ham, I. J. M., & Postma, A. (2010). Lateralization of spatial categories: A comparison of verbal and visuospatial categorical relations. *Memory and Cognition, 38*(5), 582–590.

Van der Ham, I. J. M., Postma, A., & Laeng, B. (2014). Lateralized perception: The role of attention in spatial processing. *Neuroscience and Biobehavioral Reviews, 45*, 142–148.

van der Ham, I. J. M., Raemaekers, M., van Wezel, R. J. A., Oleksiak, A., & Postma, A. (2009). Categorical and coordinate spatial relations in working memory: An fMRI study. *Brain Research, 1297*, 70–79.

van der Ham, I. J. M., van Wezel, R. J. A., Oleksiak, A., & Postma, A. (2007). The time course of hemispheric differences in categorical and coordinate spatial processing. *Neuropsychologia, 45*(11), 2492–2498.

Van der Lubbe, R. H. J., Schölvinck, M. L., Kenemans, J. L., & Postma, A. (2006). Divergence of categorical and coordinate spatial processing assessing with ERPs. *Neuropsychologia, 44*, 1547–1559.

van Polanen, V., & Davare, M. (2015). Interactions between dorsal and ventral streams for controlling skilled grasp. *Neuropsychologia, 79*, 186–191. Available from http://dx.doi.org/10.1016/j.neuropsychologia.2015.07.010.

Waller, D., & Hodgson, E. (2006). Transient and enduring spatial representations under disorientation and self-rotation. *Journal of Experimental Psychology: Learning, Memory, and Cognition, 32*(4), 867–882.

Waller, D., Montello, D. R., Richardson, A. E., & Hegarty, M. (2002). Orientation specificity and spatial updating of memories for layouts. *Journal of Experimental Psychology: Learning, Memory and Cognition*, *28*, 1051–1063.

Wang, R. F., & Spelke, E. S. (2000). Updating egocentric representations in human navigation. *Cognition*, 77(3), 215–250.

Wang, R. F., & Spelke, E. S. (2002). Human spatial representation: Insights from animals. *Trends in Cognitive Sciences*, *6*, 376–382.

Wilkinson, D., & Donnelly, N. (1999). The role of stimulus factors in making categorical and coordinate spatial judgments. *Brain and Cognition*, *39*, 171–185.

Wong-Riley, M. (1979). Changes in the visual system of monocularly sutured or enucleated cats demonstrable with cytochrome oxidase histochemistry. *Brain Research*, *171*(1), 11–28.

Zaehle, T., Jordan, K., Wüstenberg, T., Baudewig, J., Dechent, P., & Mast, F. W. (2007). The neural basis of the egocentric and allocentric spatial frame of reference. *Brain Research*, *1137*(1), 92–103.

CHAPTER 3

On Feeling and Reaching: Touch, Action, and Body Space

H. Chris Dijkerman[1,2]
[1]Experimental Psychology, Helmholtz Institute, Utrecht University, Utrecht, The Netherlands
[2]Department of Neurology, University Medical Center, Utrecht, The Netherlands

3.1 INTRODUCTION

One of the most important functions of an organism is the ability to move around the environment and to interact with objects within the environment. Spatial information is crucial here. For example, we need to know where objects are on a cluttered table in order to be able to move toward and grasp that ubiquitous cup of coffee while avoiding spilling the jug of juice. Importantly, we need to know where these items are with respect to our own body in order to perform these movements accurately. This requires spatial information about our own body parts, from proprioception and touch as well as visual information about the items in the environment. In turn somatosensory input is not just used for guiding actions, but can also directly provide spatial perceptual information about the environment through haptic exploration, as well as about our targets on our own body. These spatial somatosensory perceptual experiences are not necessarily veridical, but can be prone to specific distortions. In healthy participants, distortions in somatosensory experience may tell us something about the underlying spatial representations. However, perceptual somatosensory experience can also be disturbed in clinical populations. In this chapter I start by providing an overview of the functional organization of the somatosensory system. Somatosensory input is important for providing a representation of our body as well as for haptic exploration of external objects. Both are reviewed next. A representation of the space surrounding our body, the peripersonal space, has been linked to body representations as well as goal-directed action and is described next. Finally, spatial processes underlying the guidance of reaching and grasping are discussed.

Neuropsychology of Space.
DOI: http://dx.doi.org/10.1016/B978-0-12-801638-1.00003-3

3.2 SOMATOSENSORY PROCESSING FOR PERCEPTION AND ACTION

Over the past two decades a dominant model for visual cortical processing has been the two visual streams model, in which visual information is processed along two separate stream of cortical processing, the ventral stream and the dorsal stream (see Section 3.6 and grasping and Chapter 2). The ventral stream is supposed to be involved in visual processing for perception and recognition, while the dorsal stream processes visual input for the guidance of action (Milner & Goodale, 2008). A similar functional subdivision has been suggested for the somatosensory system, although the anatomical subdivision is much less clear (see Box 3.1)

BOX 3.1 Somatosensory Systems of the Brain

The somatosensory system is concerned with input from different submodalities such as touch, proprioception, sensitivity to hot and cold, pain and itch. Receptors within the skin, muscles, joints, and tendons convey information about these submodalities. Information from these receptors in all body parts except the face is transmitted first to the dorsal side of the spinal cord. Two ascending pathways convey the input to the brain (Fig. 3.1). The dorsal column, or medial lemniscal system carries discriminative tactile input and proprioceptive information through large myelinated fibers. The spinothalamic or anterolateral system mainly carries temperature information, pain, and affective tactile input. Both fiber systems cross to the contralateral side within the spinal cord, but at different locations. While the anterolateral system crosses about one or two spinal nerve segments above where it entered the spinal cord, the medial lemniscal system crosses much higher at the level of the medulla. Both project to different nuclei within the thalamus from which input is conveyed mainly to the primary somatosensory cortex within the anterior part of the parietal lobe. The primary somatosensory cortex contains a somatotopic maps of the contralateral half of the body. Body parts with a higher receptor density such as the hands or face are represented in a larger part of the cortical surface. Response properties within the primary somatosensory cortex closely resemble the somatosensory stimulus and its location, especially close to the thalamic input. Damage to the primary somatosensory cortex results in a loss of tactile and proprioceptive perception for the contralateral half of the body (hemianaesthesia, see Table 3.1). The insular cortex is another area that receives some somatosensory input. It is important for processing affective touch conveyed through small unmyelinated c-tactile fibers, but also

(*Continued*)

BOX 3.1 Somatosensory Systems of the Brain—cont'd

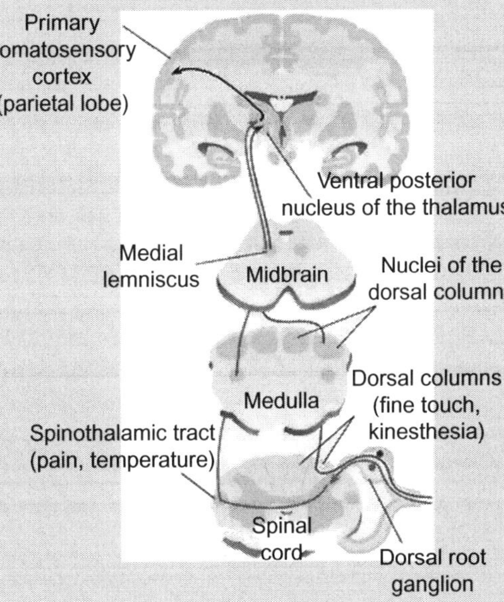

Figure 3.1 An overview of the two ascending sensory pathways, the dorsal column and the spinothalamic tracts that convey somatosensory input to the brain. *From van Stralen, H. E., & Dijkerman, H. C. (2011). Central touch disorders.* Scholarpedia *6(10), 8243.*

for pain perception and for sensitivity to hot and cold. Again, input is mainly projected contralaterally and at least for affective touch it is somatotopically represented (Bjornsdotter, Loken, Olausson, Vallbo, & Wessberg, 2009). Higher order somatosensory processing involves a more distributed network including the secondary somatosensory cortex (SII), located in the parietal operculum, the posterior parietal cortex, and the insular cortex. Responses to somatosensory input can also be found in premotor areas and in higher order visual areas such as LOC. Higher order processes can involve extracting features about and recognizing external stimuli such as objects in the environment. This mainly involves SII as well as posterior parietal areas. On other hand, somatosensory input also contains information about the body and contributes to a conscious bodily experience. Here the posterior parietal cortex, the premotor cortex, and insula play an important role. The posterior parietal cortex has been found to be involved in spatial and structural aspects of body

(*Continued*)

BOX 3.1 Somatosensory Systems of the Brain—cont'd

representations, while the insula is important for affective aspects of body representations. Activity in the premotor cortex has been linked to the feeling of body ownership (Ehrsson, Spence, & Passingham, 2004). Some authors have suggested a distinction between somatosensory processing for perception and action in higher order areas (Dijkerman & de Haan, 2007) while others suggest that a network of interrelated areas subserve various aspects of bodily experience, the body matrix (Moseley, Gallace, & Spence, 2011).

(Dijkerman & de Haan, 2007). Like the visual system, evidence for this functional dissociation comes from studies with neurological patients and from studies using illusions in healthy participants. A first piece of evidence came from studies of patients with "numbsense," a tactile equivalent of blindsight (Paillard, Michel, & Stelmach, 1983; Rossetti, Rode, & Boisson, 1995) (see also Table 3.1). These patients were unable to consciously detect tactile stimuli on their insensate hand, but were nevertheless able to localize them with above chance accuracy when making direct pointing movements toward them. Tactile information apparently could not reach the perceptual detection centers, but could have access to motor areas that involved in reaching movements. Paillard (1999) contrasted this with patient GL who suffered from peripheral deafferentation of the large myelinated fibers conveying discriminative touch and proprioceptive input to the brain. When touched with a cold stimulus, GL could localize the stimulus on a drawing of the hand (eg, intact perceptual localization), but when the hand was moved to a different location, was impaired when trying to point to the touch location. In a more recent study, Anema et al. (2009) also observed double dissociation between tactile localization when pointing directly to the target stimulus or localizing the touch on a drawing of the hand. Both patients were able to consciously detect the tactile stimulus, but nevertheless differed on their ability to localize it depending on the mode of response.

Dissociations between somatosensory processing for perceptual purposes and for the guidance of action have also been reported in healthy participants. In an early study, Westwood and Goodale (2003) showed that haptic size contrast illusions affected perceptual size estimates, but not grip aperture during grasping. Anema, Wolswijk, Ruis, and Dijkerman (2008) reported a difference in grasping and size estimation responses for

Table 3.1 An overview of different somatosensory and body-related functional deficits

Deficit	Description	Affected function
Hemianaesthesia	Loss of somatosensory function on one half of the body	Primary somatosensory function
Numbsense	Inability to detect tactile stimuli, while still being able to make movements toward them	Somatosensory perception
Somatoparaphrenia	Patients deny ownership over a body part and often attribute it to someone else	Body ownership
Misoplegia	Abnormal hatred toward a body part	Body affect
Finger agnosia	Impairment in identifying the fingers despite a preserved ability to use them	Body structure
Left–right disorientation	Impairment in the identification of the left and right sides of one's own, but also someone else's body	Body structure
Autotopagnosia	Patients are unable to point to their own body parts on verbal or nonverbal command	Body structure
Heterotopagnosia	Patients are unable to point to somebody else's body parts, while pointing to own body part is intact	Body structure
Macrosomatognosia	Perception of a body part as being larger than its actual size	Body (part) size
Microsomatognosia	Perception of a body part as being smaller than its actual size	Body (part) size
Hylognosia	An impairment in discriminating the microgeometrical features such as texture, density, or the thermal properties of an object	Haptic object recognition

(*Continued*)

Table 3.1 (Continued)

Deficit	Description	Affected function
Morphognosia	An impairment in discriminating the macrogeometrical features such as size of shape of an object	Haptic object recognition
Tactile apraxia	Impairment in performing exploratory finger and hand movements during haptic object recognition. Basic motor and somatosensory function is intact	Haptic object recognition
Apperceptive tactile agnosia/ astereognosis	Impairment in building a coherent *representation* of the object based on the integration of the micro- and/or macrogeometrical properties	Haptic object recognition
Associative tactile agnosia	Deficit in recognizing object by touch when a representation of the object is achieved, but access to semantic knowledge about the object is lost, therefore blocking recognition	Haptic object recognition

objects placed on the arm compared to objects placed on the hand. The size of the objects placed on the hand were perceptually overestimated compared to objects placed on the forearm, consistent with Weber's illusion (Weber, 1834). However, when grasping the objects, maximum grip aperture was smaller for objects placed on the hand, showing the opposite pattern to the perceptual estimations. A recent study additionally used just notable difference scores to test whether manual size estimations and grasping movements toward the objects on the hand or forearm adhered to Weber's law (note this is not the same as Weber's illusion). Weber's law suggests that "just noticeable" is a constant ratio of the original stimulus magnitude and that the sensitivity of detecting a change in any physical continuum is relative as opposed to absolute. Thus, the just noticeable difference (JND) for smaller objects should be smaller than for larger objects (Davarpanah Jazi & Heath, 2014). Indeed, Davarpanah Jazi and Heath (2014) observed that grasping responses violated Weber's law, while the manual size estimates adhered to Weber's law, at least for objects on the hand. As such the study provided support for distinct processing of haptic size cues for perceptual estimates and for the guidance of action.

Another way to assess distinct processes for the perception and action is by using illusions. Indeed, the experience of our own body is highly malleable and several bodily illusions exist. One of the most widely known illusions is the rubber hand illusion (Botvinick & Cohen, 1998) (see Box 3.2). One way to assess the effect of the rubber hand illusion is

BOX 3.2 Bodily Illusions

We experience our body continuously and this experience appears to be veridical to us. However, just like with visual and auditory perception, bodily perception can be influenced by various illusions that reflect how sensory input is processed and also the influence of stored representations of our body. Perhaps the most well-known bodily illusion is the rubber hand illusion. This illusion, discovered at a Halloween party by Matthew Botvinick, is induced by stroking a visible rubber hand placed in front of the participant synchronously with the participants own hand that is hidden from view (Fig. 3.2) (Botvinick & Cohen, 1998). This results in the experience that the felt stroking actually occurs on the rubber hand and that the rubber hand is thus part of the participant's body.

Since its discovery, the rubber hand illusion has become a standard paradigm to investigate the feeling of body ownership experimentally. It has been used to study the necessary conditions for gaining body ownership over a foreign object. For example, it has been shown that the illusion can be induced entirely by using synchronized tactile input (Ehrsson, Holmes, & Passingham, 2005), but also when tactile input is anticipated but not experienced (Ferri, Chiarelli, Merla, Gallese, & Costantini, 2013). Moreover, it can also be induced using synchronized visuomotor input (Tsakiris, Prabhu, & Haggard, 2006). It can be local, only for the stimulated finger, but not for other fingers of the same hand (Tsakiris & Haggard, 2005). The foreign objects need to resemble to some extent a hand oriented toward the body (except when viewing in a mirror) (Tsakiris & Haggard, 2005), but skin color does not matter (Farmer, Tajadura-Jimenez, & Tsakiris, 2012). The type of tactile input also needs to match that of the observed touches (Ward et al., 2015).

Moreover, it has been used to assess body ownership deficits in various clinical populations. Patient groups that show a larger than normal rubber

(Continued)

BOX 3.2 Bodily Illusions—cont'd

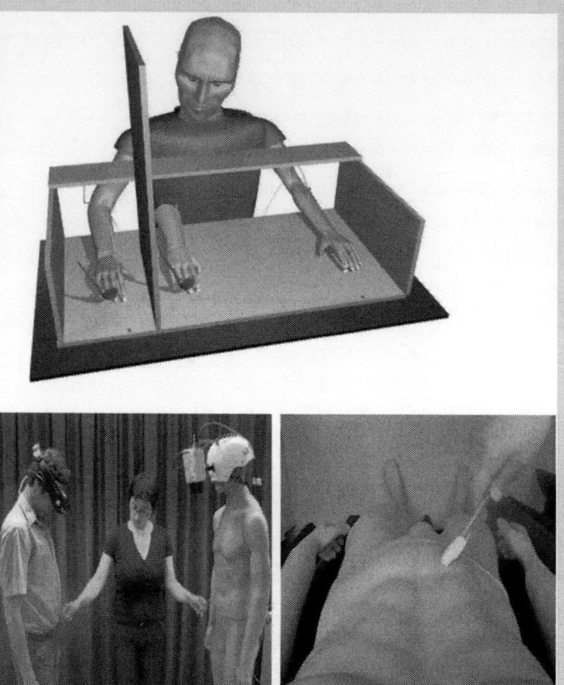

Figure 3.2 The rubber hand illusion and the full body illusion. *From Kammers, M. P. M., de Vignemont, F., Verhagen, L., & Dijkerman, H. C. (2009). The rubber hand illusion in action.* Neuropsychologia *47(1), 204–211 and Petkova, V. I., & Ehrsson, H. H. (2008). If I were you: Perceptual illusion of body swapping.* PLoS One *3(12), e3832.*

hand illusion include patients with hemiplegia after stroke (for the paralyzed hand) (Burin et al., 2015), schizophrenic patients (Thakkar, Brugger, & Park, 2009), and anorexic individuals (Eshkevari, Rieger, Longo, Haggard, & Treasure, 2014; Keizer, Smeets, Postma, van Elburg, & Dijkerman, 2014). A larger illusion has usually been linked to a reduced sense of ownership over their own body (part). Other clinical conditions are associated with a reduced rubber hand illusion. These include autistic individuals (Cascio, Foss-Feig, Burnette, Heacock, & Cosby, 2012) and also hemiplegic patients when the illusion is induced for their unaffected hand (Burin et al., 2015).

The rubber hand illusion has also inspired the development of other bodily illusions. These include the enfacement illusion in which participants watch a video of a face being stroked while simultaneously feeling face

(*Continued*)

BOX 3.2 Bodily Illusions—cont'd

stroking as well (Sforza, Bufalari, Haggard, & Aglioti, 2010), allowing them to experience ownership over the viewed face, but also a full body illusion (Petkova & Ehrsson, 2008; Slater, Spanlang, Sanchez-Vives, & Blanke, 2010). Here the participant views a different body from a first person's perspective through goggles (Fig. 3.2). The viewed body could be either a virtual body using virtual reality, or a mannequin or other person's body using a videolink to cameras attached to the other person's head. Again seeing the other body being stroked while simultaneously feeling the stroking on your own body results in the feeling that the other body belongs to you. A related illusion is the out of body illusion in which the participant views himself through a videolink from behind (Ehrsson, 2007; Lenggenhager, Tadi, Metzinger, & Blanke, 2007). Seeing your own body being stroked from the back and feeling it at the same time on your back results in the experience of being located behind your own body. Overall, these different illusions show that multisensory synchronized input is a powerful tool to modulate body ownership, at least if the viewed body (part) to some extent resembles the shape of the stimulated body (part).

Finally, other bodily illusions, that do not depend on synchronized multisensory input, exist as well. An example of such an illusion is the vibrotactile illusion in which a muscle tendon of, for example, the biceps muscle is vibrated at about 75 Hz. This creates an illusory extension of the arm (Kammers, van der Ham, & Dijkerman, 2006; Lackner, 1988). Interestingly, this experience can also affect a different body part (eg, a finger of the other hand) held by the stimulated arm (de Vignemont, Ehrsson, & Haggard, 2005; Lackner, 1988). This suggests that the vibrotactile illusion not only is an illusion based on peripheral sensory input but also affects higher order body representations.

to ask a participant to indicate *where* they feel their hand is (Botvinick & Cohen, 1998). In the illusion condition participants report the position of their hand to be shifted toward the rubber hand. However, this is only true for perceptual estimates, while reaching responses with or toward the illusion hand appear not to be influenced by the illusion (Kammers, Verhagen et al., 2009; Kammers, de Vignemont, Verhagen, & Dijkerman, 2009). This finding is consistent with the idea that multiple body representations exist, which are activated based on the task at hand. A well-known distinction is that between the body image for perceptual experience of our body and body schema for the guidance of action (Gallagher, 2005; Paillard, 1999). This idea dates back to seminal work from Head and Holmes (Head & Holmes, 1911) who actually suggested three representations, a postural schema, a superficial tactile schema, and a body image. More recently, the concept of different body representations, and if so how many, has been hotly debated (de Vignemont, 2010; Kammers, Longo, Tsakiris, Dijkerman, & Haggard, 2009). Indeed, there are several reports of bodily illusions influencing motor responses as well (Kammers, Kootker, Hogendoorn, & Dijkerman, 2009; Kammers, Longo et al., 2009; Newport, Pearce, & Preston, 2010), showing extensive interactions between somatosensory processing for perception and action. The challenge is to define the nature and specificity of the condition in which such interactions do and do not occur.

In the next section, we take a closer look at the characteristics of the spatial representations that underlie our bodily experience.

3.3 BODY SPACE

Many aspects of how we experience our body are spatial. We know where on our arm we feel an itch, what the position of our left hand is with respect to our right knee, etc. This bodily experience is multimodal in nature. We use input from our touch receptors in the skin, joint, and muscle receptors for proprioception, but also visual about the position of our body parts. Indeed, many of our bodily illusions (see Box 3.2) are induced by synchronized multisensory input about the body. Different spatial representations exist: a representation of our skin surface and a representation of our posture in joint coordinates are the most basic. However, higher order representation also exists. We have a template of the size and structure of body parts that influence our bodily perception as well. Each of these levels can also be distorted in patients with neurological of psychiatric deficits.

Here I review some of the processes that are involved in spatial processing pertaining to the body. Localizing a tactile stimulus on the body surface may be one of the most basic spatial body-related tasks we can perform. Yet, it involves a number of complex transformations (Longo, Azañón, & Haggard, 2010) (Fig. 3.3). A tactile stimulus is initially coded in somatotopic coordinates, for example, in a map of tactile receptors. However, there is no intrinsic link between this somatotopic representation and the body surface (Longo et al., 2010). For this a higher order representation is required, which according to Head and Holmes (1911) and Longo et al. (2010) would be the superficial schema. Deficits in linking somatotopic tactile input to a location on the body surface would result in

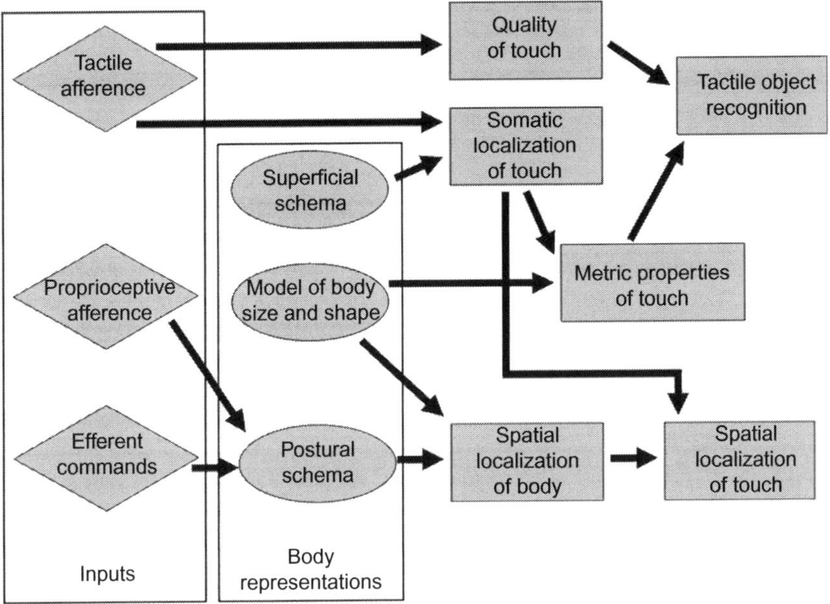

Figure 3.3 Different levels of somatosensory processing pertaining to the body. *From Longo, M. R., Azañón, E., & Haggard, P. (2010). More than skin deep: Body representation beyond primary somatosensory cortex.* Neuropsychologia *48(3), 655–668.*

patients being able to detect tactile stimuli, but making errors in localizing them. This type of deficit has been found in the earlier described study by Anema et al. (2009) and also by others (Halligan, Hunt, Marshall, & Wade, 1995).

Another aspect of body space is that we are able to localize where different body parts are with respect to each other and in external space. For this, proprioceptive input from receptors in joints, muscles, and tendons as well as tactile input about skin stretching is important. Efferent signals from the motor system may also play a role. However, while this input provides an estimate about the relative flexion or extension of body parts, it is not sufficient to localize body parts in external space (Longo et al., 2010). For this, information about the distance between joints, length and size of different body segments is needed. There are no afferent receptors that signal such features, therefore they must come from a stored representation, the postural schema (Head & Holmes, 1911; Longo et al., 2010). Thus, localizing body parts in external space would require a combination of afferent proprioceptive input and higher order stored representation. With respect to the neural correlate, evidence from neurophysiological as well as neuroimaging and patient studies suggest that particularly the posterior parietal cortex is involved in localizing body parts in external space (Graziano, Cooke, & Taylor, 2000; Pellijeff, Bonilha, Morgan, McKenzie, & Jackson, 2006; Wolpert, Goodbody, & Husain, 1998).

Being able to localize a tactile stimulus in external space would subsequently require combining postural input about the position of body parts in external space with the localization of the tactile stimulus on the body surface (Longo et al., 2010). Studies in which tactile localization in external space is required using unusual postures shows that this process takes time. Yamamoto and Kitazawa (2001) used a temporal order judgment task for tactile stimuli given to the fingertips of the left and right hand while the arms were crossed or uncrossed. Participants were very accurate when the arms were uncrossed even for short interstimulus intervals. However, when the hands were crossed, a subgroup of the participants reversed the temporal order judgment when the two tactile stimuli were delivered within 300 ms from each other. They therefore responded as if the hands were not crossed coding the tactile stimuli in a body-centered somatotopic reference frame only. A similar finding was observed when recording saccades to tactile stimuli on crossed hands (Groh & Sparks, 1996). Interestingly, this remapping of tactile stimuli to external spatial reference frame may not be possible for fingers. The Aristotle illusion (Aristotle,1924) suggests that when crossing two fingers and touching with the inside of those two fingers an external object such as a pen or even your own nose, you feel two pens/noses. The explanation for this is that this posture is so unusual that the tactile input is processed as if the fingers are uncrossed. In a more experimental setting, it has been shown that temporal order and directional judgments of two successive tactile stimuli to adjacent crossed fingers are being performed as if the fingers were uncrossed, for example, in a somatotopic reference frame (de Haan, Anema, & Dijkerman, 2012; Heed, Backhaus, & Röder, 2011). Only, after experiencing a crossed finger posture for months does remapping occur (Benedetti, 1991). Furthermore, a patient with finger agnosia, the inability to recognize and distinguish between fingers did not show any problems with tactile localization in external space when crossing fingers (Anema, Overvliet, Smeets, Brenner, & Dijkerman, 2011), presumably because of an impaired prototypical finger representation (see also below structural representations). Another aspect that is important for localizing tactile stimuli in external space is the visual input. There is considerable evidence that visual experience is essential for remapping of tactile stimuli external space to occur. Röder, Rösler, and Spence (2004) showed that temporal order judgments of congenitally blind participants are *not* affected by crossing hands. In late blind these judgments are, however. This suggests that congenitally blind participants do not use an external reference frame for when localizing tactile stimuli. Interestingly, restoring sight in a congenitally blind individual at the age of two does not result in the use of external reference frame for localizing tactile stimuli, suggesting a sensitive period for remapping of tactile stimuli to develop (Ley, Bottari, Shenoy, Kekunnaya, & Röder, 2013).

As mentioned before, peripheral somatosensory receptors do not provide information about the size of body parts (Longo et al., 2010). Nevertheless, we use body part size information when judging distances between two tactile stimuli on the body surface, or as described earlier when judging the position of body parts in external space.

Several studies suggest that visual input about the body is used to calibrate somatosensory size and distance perception. Differences in receptor density between body parts (Weinstein, 1968) results in a massively distorted somatotopic representation, with the hands and fingers being overrepresented compared, for example, to the arm and rump. This would create a problem for judgments of tactile size and distance, therefore, corrections need to be made. These corrections are based on visual information about the size of body parts (Taylor-Clarke, Jacobsen, & Haggard, 2004), however, these corrections are not perfect, resulting in minor differences in size or distance estimation depending on the stimulated body part (Weber, 1834). Thus the identical difference between two tactile stimuli is perceived as being larger for the hand (area with higher receptor density) than for the forearm (area with lower receptor density) (Weber's illusion).

Furthermore, we have an implicit representation of the size of different body parts that can be combined with tactile input for tactile size perception. This stored implicit body representation containing metric aspects of the body has been investigated in a series of studies by Longo and Haggard (2010). They asked participants to localize various landmarks of their unseen hand (eg, knuckles, fingertips) and used this localization to calculate distances between the landmarks. They argued that these distances provided information about the implicit body representation. Their results revealed a somewhat distorted implicit representation, with fingers being shorter than in reality and the width of the palm being wider. This characteristic may be related to the shape of the tactile receptive fields (Longo & Haggard, 2011). Similar distortions have also been reported for the entire body (overestimation of width, underestimation of length) (Fuentes, Longo, & Haggard, 2013). Other studies show that the characteristics of this implicit representation are indeed different from that of a visual-based explicit body image (Longo & Haggard, 2012).

Disturbances in body (part) size occur in various neurological and psychiatric conditions. Macrosomatognosia refers to the perception of a body part being larger than its actual size (Table 3.1). Patients with microsomatognosia experience their body (part) as being smaller (Frederiks, 1985). These deficits have been associated with a range of paroxysmal disorders such as migraine or seizures and often occur temporarily (Rode et al., 2012). They also have been reported for the affected hand in patients with complex regional pain syndrome (Peltz, Seifert, Lanz, Müller, & Maihöfner, 2011). Moreover, the perception of a smaller or larger body part can also be induced in healthy participants through proprioceptive illusions (de Vignemont et al., 2005) or through temporary peripheral proprioceptive deafferentation, which results in the affected body part feeling larger (Gandevia & Phegan, 1999). Damage to the central nervous also can affect body size perception. Macrosomatognosia is reported more frequently than microsomatognosia and is usually associated with parietal lesions (Frederiks, 1985). However, it has also been reported after a frontal lesion (Weijers, Rietveld, Meijer, & de Leeuw, 2013) or in Parkinson's patients (Sandyk, 1998).

The most well-known psychiatric condition in which body size distortions play a prominent role is anorexia nervosa. Indeed body image problems are a defining feature. Traditionally, investigations of body image disturbances have focused on visual body image and attitudinal aspects (Cash & Deagle, 1997; Farrell, Lee, & Shafran, 2005; Skrzypek, Wehmeier, & Remschmidt, 2001). However, more recent studies have investigated body size perception using input from other sensory modalities. Keizer and colleagues (Keizer et al., 2011; Keizer, Smeets, Dijkerman, van Elburg, & Postma, 2012) showed that anorexic participants overestimated the tactile distance between two stimuli, both on the forearm (a relatively neutral body part) and on the stomach (a sensitive body part). Moreover, anorexia patients also move as if their body is wider than in reality (Keizer et al., 2013). When walking through a door aperture, anorexia patient start rotating their shoulders for wider openings in relation to their shoulder width more than healthy participants do. This suggests that the body size distortion not only affects perceptual estimates, but also affects body size related action. Interestingly, body part size distortions appear to be reduced after inducing bodily illusions (Keizer, Smeets, Postma, van Elburg, & Dijkerman, 2014), suggesting that this distortion can be modulated.

While positional and size information about the body concerns more metric aspects of body space, other studies suggest the presence of structural representations. Structural body representation concerns the knowledge about the arrangement and form of body parts. Case studies of neurological patients with selective functional deficits reveal that such representations exist. One such impairment is autotopagnosia (Table 3.1). Patients are unable to point to their own body parts on verbal or nonverbal command (De Renzi, 1970; Sirigu, Grafman, Bressler, & Sunderland, 1991). Patients are able to name the body part and to describe its function (Guariglia, Piccardi, Allegra, & Traballesi, 2002; Sirigu et al., 1991), suggesting that semantic knowledge can be preserved (the opposite pattern has also been reported; Laiacona, Allamano, Lorenzi, & Capitani, 2006). Moreover, autotopagnosic patients can also point correctly to objects attached to the body parts (Sirigu et al., 1991), suggesting that sensorimotor function is intact as well (Buxbaum & Coslett, 2001). Impairments in body part matching across different orientations is also reported in these patients, suggesting that a structural description of the body is crucial (Buxbaum & Coslett, 2001). A related deficit is heterotopagnosia in which problems arise in pointing to somebody else's body parts when asked, while pointing to own body parts is intact (Auclair, Noulhiane, Raibaut, & Amarenco, 2009; Cleret de Langavant et al., 2012). Indeed, autotopagnosia and heterotopagnosia are double dissociated (Felician, Ceccaldi, Didic, Thinus-Blanc, & Poncet, 2003). Both disorders have been associated with left middle-temporal or parietal lesions of the dominant hemisphere (Schwoebel and Coslett, 2005), which is consistent with functional neuroimaging data of structural representations of the body (Corradi-Dell'Acqua, Hesse, Rumiati, & Fink, 2008).

Structural body representation disorders not necessarily affect the whole body, but can selectively impair the fingers, or toes. In the case of "finger agnosia" patients are impaired when asked to identify the fingers despite a preserved ability to use them (Gerstman, 1940, Kinsbourne & Warrington, 1962) (Table 3.1). It usually affects the middle three fingers of both hands (Frederiks, 1985). Although finger agnosia was initially regarded as a form of autotopagnosia (Gerstmann, 1940), the disorders appeared to be dissociated (De Renzi and Scotti, 1970). Finger gnosis has been repeatedly associated with bilateral parietal activation (Rusconi, Walsh, & Butterworth, 2005). A recent study on the neuroanatomical correlates of finger gnosis specified that left anteromedial parietal lobule plays an important role in finger identification. (Rusconi et al., 2014). Finger agnosia can be considered to be a body image deficit, as tactile input to individual fingers can be used correctly to guide movements (Anema et al., 2008). Traditionally, finger agnosia was not regarded as a unitary phenomenon, but has been described as a part of a cluster of impairments, known as the Gerstmann's syndrome (Gerstmann, 1957). Gerstmann's syndrome is characterized by four core symptoms, that is, finger agnosia, dyscalculia, dysgraphia, and left–right disorientation. The latter is also regarded as a body representation disorder and concerns the impairment in the identification of the left and right side of one's own, and also someone else's body. Gerstmann's syndrome can also occur as a developmental disorder (Kinsbourne & Warrington, 1963).

The question remains however, whether Gerstmann's syndrome is a unitary disorder, or group of independent cognitive deficits that happen to co-occur relatively frequently, for example, due to white matter disconnection (Rusconi, Pinel, Dehaene, & Kleinschmidt, 2010) or whether other deficits should be included as well (Ardila, 2014).

3.4 ACTIVE TOUCH AND HAPTIC OBJECT RECOGNITION

In daily life we often use somatosensory information not only to inform us about our own body, but also to recognize objects in our environment. When switching off the alarm clock in the morning, which is situated next to a book, or when retrieving the keys from your pocket, which you need to distinguish from the wallet that is also in your pocket. Recognizing object by touch is not a passive process. We use active hand and finger movements to extract features about the to be recognized object. This is called haptic object recognition. The term haptic is used here to show that it involves more than just passive tactile input, but a combination of tactile and proprioceptive information gained through active exploratory hand movements. Different features are important: they include size, shape, weight, texture, and the hardness of the object. Haptic object features can be classified into two categories, concerning the micro- and macrogeometrical properties of an object (Morley, Goodwin, & Darian-Smith, 1983). Microgeometrical features pertain to texture, density, or thermal properties. They involve input from receptors in the skin of the observer. Size and shape are regarded as macrogeometrical properties. They are based on tactile as well as proprioceptive input from the muscle, tendon, and joint receptors. Evidence for segregation between micro- and macrogeometrical features comes from reports of selective impairments after brain damage. An impairment in discriminating the microgeometrical features such as texture, density, or the thermal properties of an object has been named hylognosia (Denes, 1989; Stralen & Dijkerman, 2011) (see also Table 3.1). Morphognosia is an impairment in the ability to discriminate the size or the shape of an object (macrogeometrical) (see also Table 3.1). Discriminating microgeometrical features of an object is associated with activation in the parietal operculum (Binkofski et al., 1999; O'Sullivan, Roland, & Kawashima, 1994; Roland, 1987). In contrast, processing of macrogeometrical properties is associated with the anterior part of the intraparietal sulcus, suggesting that these two different types of features are segregated at a neuroanatomical level (Caselli et al., 1991; Knecht et al., 1996; Hömke et al, 2009). The idea of two separate haptic feature processing disorders, however, is not undisputed. It has been argued that impairments in perceiving macrogeometrical properties of an object is a result of impaired spatial abilities. That is, perceiving the size or shape of an object requires an analysis of the direction and extension of the exploratory hand movement, the sense of limb position in space, and tactile localization (Saetti, De Renzi, & Comper, 1999). However, some patients with morphognosia showed no spatial deficits in other (visual) modalities (Reed, Caselli, & Farah, 1996).

As mentioned above, discrimination of features and recognizing an object haptically is not a passive process but requires exploratory hand and finger movements to gather information about the object. Seminal work by Lederman and Klatzky (Lederman & Klatzky, 1987, 1993) has shown that these exploratory hand movements are not random but directed for extracting the most relevant features. They described six exploratory procedures each aimed at extracting a specific object feature (Fig. 3.4). Thus, lateral motion is used to extract texture information, while unsupported holding can be used to get information about the object's weight (Lederman & Klatzky, 1993). Moreover, certain exploratory procedures, such as enclosure, provide information about more than one object feature and are relatively fast to perform. This exploratory procedure is therefore often the first choice when haptically trying to recognize an unknown object (Lederman & Klatzky, 1993). Interestingly,

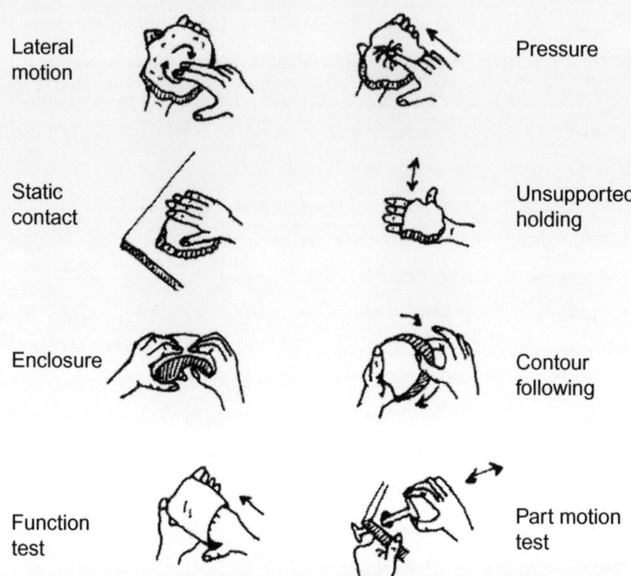

Figure 3.4 Different exploratory procedures for haptic object recognition. *From Lederman, S. J., & Klatzky, R. L. (1987). Hand movements: A window into haptic object recognition.* Cognitive Psychology *19(3), 342–368.*

automatic techniques are now being developed to recognize different exploratory procedures, something which so far had to be done manually (Jansen, Bergmann Tiest, & Kappers, 2015).

Deficits in performing exploratory hand movement, while basic sensorimotor function is intact, are called "tactile apraxia" (see also Table 3.1), in which difficulties arise in adjusting hand movements to the characteristics of an object. Tactile apraxia is often linked to lesions in superior posterior parietal areas (Binkofski, Kunesch, Classen, Seitz, & Freund, 2001). Difficulties in the haptic exploration of an object can lead to problems in recognition of that object (Valenza et al., 2001), although this is not necessary (Caselli, 1991). Indeed, problems in object recognition can have different causes. Below, the haptic recognition of objects and their associated disorders are discussed, but first haptic perception of another spatial feature, orientation, is reviewed.

3.4.1 Haptic Processing of Orientation Information

Haptic perception of spatial features is not always veridical. Perhaps this is most evident for the processing of haptic spatial orientation. In a series of

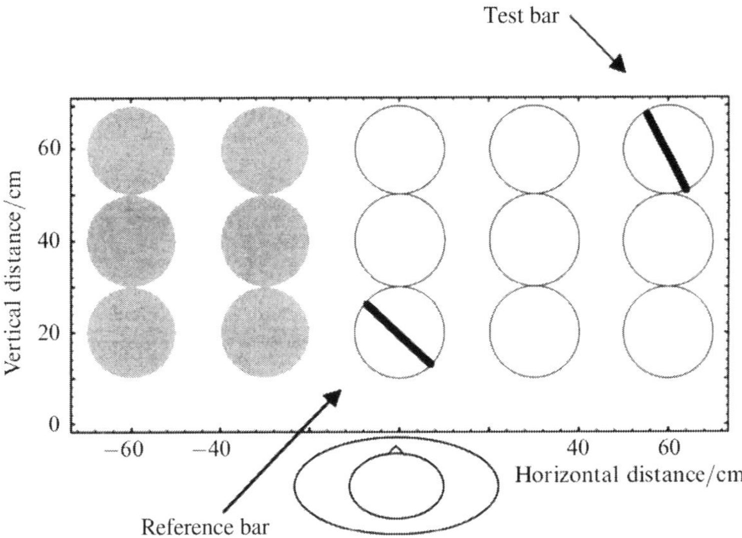

Figure 3.5 Setup of the parallel setting task. Blindfolded participants are required to haptically explore the reference bar and to rotate the test bar until both have the same orientation. *From Kappers, A. M., & Koenderink, J. J. (1999). Haptic perception of spatial relations.* Perception *28(6), 781–795.*

studies, Kappers and colleagues presented blindfolded participants with two metal bars that could rotate (Kappers & Koenderink, 1999). The reference bar was presented at one location in the workspace (Fig. 3.5), while the test bar was placed at a different location. Participants were asked to feel the orientation of the reference bar and to rotate the test bar until their orientations matched. Participants made large orientation errors (up to 40 degrees). These orientation errors depended on the horizontal distance between the two bars. Subsequent studies suggest that these errors appear to be a consequence of using hand-centered egocentric reference frames. That is, when judging the orientation of the bars participants relate it to the orientation of the hand with which the bar is felt. The orientation of the hand depends very much on where in the workspace the bar is positioned. When feeling a bar positioned on the right of the body midline, the hand is more in a clockwise orientation, while for bars on the left the hand is rotated anticlockwise. Interestingly, introducing a delay between presenting the reference bar and the test bar resulted in smaller errors, presumably because the participants started using a more allocentric reference frame for their responses (Zuidhoek, Kappers, Van Der Lubbe, & Postma, 2003). Similarly, when noninformative visual information is provided that allowed participants to favor coding in extrinsic coordinates it also resulted in improved performance (Newport, Rabb, & Jackson, 2002). Further corroborative evidence comes from a study with congenitally and late blind participants. Introducing a delay between the presentation of the reference and test bars resulted in an improvement in parallel setting for the late blind participants, but not for the congenitally blind participants (Postma, Zuidhoek, Noordzij, & Kappers, 2008). This suggests that visual experience is crucial for building the allocentric representation used during the delayed parallel setting task (see also chapter: On Inter and Intrahemispheric Differences in Visuospatial Perception).

3.4.2 Haptic Object Recognition

Besides intact somatosensory processing of features extracted using exploratory hand movements, recognizing objects by touch requires that multiple somatosensory signals are combined in a representation of an object. Information about the texture, shape, weight, and hardness needs to be gathered and integrated. Subsequently, semantic properties about the object (its use and function) are retrieved from memory. A deficit in building the object representation or in accessing the semantic properties results in "tactile agnosia" (Caselli, 1991; Denes, 1989; Endo, Miyasaka, Makishita, Yanagisawa, & Sugishita, 1992; Platz, 1996; Reed et al., 1996). In tactile agnosia, basic somatosensory processing is intact. Patients are also able to recognize objects through other sensory modalities. The problem in recognizing objects arises at higher levels. First, the problem could be one of building a coherent *representation* of the object based on the integration of the micro- and/or macrogeometrical properties. This is called tactile apperceptive agnosia or astereognosis (see also Table 3.1). These patients are unable to make an accurate drawing of the object they have explored haptically. Clinical reports of apperceptive agnosia without primary somatosensory or motor deficits are rare and are often linked to right hemispheric damage. Since the right hemisphere is associated with spatial perception, some authors have suggested that higher order tactile disorders are merely a consequence of impairments in spatial skills (Saetti et al., 1999; Semmes, 1965). Indeed, somatosensory impairments often occur together with deficits in higher order spatial processing such as hemispatial neglect (Vallar, 1997). However, other studies reported that tactile agnosia can exist without spatial deficits (Caselli, 1991; Reed et al., 1996).

Tactile associative agnosia is the second type of haptic object recognition deficit and occurs when a representation of an object is achieved (the patient can draw the haptically explored object), but access to semantic knowledge about the object is lost, therefore blocking recognition. Veronelli, Ginex, Dinacci, Cappa, and Corbo (2014) reported a case of pure associative agnosia of the left hand following a right hemorrhagic lesion limited to the post-central and supra-marginal gyri. This patient was unable to recognize objects only with the left hand, with a preserved tactile discrimination or visuotactile matching of objects. Indeed, patients with associative tactile agnosia can describe the object (eg, a soft round object in case of a ball) but are unable to indicate either the use or the name of the object. For this, semantic information from memory storage about this object is needed. Providing semantic cues about an object improves haptic recognition performance, suggesting that top-down mechanisms are involved in haptic processing (Bohlhalter, Fretz, & Weder, 2002).

3.5 PERIPERSONAL SPACE

It is now well-known that, in addition to body space, the area surrounding our body, in which objects are located that can be grasped or explored haptically, is represented separately as well. Peripersonal space representations are multimodal by nature, with visual (and also auditory) stimuli near a body part being coded together with tactile stimuli on that body part. Evidence for this idea comes from neurophysiological, neuropsychological, and behavioral studies.

Neurophysiological studies suggest that neurons in posterior parietal (area 7a, VIP) and (dorsal) premotor areas respond to tactile stimuli on the skin as well as to visual stimuli nearby (Bremmer, Schlack, Duhamel, Graf, & Fink, 2001; Duhamel, Colby, & Goldberg, 1998; Graziano & Cooke, 2006; Graziano et al., 2000; Rizzolatti, Luppino, & Matelli, 1998; Rizzolatti, Scandolara, Matelli, & Gentilucci, 1981a) (Fig. 3.6). These bimodal neurons may show actual multimodal integration, in that they do respond in a nonlinear fashion when input from both modalities is present (Avillac, Ben Hamed, & Duhamel, 2007; Makin, Holmes, & Ehrsson, 2008). Their receptive fields have been found to be related mainly to the head and hand/arm and often code stimuli in body part-centered or head-centered coordinates (Bremmer et al., 2001) and, are sensitive to motion (approaching or moving away) (Bremmer et al., 2001; Duhamel et al., 1998) particularly to looming objects (Graziano & Cooke, 2006) and optic

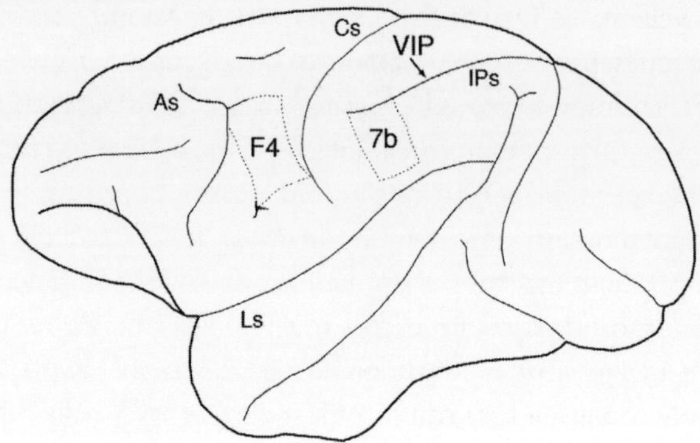

Figure 3.6 Cortical areas involved in multisensory coding of peripersonal space in the primate brain. *From di Pellegrino, G., & Làdavas, E. (2015). Peripersonal space in the brain.* Neuropsychologia, *66, 126–133.*

flow during self-motion (Bremmer, Duhamel, Ben Hamed, & Graf, 2002; Graziano & Cooke, 2006). Moreover, they have been linked to a safety zone around the body and to defensive actions (Cooke and Graziano, 2004; Graziano, 2009; Graziano and Cooke, 2006). They respond to a realistic model of the hand and distinguish between the left and right arm (Graziano, 2000).

In humans, functional imaging reveals intraparietal sulcus and lateral occipital complex (LOC) activation for stimuli approaching the hand in near compared to far space (Makin, Holmes, & Zohary, 2007). In a more recent study, using a similar behavioral paradigm in combination with adaptation fMRI, Brozzoli also found involvement of anterior and inferior parietal regions when an object was approaching the hand in peripersonal space (Brozzoli, Gentile, Petkova, & Ehrsson, 2011). In addition, ventral and dorsal premotor adaptation was observed. Together these functional neuroimaging studies suggest that similar neural mechanisms coding a multimodal representation of peripersonal space may be present in humans as those reported based on neurophysiological studies in nonhuman primates.

In addition to the neurophysiological and neuroimaging findings reported above, there has been ample evidence for a visuotactile representation of peripersonal space from behavioral studies. In particular, crossmodal attentional cueing has shown that facilitation occurs when a visual cue near the hand is followed by a tactile stimulus on the hand (Driver and Spence, 1998; Spence, Lloyd, McGlone, Nicholls & Driver, 2000; Spence, Pavani, & Driver, 2000). This is the case for endogenous

(Eimer, van Velzen, & Driver, 2002; Spence, Pavani et al., 2000) as well as exogenous cues (Eimer and Driver, 2001; Kennett, Eimer, Spence, & Driver, 2001; Trenner et al., 2008). Similar effects have been reported for extinction after unilateral brain damage. These patients are impaired in detecting tactile stimuli on the contralesional side when accompanied by a visual stimulus on the ipsilesional side (Ladavas & Farne, 2004; Ladavas & Serino, 2008). Extinction is more pronounced when the visual stimulus is near the homologue body part on the ipsilesional side (Ladavas & Serino, 2008; Ladavas, di Pellegrino, Farne, & Zeloni, 1998). This is not the case when the visual stimulus was on the ipsilesional side far away from the body, nor when it was near a different part of the body (eg, face instead of hand) (Farne, Dematte, & Ladavas, 2005). Moreover, it moves with hand position (di Pellegrino, Ladavas, & Farne, 1997). Again, this suggests body part-centered coding, although other studies may suggest a more flexible coding in cross-modal extinction (Costantini, Bueti, Pazzaglia, & Aglioti, 2007; Tinazzi, Ferrari, Zampini, & Aglioti, 2000).

Recent studies suggest that a possible mechanism responsible for coding of peripersonal space may be visuotactile prediction (Clery, Guipponi, Odouard, Wardak, & Ben Hamed, 2015; Kandula, Hofman, & Dijkerman, 2014). That is, visual stimuli near the body are often followed by tactile stimuli on the body, therefore a tactile stimulus can automatically be anticipated following a nearby visual stimulus. Indeed, tactile processing is enhanced at the location and time predicted by an approaching visual stimulus (Clery et al., 2015; Gray & Tan, 2002; Kandula et al., 2014).

An important question is which function peripersonal spatial representation subserves. Several suggestions have been made, indeed prompting some research to suggest that different peripersonal space representations exist (De Vignemont & Iannetti, 2014). Originally peripersonal space was linked to preparation of motor acts (Rizzolatti, Scandolara, Matelli, & Gentilucci, 1981b). Indeed in more recent behavioral studies with human participants, peripersonal space has been linked to goal-directed sensorimotor responses (Brozzoli, Makin, Cardinali, Holmes, & Farne, 2012). Brozzoli et al. showed that visuotactile integration is also important when grasping toward neutral objects such as rectangular objects. They combined a cross-modal congruency task with visuomotor prehension and showed stronger congruency effects during the grasping movement than before (Brozzoli, Cardinali, Pavani, & Farne, 2010). Makin, Holmes, Brozzoli, and Farnè (2012) have suggested that bimodal hand-centered representations in particularly the premotor cortex are involved in rapid online control of action, following target perturbations. This contrasts to eye-centered coding of the target, which provides a more accurate representation of the object and hand position that may be used when more time is available.

As mentioned before, peripersonal space has also been considered as a safety zone around the body (see above) and thus has been linked to defensive actions. Graziano and colleagues reported that stimulation of the same neurones involved in visuotactile coding of peripersonal space evoke defensive actions like raising or withdrawing an arm (Graziano, 2009; Graziano & Cooke, 2006). In humans, responses to tactile stimuli seem to be enhanced when accompanied by threatening visual stimuli in peripersonal space such as spiders, snakes, or growling dogs (Poliakoff, Miles, Li, & Blanchette, 2007; Taffou & Viaud-Delmon, 2014; de Haan, Smit, Van der Stigchel, & Dijkerman, 2016).

Another aspect of peripersonal space coding that has received considerable attention recently is its social function. Various studies have provided direct evidence for the notion that visual social cues influence visuotactile representations of peripersonal space. Soto-Faraco assessed the role of visual social attention on tactile perception. They observed that eye gaze cued attention toward the location of a tactile target and resulted in improved perception at the cued location. This is consistent with the idea that attention is used to bias perceptual inference to optimize prediction (Soto-Faraco, Sinnett, Alsius, & Kingstone, 2005). A study by Heed, Habets, Sebanz, and Knoblich (2010) investigated visuotactile cross-modal congruency effects while another person was simultaneously performing a similar task. Cross-modal cueing effects were influenced by the partner, but only when he was situated near the participant and performed the same task. This suggests a direct link between social contextual factors and peripersonal space. A direct test of the effect of social cues on peripersonal space boundaries was performed by Teneggi et al. (2013). They used a recently developed method for determining peripersonal space boundary based on the effect of approaching auditory stimuli on tactile responses (Canzoneri, Magosso, & Serino, 2012) and tested whether the presence of a confederate standing nearby and facing the participant would affect this boundary. Their results showed that the peripersonal space boundary becomes smaller in such a situation. Follow-up experiments showed a merging of the peripersonal space of the two people during an economic game but only if they performed cooperatively. This suggests that peripersonal space boundaries can be modulated by the social context in which people interact. Another recent study by Maister, Cardini, Zamariola, Serino, and Tsakiris (2015) used a bodily illusion, the enfacement illusion, in which the participant and a confederate were touched simultaneously on the same cheek. The illusion induces a shared sensory experience between confederate and participant. Using the same audiotactile method to map peripersonal space boundary as Teneggi et al. (2013), Maister et al. (2015) showed that the participants were now also sensitive to audiotactile integration within the peripersonal space of the confederate. They further showed this did not happen in the space between the participant and the confederate. Thus, a remapping rather than an extension of peripersonal space had occurred. Overall, these studies show that social interactions modulate peripersonal space, however, some discrepancies remain with respect to the precise effects observed.

To summarize, a multimodal representation exists of the space surrounding our body, the peripersonal space. This representation has been found to be important for various functions, including defensive action, goal-directed visuomotor behavior, and social interactions. In the next section I will review the functional and neural mechanisms underlying one of these functions, visuomotor behavior.

3.6 VISUOMOTOR REACHING AND GRASPING

Spatial information required for goal-directed arm movements is provided by the visual as well as the somatosensory system. Both can provide input about the target toward which the hand moves as well as about the moving arm itself. Visual input about the target is processed in the posterior parietal areas along the visual dorsal stream (see also Chapter 2). Early neurophysiological single cell recordings in awake monkey have suggested that there are separate visuomotor channels for different types of visuomotor acts, for example, for reaching, grasping, saccadic, and smooth pursuit eye movements (Hyvärinen & Poranen, 1974; Milner & Dijkerman, 1998). Here we focus on hand and arm movements, as eye movements are discussed in Chapter 5. The distinct neural channels of visuomotor processing for reaching and grasping have been corroborated in more recent functional neuroimaging studies showing that grasping involves the human homologue of AIP, while reaching involves the superior parieto-occipital cortex (SPOC) (Gallivan, Cavina-Pratesi, & Culham, 2009). Indeed, several authors have suggested that reaching and grasping movements require different types of visual information. Reaching movements are dependent on spatial *location* data, while grasping movement involve nonspatial *size* input. Milner and Goodale (1995) argued that the involvement of the posterior parietal cortex in visually guided grasping is an important piece of evidence for the idea that the dorsal stream is not necessarily a spatial visual processing stream, but rather processes visual input for the guidance of action. Other evidence for the idea of separate visuomotor channels for reaching and grasping comes from studies of patients with optic ataxia (see also Chapter 3). Jeannerod, Decety, and Michel (1994) and Jakobson, Archibald, Carey, and Goodale (1991) described patients who had a selective visuomotor deficit for grasping, while reaching to specific locations appeared to be intact. fMRI studies also suggest that different routes within the visual dorsal stream are involved in reaching and grasping. Earlier neuroanatomical studies in monkeys suggested a distinction between dorsolateral and dorsomedial routes (Rizzolatti & Matelli, 2003). The dorsolateral route involved area the anterior part of the intraparietal sulcus (area AIP) (Fig. 3.7) projecting to the ventral portion of the premotor cortex. Based on neurophysiological studies, this route is considered to be involved in the sensory guidance of grasping movements. The dorsomedial route involves area V6A in monkeys or the superior parieto-occipital cortex in humans and is considered to process visual information for the guidance of reaching movements (Culham, Cavina-Pratesi, & Singhal, 2006; Rizzolatti & Matelli, 2003). However, the idea of separate visuomotor channels for reaching and grasping has been challenged based on evidence from different fields of study. First, recent neurophysiological studies suggest that the dorsolateral and dorsomedial routes have different functional properties than a distinction between reaching and grasping. Fattori, Breveglieri, Raos, Bosco, and Galletti (2012) observed grasping related activity in the dorsomedial area V6A. This is further substantiated by fMRI and combined EEG/TMS studies in humans (Verhagen et al., 2008, 2012). These studies suggest that both dorsolateral and dorsomedial routes are involved in visuomotor grasping but in a hierarchical manner. Area AIP within the dorsolateral route generates a fast motor plan based on available spatial and pictorial cues.

This information is then conveyed to the dorsomedial route which specifies motor parameters controlling arm, wrist, and finger movements with respect to object configuration just before movement onset (Verhagen et al., 2013).

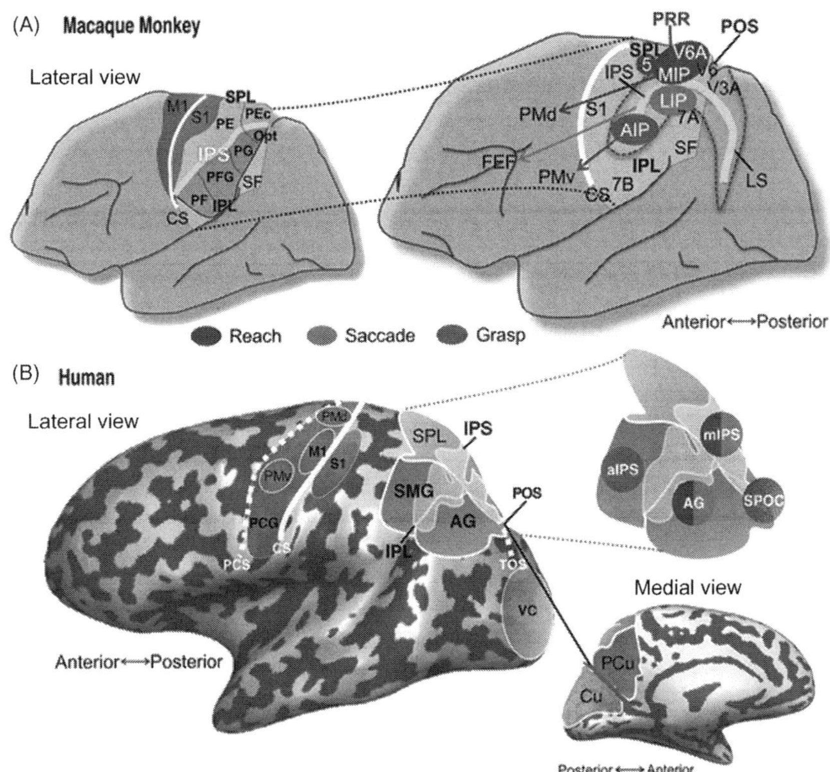

Figure 3.7 Posterior parietal areas involved in visuomotor control. *AIP*, Anterior part of the intraparietal sulcus (involved in grasping) and *MIP*, medial part of the intraparietal sulcus. *From Vesia, M., & Crawford, J. D. (2012). Specialization of reach function in human posterior parietal cortex.* Experimental Brain Research *221(1), 1–18.*

Other evidence against the idea of separate processing for reaching and grasping comes from behavioral studies. Smeets and Brenner (1999) suggested that grasping involves positioning the index finger and thumb on appropriate positions on the surface of the object, depending on characteristics such as object shape, fragility, reaching movement, and required accuracy. Grasping occurs by controlling index finger and thumb movements more or less independently and making sure that they approach the appropriate positions approximately orthogonal to the object surface. Thus, here grasping movements can be seen as two fingered pointing movements that also depend on spatial location data.

While grasping and reaching movements are both aimed toward an object in external space, in everyday behavior it is at least as important that we also avoid bumping into and knocking over objects that are in the way during a reaching/grasping movement. The next section reviews the literature on spatial processing during obstacle avoidance.

3.7 OBSTACLE AVOIDANCE

Two different types of processes have been considered to be relevant when grasping a target object when other objects are present. First, the nontarget object may act as a potential target. That is, the presence of the nontarget may induce competing motor responses toward these nontargets that need to be inhibited (see also chapter 5) (Howard & Tipper, 1997). This is based on the idea that in the posterior parietal cortex and in motor areas reach direction selective neurones exist that may be activated by stimuli in the environment. Any overlap between activations for target and nontarget leads to inhibition of the latter, resulting to reaching movements that deviate away from the nontargets. Indeed the presence of nontargets in the workspace leads to more activation in posterior parietal cortex in humans (Chapman et al., 2007). This deviation away can be observed even when the nontarget stimuli are not physical objects but, for example, LEDs. This is essentially a problem of *target selection*.

A second process that may be involved is that the visuomotor response is programmed in such a way as to avoid contact with the nontarget obstacle, for example, by maintaining a minimum distance (Tresilian, 1998). Evidence in line with this account comes from several studies reporting an increase in movement time when nontargets are present (Biegstraaten, Smeets, & Brenner, 2003; Jackson, Jackson, & Rosicky, 1995; Mon-Williams, Tresilian, Coppard, & Carson, 2001), suggesting that the grasping movement is slowed down to increase spatial accuracy and avoid potential collisions. These adjustments are not a general response to the presence of nontarget objects (Mon-Williams et al., 2001), on the contrary, the effect is specific to the layout of the workspace in that nontarget objects only elicit an avoidance response when the preferred distance to them is too small. Thus here obstacle avoidance is considered to be an aspect of action specification.

A more recent proposal combines both models and suggests that target selection and action specification run in parallel influencing each other and involving similar neural substrates in parietal and premotor areas (Cisek & Kalaska, 2010). It is therefore suggested that both are required and effects reported might not be uniquely attributable to either attentional allocation during target selection or movement planning.

Several features of the nontarget object appear to influence obstacle avoidance. First, evidently the position of the nontarget object is important. When the nontarget is closer to the path the hand would travel without obstacle larger deviations in the reaching trajectory occur. A recent study by Menger, Dijkerman, and Stigchel (2014) systematically varied nontarget positions during goal-directed grasping movements (Fig. 3.8). They observed various effects. First, objects on the outside of the reaching arm result in larger deviations, presumably because of the avoidance movement taking not only the hand, but also the attached arm trajectory into account (Menger, Van der Stigchel, & Dijkerman, 2012). Second, nontarget objects close to the starting position cause more deviation than those closer to the target object.

Importantly, it is not so much the absolute position of the nontarget obstacle that is relevant for programming an appropriate reaching response, but a combination of the distance and direction of this object, with the direction appearing to play a larger role. Other features of the nontarget object that appear to influence the grasping movement are

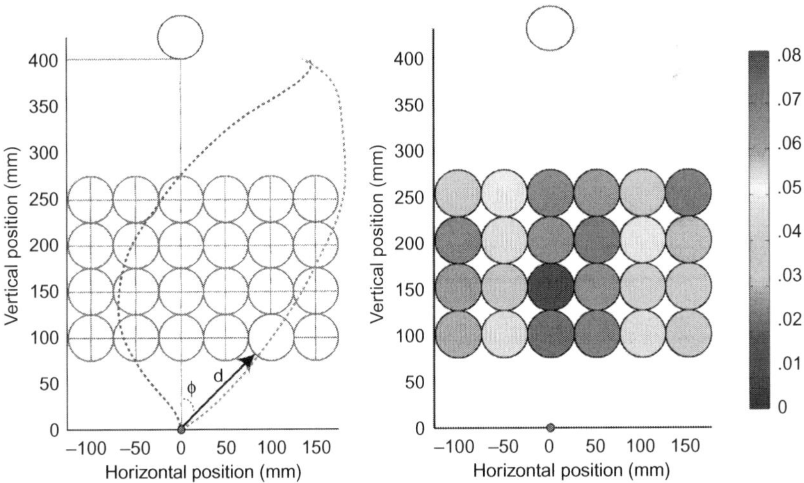

Figure 3.8 Effects of nontarget position on deviation of hand during reaching. Left: the layout of the different nontarget position (note only one nontarget was present in a particular trial) and example. Right: a schematic depiction of the amount of deviation (warmer colors mean more deviation). *From Menger, R., Dijkerman, H. C., & Van der Stigchel, S. (2014). On the relation between nontarget object location and avoidance responses.* Journal of Vision *14(9), 1–14.*

its size (height) and orientation (Alberts, Saling, & Stelmach, 2002; Chapman & Goodale, 2008; Saling, Alberts, Stelmach, & Bloedel, 1998). These features are all arguably processed by the visual dorsal stream. Indeed, patients suffering from optic ataxia following posterior parietal lesions are impaired in adjusting their reaching trajectory to the position of the nontarget objects (Schindler et al., 2004), while visual form agnosic patients with ventral stream lesions do adjust their reaching movements to the position of the obstacle (Rice et al., 2006). However, several authors have suggested that object identity should influence obstacle avoidance as well, as the consequences of a potential collision may influence the safety margin and these consequences can only be estimated when the identity of the obstacle is known. This idea was tested by de Haan, Van der Stigchel, Nijnens, and Dijkerman (2014). They asked participants to make reach-to-grasp movements while a glass was situated in the workspace. The glass could be empty or filled with water. Thus the spatial configuration of the obstacle was identical, while the possible consequences of collision with the obstacle differed. Indeed, the participants' reaching trajectories veered away more from the filled compared to the empty glass, showing that object recognition can influence avoidance behavior. However, even simpler nonspatial ventral stream related features can also influence reaching trajectories in an obstacle avoidance paradigm. Menger, Dijkerman, and Van der Stigchel (2013) showed that similarity in color between target and nontarget resulted in a larger deviation in reaching trajectory. This result is entirely consistent with the attentional target specification account of reaching trajectories in obstacle avoidance. Nevertheless, other studies (Menger et al., 2012) showed that nonattentional factors such as the posture of the reaching hand at the start of the movement also influence reaching trajectories, indicating that both target selection and movement specification are important, as suggested by Cisek and Kalaska (2010).

3.8 REFERENCE FRAMES IN VISUOMOTOR CONTROL

When reaching toward an object or when avoiding an obstacle while moving, it is important to know the location of the object with respect to the actor in order to program an accurate reaching movement. Indeed, it is widely acknowledged that sensory processing for the guidance of action occurs in egocentric coordinates. Milner and Goodale (1995) have suggested that the visuomotor dorsal stream processes visual information in entirely egocentric coordinates. In contrast, visual information processed in the ventral stream is essential for allocentric spatial representations, as identity information is required to tag individual items when localizing them with respect to each other (Milner, Dijkerman, & Carey, 1999). The well-studied visual form agnosic patient DF was demonstrated to have impaired allocentric coding, while egocentric coding remained intact (Carey, Dijkerman, Murphy, Goodale, & Milner, 2006; Dijkerman, Milner, & Carey, 1998; Schenk, 2006); however, allocentric categorical judgments were possible (Carey, Dijkerman, & Milner, 2009; see also Ruotolo, van der Ham, Postma, Ruggiero, & Iachini, 2015, Chapter 2). Similarly, introducing a delay between visual stimulus presentation and reaching response also results in healthy participants basing their reaching response on an allocentric rather than egocentric representation (Rossetti, 1998). As the visual dorsal stream is involved in the moment to moment calculation of the spatial position of the target, as target as well as observer tend to move around, introducing a delay presumably results in the use of ventral stream-based allocentric representations.

While it is clear that visuomotor responses depend on egocentric processing of items in the workspace, which type of egocentric representations is used has been a topic of much further investigation. The problem is that visual input about the stimulus is originally registered in retinotopic coordinates, while ultimately the reaching responses need to be computed in hand- or arm-centered coordinates. How does the brain solve this problem? Two different mechanisms have been proposed: First, using proprioceptive information about the position of the eye in the socket, retinotopic coordinates are transformed into head-centered coordinates. Adding proprioceptive input about the position of the head with respect to the trunk allows calculation of the position of the target with respect to the trunk. Finally proprioceptive input about the hand with respect to the trunk results in a hand-centered localization of the target object (Andersen, 1997). An alternative and more recent proposal is that that both target and effector (the hand) are localized in the same coordinate system. Indeed, there is considerable evidence that both hand and target are coded in eye-centered reference frames in the posterior parietal cortex.

Neurophysiological studies in monkeys show that targets and the hand are coding with respect to the eye (Batista, Buneo, Snyder, & Andersen, 1999; Buneo, Jarvis, Batista, & Andersen, 2002). Evidence for gaze-centered coding of reach targets in humans comes from patients with optic ataxia. These patients show errors when reaching for targets in their peripheral vision, while basic visual and motor function is intact. Several studies have shown that these reaching errors are linked to the direction of gaze, suggesting a gaze-centered coding of the target position (Dijkerman et al., 2006; Khan, Pisella, Rossetti, Vighetto, & Crawford, 2005; Khan, Pisella, Vighetto, et al., 2005). However, it is also clear that body- and hand-centered coding of targets exist as well. This has been shown using neurophysiology in monkeys (Buneo et al., 2002; Graziano & Gross, 1998; Hadjidimitrakis, Bertozzi, Breveglieri, Fattori, & Galletti, 2013). Neuroimaging studies with healthy participants also suggest that in the posterior parietal cortex and in the premotor cortex both gaze-centered coding and body part (hand)-centered coding exist (Beurze, Toni, Pisella, & Medendorp, 2010; Beurze, Van Pelt, & Medendorp, 2006). Transformation between the two reference frames may be achieved by vectorially subtracting hand location from target location which are both coded in eye-centered coordinates (Beurze et al., 2010; Buneo et al., 2002). Furthermore, reference frames may be used flexibly (Leoné, Henriques, Medendorp, & Toni, 2015), depending on the sensory context. That is, combined gaze- and body-centered reference frames may be used when reaching for visual targets, while for unseen proprioceptive targets body-centered reference frames may dominate (Bernier & Grafton, 2010).

The research on reference frames exemplifies the importance of both visual and somatosensory input during goal-directed movements. The next section discusses how visual and somatosensory input are combined.

3.9 HOW VISION AND SOMATOSENSORY INPUT ARE COMBINED DURING REACHING BEHAVIOR

Goal-directed movements inevitably require input from multiple sensory modalities. The most widely studied situation is where a visual target is shown toward which the participant moves. The somatosensory system then provides information about the location and configuration of the moving arm. Alternatively, information about the target location can be proprioceptive or tactile as well (see Section 3.2) and visual information about the moving hand can also be available.

Overall, there is considerable evidence to suggest that both the dorso-lateral and the dorsomedial visual streams contain neurones involved in multimodal coding of body-related and arm-related configurations used for the guidance of action. For example, nonvisual neurones responding to somatosensory as well as bimodal stimulation have been found in primate area V6A (Breveglieri, Kutz, Fattori, Gamberini, & Galletti, 2002; Galletti, Kutz, Gamberini, Breveglieri, & Fattori, 2003), which is part of the dorsomedial route. The same is true for area PEc, which lies just anterior to V6A (Breveglieri, Galletti, Monaco, & Fattori, 2008). Area AIP also responses to visual as well as somatosensory input. However, here it might be related more to tactile contact at the end of the grasping movement (Gardner et al., 2007; Grefkes, Weiss, Zilles, & Fink, 2002). Tactile input during contact with the target object at the end of grasping movements indeed is important for the absolute calibration between object features and the required motor output (Davarpanah, Hosang, & Heath, 2015; Heath & Holmes, 2015). Without tactile feedback the motor system relies on relative size cues to program hand opening during grasping. This is shown by studies with healthy participants in which removal of tactile feedback at the end of the movement changes the way maximum hand opening during the grasping movement relates to object width. Moreover, visual form agnosic patient DF, whose lesion affects ventral stream processing of size and shape cues, is highly dependent on tactile input at the end of the movement for normal grip scaling during goal-directed prehension movements (Schenk, 2012). This tactile input has been observed to be necessary to engage the visual dorsal stream (Whitwell, Milner, Cavina-Pratesi, Byrne, & Goodale, 2014).

Combining visual with somatosensory input can also be important when reaching for multisensory spatial targets. Traditionally, visual input is considered to provide more precise spatial information. Reaching errors to visual targets are often smaller than those to proprioceptive targets (von Hofsten & Rösblad, 1988). Indeed, proprioceptive localization tends to drift over time. Providing temporary visual input results in a reduction of this drift (Wann & Ibrahim, 1992). However, more recent studies show that differences in precision of localizing visual and proprioceptive targets depend on certain aspects of the task. First van Beers, Wolpert, and Haggard (2002) showed that proprioceptive target are localized more accurately than visual targets when they vary in depth. Second, when visual input is limited, proprioceptive input may increase precision of localization (Monaco et al., 2010). Overall, these findings are consistent with the idea that localization input is processed in statistically optimal integration from multiple modalities with the more reliably input receiving a higher weighting. This can even explain the patterns of proprioceptive drift and visual correction reported in the earlier experiment by

Wann & Ibrahim (Smeets, van den Dobbelsteen, de Grave, van Beers, & Brenner, 2006). This idea is similar to multimodal object perception (Ernst & Banks, 2002) (for more information about multisensory processes see also Chapter 4).

3.10 CONCLUSION

The aim of this chapter was to provide an overview of the spatial processes that are important for bodily experience and for sensory-guided action. Three different aspects were discussed in particular. First, spatial aspects of somatosensory processing were reviewed. Somatosensory input can provide information about external stimuli in the environment as well as about our own body. Both have been reviewed, including deficits in spatial aspects of somatosensory processing. A second topic has been the representation of the space surrounding our body, the peripersonal space. Final, the sensory processes, visual and nonvisual, that are important for reaching and grasping movements have been reviewed. The functional as well as neural organization underlying sensory-guided action was discussed. Although these three aspects are discussed separately, it is clear that they are interdependent. Thus reaching and grasping movements depend on somatosensory input about the spatial configuration of the hand and arm. Similarly, visuotactile representations of peripersonal space may be particularly relevant for reaching and grasping movements. And body representations such as the body schema have been linked to peripersonal space (Cardinali, Brozzoli, & Farne, 2009). This is also reflected in the underlying neural mechanisms, which mostly entail various frontoparietal networks for all three functions.

Furthermore, recent studies suggest that each of these three functions is also relevant for and influenced by other cognitive, social, and affective representations. Examples are the earlier mentioned social influences on peripersonal space boundaries, and also the role of body postures on emotion perception (de Gelder, 2006) and the link between body ownership and affective processing (van Stralen et al., 2014). Future research will no doubt further delineate the interactions between these different functions.

Final, for all these functions, neuropsychological studies of patients with selective deficits have been instrumental in delineating the neurocognitive architecture of these functions. This is true for visually guided actions (optic ataxia), body representation (eg, autotopagnosia), as well as peripersonal space (cross-modal extinction). These neuropsychological studies are invariably combined with evidence from other methodologies (neurophysiological, psychophysics, or neuroimaging). Nevertheless, neuropsychological studies have provided crucial evidence for functional models. I have no doubt this will continue to be the case.

REFERENCES

Alberts, J. L., Saling, M., & Stelmach, G. E. (2002). Alterations in transport path differentially affect temporal and spatial movement parameters. *Experimental Brain Research, 143*(4), 417–425.

Andersen, R. A. (1997). Multimodal integration for the representation of space in the posterior parietal cortex. *Philosophical Transactions of the Royal Society of London. Series B, Biological Sciences, 352*(1360), 1421–1428.

Anema, H. A., Overvliet, K. E., Smeets, J. B. J., Brenner, E., & Dijkerman, H. C. (2011). Integration of tactile input across fingers in a patient with finger agnosia. *Neuropsychologia, 49*(1), 138–146.

Anema, H. A., van Zandvoort, M. J. E., de Haan, E. H. F., Kappelle, L. J., de Kort, P. L. M., Jansen, B. P. W., & Dijkerman, H. C. (2009). A double dissociation between somatosensory processing for perception and action. *Neuropsychologia, 47*(6), 1615–1620.

Anema, H. A., Wolswijk, V. W. J., Ruis, C., & Dijkerman, H. C. (2008). Grasping Weber's illusion: The effect of receptor density differences on grasping and matching. *Cognitive Neuropsychology, 25*(7), 951–967.

Ardila, A. (2014). A proposed reinterpretation of Gerstmann's syndrome. *Archives of Clinical Neuropsychology, 29*(November), 828–833.

Aristotle (1924). *Metaphysics (W. D. Ross, Trans.).* Oxford: Oxford University Press.

Auclair, L., Noulhiane, M., Raibaut, P., & Amarenco, G. (2009). Where are your body parts? A pure case of heterotopagnosia following left parietal stroke. *Neurocase: Case Studies in Neuropsychology, Neuropsychiatry, and Behavioural Neurology, 15*(6), 459–465.

Avillac, M., Ben Hamed, S., & Duhamel, J. R. (2007). Multisensory integration in the ventral intraparietal area of the macaque monkey. *The Journal of Neuroscience, 27*(8), 1922–1932.

Batista, A. P., Buneo, C. A., Snyder, L. H., & Andersen, R. A. (1999). Reach plans in eye-centered coordinates. *Science (New York, NY), 285*(5425), 257–260.

Benedetti, F. (1991). Perceptual learning following a long-lasting tactile reversal. *Journal of Experimental Psychology: Human Perception and Performance, 17*(1), 267–277.

Bernier, P.-M., & Grafton, S. T. (2010). Human posterior parietal cortex flexibly determines reference frames for reaching based on sensory context. *Neuron, 68*(4), 776–788.

Beurze, S. M., Toni, I., Pisella, L., & Medendorp, W. P. (2010). Reference frames for reach planning in human parietofrontal cortex. *Journal of Neurophysiology, 104*(July 2010), 1736–1745.

Beurze, S. M., Van Pelt, S., & Medendorp, W. P. (2006). Behavioral reference frames for planning human reaching movements. *Journal of Neurophysiology, 96*(1), 352–362.

Biegstraaten, M., Smeets, J. B. J., & Brenner, E. (2003). The influence of obstacles on the speed of grasping. *Experimental Brain Research, 149*(4), 530–534.

Binkofski, F., Buccino, G., Stephan, K. M., Rizzolatti, G., Seitz, R. J., & Freund, H. J. (1999). A parieto-premotor network for object manipulation: Evidence from neuroimaging. *Experimental Brain Research, 128*(1–2), 210–213.

Binkofski, F., Kunesch, E., Classen, J., Seitz, R. J., & Freund, H. J. (2001). Tactile apraxia: Unimodal apractic disorder of tactile object exploration associated with parietal lobe lesions. *Brain, 124*(Pt 1), 132–144.

Bjornsdotter, M., Loken, L., Olausson, H., Vallbo, Å., & Wessberg, J. (2009). Somatotopic organization of gentle touch processing in the posterior insular cortex. *The Journal of Neuroscience, 29*(29), 9314–9320.

Bohlhalter, S., Fretz, C., & Weder, B. (2002). Hierarchical versus parallel processing in tactile object recognition: A behavioural-neuroanatomical study of aperceptive tactile agnosia. *Brain: A Journal of Neurology, 125*(Pt 11), 2537–2548.

Botvinick, M., & Cohen, J. (1998). Rubber hands "feel" touch that eyes see. *Nature, 391* (6669), 756.

Bremmer, F., Duhamel, J. R., Ben Hamed, S., & Graf, W. (2002). Heading encoding in the macaque ventral intraparietal area (VIP). *The European Journal of Neuroscience, 16* (8), 1554–1568.

Bremmer, F., Schlack, A., Duhamel, J. R., Graf, W., & Fink, G. R. (2001). Space coding in primate posterior parietal cortex. *Neuroimage, 14*(1 Pt 2), S46–S51.

Breveglieri, R., Galletti, C., Monaco, S., & Fattori, P. (2008). Visual, somatosensory, and bimodal activities in the macaque parietal area PEc. *Cerebral Cortex (New York, NY: 1991), 18*(4), 806–816.

Breveglieri, R., Kutz, D. F., Fattori, P., Gamberini, M., & Galletti, C. (2002). Somatosensory cells in the parieto-occipital area V6A of the macaque. *Neuroreport, 13* (16), 2113–2116.

Brozzoli, C., Cardinali, L., Pavani, F., & Farne, A. (2010). Action-specific remapping of peripersonal space. *Neuropsychologia, 48*(3), 796–802.

Brozzoli, C., Gentile, G., Petkova, V. I., & Ehrsson, H. H. (2011). FMRI adaptation reveals a cortical mechanism for the coding of space near the hand. *The Journal of Neuroscience, 31*(24), 9023–9031.

Brozzoli, C., Makin, T. R., Cardinali, L., Holmes, N., & Farne, A. (2012). Chapter 23 peripersonal space: A multisensory interface for body–object interactions. In M. Murray, & M. Wallace (Eds.), *The neural bases of multisensory processes* (pp. 1–13). Boca Raton, FL: CRC Press.

Buneo, C. A., Jarvis, M. R., Batista, A. P., & Andersen, R. A. (2002). Direct visuomotor transformations for reaching. *Nature, 416*(6881), 632–636.

Burin, D., Livelli, A., Garbarini, F., Fossataro, C., Folegatti, A., Gindri, P., & Pia, L. (2015). Are movements necessary for the sense of body ownership? Evidence from the rubber hand illusion in pure hemiplegic patients. *PLoS One, 10*(3), e0117155.

Buxbaum, L. J., & Coslett, H. B. (2001). Specialised structural descriptions for human body parts: Evidence from autotopagnosia. *Cognitive Neuropsychology, 18*(4), 289–306.

Canzoneri, E., Magosso, E., & Serino, A. (2012). Dynamic sounds capture the boundaries of peripersonal space representation in humans. *PLoS One*, 7(9), e44306.

Cardinali, L., Brozzoli, C., & Farne, A. (2009). Peripersonal space and body schema: Two labels for the same concept? *Brain Topography, 21*(3-4), 252–260.

Carey, D. P., Dijkerman, H. C., & Milner, A. D. (2009). Pointing to two imaginary targets at the same time: Bimanual allocentric and egocentric localization in visual form agnosic D.F. *Neuropsychologia, 47*(6), 1469–1475.

Carey, D. P., Dijkerman, H. C., Murphy, K. J., Goodale, M. A., & Milner, A. D. (2006). Pointing to places and spaces in a patient with visual form agnosia. *Neuropsychologia, 44*(9), 1584–1594.

Cascio, C. J., Foss-Feig, J. H., Burnette, C. P., Heacock, J. L., & Cosby, A. A. (2012). The rubber hand illusion in children with autism spectrum disorders: Delayed influence of combined tactile and visual input on proprioception. *Autism: The International Journal of Research and Practice, 16*, 406–419.

Caselli, R. J. (1991). Rediscovering tactile agnosia. *Mayo Clinic Proceedings. Mayo Clinic*, *66*(2), 129–142.

Cash, T. F., & Deagle, E. A. (1997). The nature and extent of body-image disturbances in anorexia nervosa and bulimia nervosa: a meta-analysis. *The International Journal of Eating Disorders*, *22*(2), 107–125.

Chapman, C. S., & Goodale, M. A. (2008). Missing in action: The effect of obstacle position and size on avoidance while reaching. *Experimental Brain Research*, *191*(1), 83–97.

Chapman, H., Pierno, A. C., Cunnington, R., Gavrilescu, M., Egan, G., & Castiello, U. (2007). The neural basis of selection-for-action. *Neuroscience Letters*, *417*(2), 171–175.

Cisek, P., & Kalaska, J. F. (2010). Neural mechanisms for interacting with a world full of action choices. *Annual Review of Neuroscience*, *33*(1), 269–298.

Cleret de Langavant, L., Trinkler, I., Remy, P., Thirioux, B., McIntyre, J., Berthoz, A., ... Bachoud-Lévi, A.-C. (2012). Viewing another person's body as a target object: A behavioural and PET study of pointing. *Neuropsychologia*, *50*(8), 1801–1813.

Clery, J., Guipponi, O., Odouard, S., Wardak, C., & Ben Hamed, S. (2015). Impact prediction by looming visual stimuli enhances tactile detection. *Journal of Neuroscience*, *35* (10), 4179–4189.

Cooke, D. F., & Graziano, M. S. (2004). Sensorimotor integration in the precentral gyrus: Polysensory neurons and defensive movements. *Journal of Neurophysiology*, *91*(4), 1648–1660.

Corradi-Dell'Acqua, C., Hesse, M. D., Rumiati, R. I., & Fink, G. R. (2008). Where is a nose with respect to a foot? The left posterior parietal cortex processes spatial relationships among body parts. *Cerebral Cortex*, *18*(December), 2879–2890.

Costantini, M., Bueti, D., Pazzaglia, M., & Aglioti, S. M. (2007). Temporal dynamics of visuo-tactile extinction within and between hemispaces. *Neuropsychology*, *21*(2), 242–250.

Culham, J. C., Cavina-Pratesi, C., & Singhal, A. (2006). The role of parietal cortex in visuomotor control: What have we learned from neuroimaging? *Neuropsychologia*, *44*(13), 2668–2684.

Davarpanah, S., Hosang, S., & Heath, M. (2015). Neuropsychologia memory delay and haptic feedback influence the dissociation of tactile cues for perception and action. *Neuropsychologia*, *71*, 91–100.

Davarpanah Jazi, S., & Heath, M. (2014). Weber's law in tactile grasping and manual estimation: Feedback-dependent evidence for functionally distinct processing streams. *Brain and Cognition*, *86*, 32–41.

de Gelder, B. (2006). Towards the neurobiology of emotional body language. *Nature Reviews Neuroscience*, 7(3), 242–249.

de Haan, A. M., Anema, H. A., & Dijkerman, H. C. (2012). Fingers crossed! An investigation of somatotopic representations using spatial directional judgements. *PLoS One*, 7(9), e45408.

de Haan, A. M., Van der Stigchel, S., Nijnens, C. M., & Dijkerman, H. C. (2014). The influence of object identity on obstacle avoidance reaching behaviour. *Acta Psychologica*, *150*, 94–99.

de Haan, A. M., Smit, M., Van der Stigchel, S., & Dijkerman, H. C. (2016). Approaching threat modulates visuotactile interactions in peripersonal space. *Experimental Brain Research*, . http://doi.org/10.1007/s00221-016-4571-2.

De Renzi, E., & Scotti, G. (1970). Autotopagnosia: Fiction or Reality? *Archives of Neurology*, *23*(3), 221.

de Vignemont, F. (2010). Body schema and body image—Pros and cons. *Neuropsychologia*, *48*(3), 669–680.

de Vignemont, F., Ehrsson, H. H., & Haggard, P. (2005). Bodily illusions modulate tactile perception. *Current Biology*, *15*(14), 1286–1290.

De Vignemont, F., & Iannetti, G. D. (2014). Neuropsychologia: How many peripersonal spaces? *Neuropsychologia*, 1–8.

Denes, G. (1989). Disorders of body awareness and body knowledge. In F. Boller, & J. Grafman (Eds.), *Handbook of neuropsychology* (pp. 207–225). Amsterdam: Elsevier Science Publishers.

di Pellegrino, G., & Làdavas, E. (2015). Peripersonal space in the brain. *Neuropsychologia*, *66*, 126–133.

di Pellegrino, G., Ladavas, E., & Farne, A. (1997). Seeing where your hands are. *Nature*, *388*(6644), 730.

Dijkerman, H. C., & de Haan, E. H. (2007). Somatosensory processes subserving perception and action. *The Behavioral and Brain Sciences*, *30*(2), 139–189.

Dijkerman, H. C., McIntosh, R. D., Anema, H. A., de Haan, E. H. F., Kappelle, L. J., & Milner, A. D. (2006). Reaching errors in optic ataxia are linked to eye position rather than head or body position. *Neuropsychologia*, *44*(13), 2766–2773.

Dijkerman, H. C., Milner, A. D., & Carey, D. P. (1998). Grasping spatial relationships: Failure to demonstrate allocentric visual coding in a patient with visual form agnosia. *Consciousness and Cognition*, 7(3), 424–437.

Driver, J., & Spence, C. (1998). Crossmodal attention. *Current Opinion in Neurobiology*, *8* (2), 245–253.

Duhamel, J. R., Colby, C. L., & Goldberg, M. E. (1998). Ventral intraparietal area of the macaque: Congruent visual and somatic response properties. *Journal of Neurophysiology*, *79*(1), 126–136.

Ehrsson, H. H. (2007). The experimental induction of out-of-body experiences. *Science (New York, NY)*, *317*(5841), 1048.

Ehrsson, H. H., Holmes, N. P., & Passingham, R. E. (2005). Touching a rubber hand: Feeling of body ownership is associated with activity in multisensory brain areas. *The Journal of Neuroscience*, *25*(45), 10564–10573.

Ehrsson, H. H., Spence, C., & Passingham, R. E. (2004). That's my hand! Activity in premotor cortex reflects feeling of ownership of a limb. *Science (New York, NY)*, *305* (5685), 875–877.

Eimer, M., & Driver, J. (2001). Crossmodal links in endogenous and exogenous spatial attention: Evidence from event-related brain potential studies. *Neuroscience and Biobehavioral Reviews*, *25*(6), 497–511.

Eimer, M., van Velzen, J., & Driver, J. (2002). Cross-modal interactions between audition, touch, and vision in endogenous spatial attention: ERP evidence on preparatory states and sensory modulations. *Journal of Cognitive Neuroscience*, *14*(2), 254–271.

Endo, K., Miyasaka, M., Makishita, H., Yanagisawa, N., & Sugishita, M. (1992). Tactile agnosia and tactile aphasia: Symptomatological and anatomical differences. *Cortex*, *28*(3), 445–469.

Ernst, M. O., & Banks, M. S. (2002). Humans integrate visual and haptic information in a statistically optimal fashion. *Nature*, *415*(6870), 429–433.

Eshkevari, E., Rieger, E., Longo, M. R., Haggard, P., & Treasure, J. (2014). Persistent body image disturbance following recovery from eating disorders. *International Journal of Eating Disorders*, *47*, 400–409.

Farmer, H., Tajadura-Jiménez, A., & Tsakiris, M. (2012). Beyond the colour of my skin: How skin colour affects the sense of body-ownership. *Consciousness and Cognition*, *21* (3), 1242–1256.

Farne, A., Dematte, M. L., & Ladavas, E. (2005). Neuropsychological evidence of modular organization of the near peripersonal space. *Neurology*, *65*(11), 1754–1758.

Farrell, C., Lee, M., & Shafran, R. (2005). Assessment of body size estimation: a review. *European Eating Disorders Review*, *13*, 75–88.

Fattori, P., Breveglieri, R., Raos, V., Bosco, A., & Galletti, C. (2012). Vision for action in the macaque medial posterior parietal cortex. *Journal of Neuroscience, 32*(9), 3221–3234.
Felician, O., Ceccaldi, M., Didic, M., Thinus-Blanc, C., & Poncet, M. (2003). Pointing to body parts: A double dissociation study. *Neuropsychologia, 41*(10), 1307–1316.
Ferri, F., Chiarelli, A. M., Merla, A., Gallese, V., & Costantini, M. (2013). The body beyond the body: Expectation of a sensory event is enough to induce ownership over a fake hand. *Proceedings. Biological Sciences/The Royal Society, 280*(June), 20131140.
Frederiks, J. A. (1985). Macrosomatognosia and microsomatognosia. *Psychiatria, Neurologia, Neurochirurgia, 66*, 531–536.
Fuentes, C. T., Longo, M. R., & Haggard, P. (2013). Body image distortions in healthy adults. *Acta Psychologica, 144*(2), 344–351.
Gallagher, S. (2005). *How the body shapes the mind.* Oxford: Oxford University Press.
Galletti, C., Kutz, D. F., Gamberini, M., Breveglieri, R., & Fattori, P. (2003). Role of the medial parieto-occipital cortex in the control of reaching and grasping movements. *Experimental Brain Research, 153*(2), 158–170.
Gallivan, J. P., Cavina-Pratesi, C., & Culham, J. C. (2009). Is that within reach? fMRI reveals that the human superior parieto-occipital cortex encodes objects reachable by the hand. *The Journal of Neuroscience, 29*(14), 4381–4391.
Gandevia, S. C., & Phegan, C. M. (1999). Perceptual distortions of the human body image produced by local anaesthesia, pain and cutaneous stimulation. *The Journal of Physiology, 514*(Pt 2), 609–616.
Gardner, E. P., Babu, K. S., Reitzen, S. D., Ghosh, S., Brown, A. S., Chen, J., ... Ro, J. Y. (2007). Neurophysiology of prehension. I. Posterior parietal cortex and object-oriented hand behaviors. *Journal of Neurophysiology, 97*(1), 387–406.
Gerstmann, J. (1940). Syndrome of finger agnosia, disorientation for right and left, agraphia and aculculia. *Archives of Neurology and Psychiatry, 44*, 398–407.
Gerstmann, J. (1957). Some notes on the Gerstmann syndrome. *Neurology, 7*(12), 866–869.
Gray, R., & Tan, H. Z. (2002). Dynamic and predictive links between touch and vision. *Experimental Brain Research, 145*(1), 50–55.
Graziano, M. S. A. (2000). Coding the location of the arm by sight. *Science (New York, NY), 290*(5497), 1782–1786.
Graziano, M. S. (2009). *The intelligent movement machine.* New York: Oxford University Press.
Graziano, M. S., & Cooke, D. F. (2006). Parieto-frontal interactions, personal space, and defensive behavior. *Neuropsychologia, 44*(6), 845–859.
Graziano, M. S., & Gross, C. G. (1998). Spatial maps for the control of movement. *Current Opinion in Neurobiology, 8*(2), 195–201.
Graziano, M. S., Cooke, D. F., & Taylor, C. S. (2000). Coding the location of the arm by sight. *Science (New York, NY), 290*(5497), 1782–1786.
Grefkes, C., Weiss, P. H., Zilles, K., & Fink, G. R. (2002). Crossmodal processing of object features in human anterior intraparietal cortex: An fMRI study implies equivalencies between humans and monkeys. *Neuron, 35*(1), 173–184.
Groh, J. M., & Sparks, D. L. (1996). Saccades to somatosensory targets. III. Eye-position-dependent somatosensory activity in primate superior colliculus. *Journal of Neurophysiology, 75*(1), 439–453.
Guariglia, C., Piccardi, L., Allegra, M. C. P., & Traballesi, M. (2002). Is autotopoagnosia real? EC says yes: A case study. *Neuropsychologia, 40*, 1744–1749.
Hadjidimitrakis, K., Bertozzi, F., Breveglieri, R., Fattori, P., & Galletti, C. (2013). Body-centered, mixed, but not hand-centered coding of visual targets in the medial posterior parietal cortex during reaches in 3D space. *Cerebral Cortex*, 1–12.

Halligan, P. W., Hunt, M., Marshall, J. C., & Wade, D. T. (1995). Sensory detection without localization. *Neurocase: Case Studies in Neuropsychology, Neuropsychiatry, and Behavioural Neurology, 1*, 259–266.

Head, H., & Holmes, G. (1911). Sensory disturbances from cerebral lesions. *Brain, 34*(2-3), 102–254.

Heath, M., & Holmes, S.A. (2015). An inverse grip starting posture gives rise to time-dependent adherence to Weber' s law: A reply to Ganel et al. (2014), *Journal of Vision, 15*(6), 1–4.

Heed, T., Backhaus, J., & Röder, B. (2011). Integration of hand and finger location in external spatial coordinates for tactile localization. *Journal of Experimental Psychology: Human Perception and Performance.*

Heed, T., Habets, B., Sebanz, N., & Knoblich, G. (2010). Others' actions reduce cross-modal integration in peripersonal space. *Current Biology, 20*(15), 1345–1349.

Hömke, L., Amunts, K., Bönig, L., Fretz, C., Binkofski, F., Zilles, K., & Weder, B. (2009). Analysis of lesions in patients with unilateral tactile agnosia using cytoarchitectonic probabilistic maps. *Human Brain Mapping, 30*(5), 1444–1456.

Howard, L. A., & Tipper, S. P. (1997). Hand deviations away from visual cues: Indirect evidence for inhibition. *Experimental Brain Research, 113*, 144–152.

Hyvärinen, J., & Poranen, A. (1974). Function of parietal associative area 7 as revealed from cellular discharges in alert monkeys. *Brain, 97*, 673–692.

Jackson, S. R., Jackson, G. M., & Rosicky, J. (1995). Are non-relevant objects represented in working memory? The effect of non-target objects on reach and grasp kinematics. *Experimental Brain Research, 102*(3), 519–530.

Jakobson, L. S., Archibald, Y. M., Carey, D. P., & Goodale, M. A. (1991). A kinematic analysis of reaching and grasping movements in a patient recovering from optic ataxia. *Neuropsychologia, 29*, 803–809.

Jansen, S. E. M., Bergmann Tiest, W. M., & Kappers, A. M. L. (2015). Haptic exploratory behavior during object discrimination: A novel automatic annotation method. *PLoS One, 10*(2), e0117017.

Jeannerod, M., Decety, J., & Michel, F. (1994). Impairment of grasping movements following posterior parietal lesion. *Neuropsychologia, 32*, 369–380.

Kammers, M. P., Kootker, J. A., Hogendoorn, H., & Dijkerman, H. C. (2010). How many motoric body representations can we grasp? *Experimental Brain Research, 202*(1), 203–212.

Kammers, M. P., Verhagen, L., Dijkerman, H. C., Hogendoorn, H., De Vignemont, F., & Schutter, D. J. (2009). Is this hand for real? Attenuation of the rubber hand illusion by transcranial magnetic stimulation over the inferior parietal lobule. *Journal of Cognitive Neuroscience, 21*(7), 1311–1320.

Kammers, M. P. M., de Vignemont, F., Verhagen, L., & Dijkerman, H. C. (2009). The rubber hand illusion in action. *Neuropsychologia, 47*(1), 204–211.

Kammers, M. P. M., Longo, M. R., Tsakiris, M., Dijkerman, H. C., & Haggard, P. (2009). Specificity and coherence of body representations. *Perception, 38*(12), 1804–1820.

Kammers, M. P. M., van der Ham, I. J. M., & Dijkerman, H. C. (2006). Dissociating body representations in healthy individuals: Differential effects of a kinaesthetic illusion on perception and action. *Neuropsychologia, 44*(12), 2430–2436.

Kandula, M., Hofman, D., & Dijkerman, H. C. (2015). Visuo-tactile interactions are dependent on the predictive value of the visual stimulus. *Neuropsychologia, 70.*

Kappers, A. M., & Koenderink, J. J. (1999). Haptic perception of spatial relations. *Perception, 28*(6), 781–795.

Keizer, A., Smeets, M. A. M., Dijkerman, H. C., Uzunbajakau, S. A., van Elburg, A., & Postma, A. (2013). Too fat to fit through the door: First evidence for disturbed body-scaled action in anorexia nervosa during locomotion. *PLoS One, 8*(5), e64602.

Keizer, A., Smeets, M. A. M., Dijkerman, H. C., van den Hout, M., Klugkist, I., van Elburg, A., & Postma, A. (2011). Tactile body image disturbance in anorexia nervosa. *Psychiatry Research, 190*(1), 115–120.

Keizer, A., Smeets, M. A. M., Dijkerman, H. C., van Elburg, A., & Postma, A. (2012). Aberrant somatosensory perception in anorexia nervosa. *Psychiatry Research, 200* (2–3), 530–537.

Keizer, A., Smeets, M. A. M., Postma, A., van Elburg, A., & Dijkerman, H. C. (2014). Does the experience of ownership over a rubber hand change body size perception in anorexia nervosa patients? *Neuropsychologia, 62*, 26–37.

Kennett, S., Eimer, M., Spence, C., & Driver, J. (2001). Tactile-visual links in exogenous spatial attention under different postures: Convergent evidence from psychophysics and ERPs. *Journal of Cognitive Neuroscience, 13*(4), 462–478.

Khan, A. Z., Pisella, L., Rossetti, Y., Vighetto, A., & Crawford, J. D. (2005). Impairment of gaze-centered updating of reach targets in bilateral parietal-occipital damaged patients. *Cerebral Cortex, 15*(10), 1547–1560.

Khan, A. Z., Pisella, L., Vighetto, A., Cotton, F., Luaute, J., Boisson, D., ... Rossetti, Y. (2005). Optic ataxia errors depend on remapped, not viewed, target location. *Nature Neuroscience, 8*(4), 418–420.

Kinsbourne, M., & Warrington, E. K. (1962). A study of finger agnosia. *Brain, 85*, 47–66.

Kinsbourne, M., & Warrington, E. K. (1963). The developmental Gerstmann syndrome. *Archives of Neurology, 8*, 490–501.

Knecht, S., Kunesch, E., & Schnitzler, A. (1996). Parallel and serial processing of haptic information in man: Effects of parietal lesions on sensorimotor hand function. *Neuropsychologia, 37*, 669–687.

Klatzky, R. L., & Lederman, S. J. (1990). Intelligent exploration by the human hand. In V. Subramanian, & T. Iberall (Eds.), *Dextrous robot hands* (pp. 66–81). New York: Springer.

Lackner, J. R. (1988). Some proprioceptive influences on the perceptual representation of body shape and orientation. *Brain, 111*(Pt 2), 281–297.

Ladavas, E., & Farne, A. (2004). Visuo-tactile representation of near-the-body space. *Journal of Physiology, Paris, 98*(1-3), 161–170.

Ladavas, E., & Serino, A. (2008). Action-dependent plasticity in peripersonal space representations. *Cognitive Neuropsychology, 25*(7-8), 1099–1113.

Ladavas, E., di Pellegrino, G., Farne, A., & Zeloni, G. (1998). Neuropsychological evidence of an integrated visuotactile representation of peripersonal space in humans. *Journal of Cognitive Neuroscience, 10*(5), 581–589.

Laiacona, M., Allamano, N., Lorenzi, L., & Capitani, E. (2006). A case of impaired naming and knowledge of body parts. Are limbs a separate sub-category? *Neurocase: Case Studies in Neuropsychology, Neuropsychiatry, and Behavioural Neurology, 12*(5), 307–316.

Lederman, S. J., & Klatzky, R. L. (1987). Hand movements: A window into haptic object recognition. *Cognitive Psychology, 19*(3), 342–368.

Lederman, S. J., & Klatzky, R. L. (1993). Extracting object properties through haptic exploration. *Acta Psychologica, 84*(1), 29–40.

Lenggenhager, B., Tadi, T., Metzinger, T., & Blanke, O. (2007). Video ergo sum: Manipulating bodily self-consciousness. *Science (New York, NY), 317*(5841), 1096–1099.

Leoné, F. T. M., Henriques, D. Y. P., Medendorp, W. P., & Toni, I. (2015). Flexible reference frames for grasp planning in human parietofrontal cortex. *Cortex, Human Parietofrontal, 2*(June), 1–15.

Ley, P., Bottari, D., Shenoy, B. H., Kekunnaya, R., & Röder, B. (2013). Partial recovery of visual–spatial remapping of touch after restoring vision in a congenitally blind man. *Neuropsychologia, 51*(6), 1119–1123.

Longo, M. R., & Haggard, P. (2010). An implicit body representation underlying human position sense. *Proceedings of the National Academy of Sciences of the United States of America, 107*, 11727–11732.

Longo, M. R., & Haggard, P. (2011). Weber's illusion and body shape: Anisotropy of tactile size perception on the hand. *Journal of Experimental Psychology: Human Perception and Performance, 37*(3), 720–726.

Longo, M. R., & Haggard, P. (2012). Implicit body representations and the conscious body image. *Acta Psychologica, 141*(2), 164–168.

Longo, M. R., Azañón, E., & Haggard, P. (2010). More than skin deep: Body representation beyond primary somatosensory cortex. *Neuropsychologia, 48*(3), 655–668.

Maister, L., Cardini, F., Zamariola, G., Serino, A., & Tsakiris, M. (2015). Your place or mine: Shared sensory experiences elicit a remapping of peripersonal space. *Neuropsychologia, 70*, 455–461.

Makin, T. R., Holmes, N. P., & Ehrsson, H. H. (2008). On the other hand: Dummy hands and peripersonal space. *Behavioural Brain Research, 191*(1), 1–10.

Makin, T. R., Holmes, N. P., & Zohary, E. (2007). Is that near my hand? Multisensory representation of peripersonal space in human intraparietal sulcus. *The Journal of Neuroscience, 27*(4), 731–740.

Makin, T. R., Holmes, N. P., Brozzoli, C., & Farnè, A. (2012). Keeping the world at hand: Rapid visuomotor processing for hand-object interactions. *Experimental Brain Research, 219*(4), 421–428.

Menger, R., Dijkerman, H. C., & Van der Stigchel, S. (2013). The effect of similarity: Non-spatial features modulate obstacle avoidance. *PLoS One, 8*(4), e59294.

Menger, R., Dijkerman, H. C., & Van der Stigchel, S. (2014). On the relation between nontarget object location and avoidance responses. *Journal of Vision, 14*(9), 1–14.

Menger, R., Van der Stigchel, S., & Dijkerman, H. C. (2012). How obstructing is an obstacle? The influence of starting posture on obstacle avoidance. *Acta Psychologica, 141*(1), 1–8.

Milner, A. D., & Dijkerman, H. C. (1998). Visual processing in the primate parietal lobe. In A. D. Milner (Ed.), *Comparative neuropsychology* (pp. 70–94). Oxford: Oxford University Press.

Milner, A. D., & Goodale, M. A. (1995). *The visual brain in action*. Oxford: Oxford University Press.

Milner, A. D., & Goodale, M. A. (2008). Two visual systems re-viewed. *Neuropsychologia, 46*(3), 774–785.

Milner, A. D., Dijkerman, H. C., & Carey, D. P. (1999). Visuospatial processing in a pure case of visual-form agnosia. In N. Burgess, K. J. Jeffery, & J. O. O'Keefe (Eds.), *The hippocampal and parietal foundations of spatial cognition* (pp. 443–466). Oxford: Oxford University Press.

Monaco, S., Króliczak, G., Quinlan, D. J., Fattori, P., Galletti, C., Goodale, M. A., & Culham, J. C. (2010). Contribution of visual and proprioceptive information to the precision of reaching movements. *Experimental Brain Research, 202*(1), 15–32.

Mon-Williams, M., Tresilian, J. R., Coppard, V. L., & Carson, R. G. (2001). The effect of obstacle position on reach-to-grasp movements. *Experimental Brain Research, 137*(3-4), 497–501.

Morley, J. W., Goodwin, A. W., & Darian-Smith, I. (1983). Tactile discrimination of gratings. *Experimental Brain Research, 49*(2), 291–299.

Moseley, G. L., Gallace, A., & Spence, C. (2012). Bodily illusions in health and disease: Physiological and clinical perspectives and the concept of a cortical "body matrix". *Neuroscience and Biobehavioral Reviews, 36*(1), 34–46.

Newport, R., Pearce, R., & Preston, C. (2010). Fake hands in action: Embodiment and control of supernumerary limbs. *Experimental Brain Research, 204*(3), 385–395.

Newport, R., Rabb, B., & Jackson, S. R. (2002). Noninformative vision improves haptic spatial perception. *Current Biology: CB, 12*(19), 1661–1664.

O'Sullivan, B. T., Roland, P. E., & Kawashima, R. (1994). A PET study of somatosensory discrimination in man. *Microgeometry Versus Macrogeometry, 6*, 137–148.

Paillard, J. (1999). Body schema and body image—A double dissociation in deafferented patients. In G.N. Gantchev, S. Mori, & J. Massion (Eds.), *Motor control, today and tomorrow* (pp. 198–214). Sofia: Academic Publishing House.

Paillard, J., Michel, F., & Stelmach, G. (1983). Localization without content. A tactile analogue of "blind sight". *Archives of Neurology, 40*(9), 548–551.

Pellijeff, A., Bonilha, L., Morgan, P. S., McKenzie, K., & Jackson, S. R. (2006). Parietal updating of limb posture: An event-related fMRI study. *Neuropsychologia, 44*(13), 2685–2690.

Peltz, E., Seifert, F., Lanz, S., Müller, R., & Maihöfner, C. (2011). Impaired hand size estimation in CRPS. *The Journal of Pain, 12*(10), 1095–1101.

Petkova, V. I., & Ehrsson, H. H. (2008). If I were you: Perceptual illusion of body swapping. *PLoS One, 3*(12), e3832.

Platz, T. (1996). Tactile agnosia. Casuistic evidence and theoretical remarks on modality-specific meaning representations and sensorimotor integration. *Brain, 119*(Pt 5), 1565–1574.

Poliakoff, E., Miles, E., Li, X., & Blanchette, I. (2007). The effect of visual threat on spatial attention to touch. *Cognition, 102*(3), 405–414.

Postma, A., Zuidhoek, S., Noordzij, M. L., & Kappers, A. M. L. (2008). Haptic orientation perception benefits from visual experience: Evidence from early-blind, late-blind, and sighted people. *Perception & Psychophysics, 70*(7), 1197–1206.

Reed, C. L., Caselli, R. J., & Farah, M. J. (1996). Tactile agnosia: Underlying impairment and implications for normal tactile object recognition. *Brain, 119*, 875–888.

Rice, N. J., McIntosh, R. D., Schindler, I., Mon-Williams, M., Demonet, J. F., & Milner, A. D. (2006). Intact automatic avoidance of obstacles in patients with visual form agnosia. *Experimental Brain Research, 174*(1), 176–188.

Rizzolatti, G., & Matelli, M. (2003). Two different streams form the dorsal visual system: Anatomy and functions. *Experimental Brain Research, 153*(2), 146–157.

Rizzolatti, G., Luppino, G., & Matelli, M. (1998). The organization of the cortical motor system: New concepts. *Electroencephalography and Clinical Neurophysiology, 106*(4), 283–296.

Rizzolatti, G., Scandolara, C., Matelli, M., & Gentilucci, M. (1981a). Afferent properties of periarcuate neurons in macaque monkeys. I. Somatosensory responses. *Behavioural Brain Research, 2*(2), 125–146.

Rizzolatti, G., Scandolara, C., Matelli, M., & Gentilucci, M. (1981b). Afferent properties of periarcuate neurons in macaque monkeys. II. Visual responses. *Behavioural Brain Research, 2*(2), 147–163.

Rode, G., Vallar, G., Revol, P., Tilikete, C., Jacquin-Courtois, S., Rossetti, Y., & Farne, A. (2012). Facial macrosomatognosia and pain in a case of Wallenberg's syndrome: Selective effects of vestibular and transcutaneous stimulations. *Neuropsychologia, 50*(2), 245–253.

Röder, B., Rösler, F., & Spence, C. (2004). Early vision impairs tactile perception in the blind. *Current Biology, 14*, 121–124.

Roland, P. E. (1987). Somatosensory detection of microgeometry, macrogeometry and kinesthesia after localized lesions of cerebral hemispheres in man. *Brain Research Reviews, 12*, 43–94.

Rossetti, Y. (1998). Implicit short-lived motor representations of space in brain damaged and healthy subjects. *Consciousness and Cognition, 7*, 520–558.

Rossetti, Y., Rode, G., & Boisson, D. (1995). Implicit processing of somaethetic information: A dissociation between where and how. *Neuroreport, 6*, 506–510.

Ruotolo, F., van der Ham, I., Postma, A., Ruggiero, G., & Iachini, T. (2015). How coordinate and categorical spatial relations combine with egocentric and allocentric reference frames in a motor task: Effects of delay and stimuli characteristics. *Behavioural Brain Research*, *284*, 1–12.

Rusconi, E., Pinel, P., Dehaene, S., & Kleinschmidt, A. (2010). The enigma of Gerstmann's syndrome revisited: A telling tale of the vicissitudes of neuropsychology. *Brain: A Journal of Neurology*, *133*(Pt 2), 320–332.

Rusconi, E., Walsh, V., & Butterworth, B. (2005). Dexterity with numbers: rTMS over left angular gyrus disrupts finger gnosis and number processing. *Neuropsychologia*, *43* (11), 1609–1624.

Saetti, M. C., De Renzi, E., & Comper, M. (1999). Tactile morphagnosia secondary to spatial deficits. *Neuropsychologia*, *37*(9), 1087–1100.

Saling, M., Alberts, J., Stelmach, G. E., & Bloedel, J. R. (1998). Reach-to-grasp movements during obstacle avoidance. *Experimental Brain Research*, *118*(2), 251–258.

Sandyk, R. (1998). Reversal of a body image disorder (macrosomatognosia) in Parkinson's disease by treatment with AC pulsed electromagnetic fields. *International Journal of Neuroscience*, *93*(1-2), 43–54.

Schenk, T. (2006). An allocentric rather than perceptual deficit in patient D.F. *Nature Neuroscience*, *9*(11), 1369–1370.

Schenk, T. (2012). No dissociation between perception and action in patient DF when haptic feedback is withdrawn. *The Journal of Neuroscience*, *32*(6), 2013–2017.

Schindler, I., Rice, N. J., McIntosh, R. D., Rossetti, Y., Vighetto, A., & Milner, A. D. (2004). Automatic avoidance of obstacles is a dorsal stream function: Evidence from optic ataxia. *Nature Neuroscience*, 7(7), 779–784.

Schwoebel, J., & Coslett, H. B. (2005). Evidence for multiple, distinct representations of the human body. *J Cogn Neurosci*, *17*(4), 543–553.

Semmes, J. (1965). A non-tactual factor in astereognosis. *Neuropsychologia*, *3*, 295–315.

Sforza, A., Bufalari, I., Haggard, P., & Aglioti, S. M. (2010). My face in yours: Visuo-tactile facial stimulation influences sense of identity. *Social Neuroscience*, *5*(October 2014), 148–162.

Sirigu, A., Grafman, J., Bressler, K., & Sunderland, T. (1991). Multiple representations contribute to body knowledge processing. Evidence from a case of autotopagnosia. *Brain*, *114*, 629–642.

Skrzypek, S., Wehmeier, P. M., & Remschmidt, H. (2001). Body image assessment using body size estimation in recent studies on anorexia nervosa. A brief review. *European Child & Adolescent Psychiatry*, *10*(4), 215–221.

Slater, M., Spanlang, B., Sanchez-Vives, M. V., & Blanke, O. (2010). First person experience of body transfer in virtual reality. *PLoS One*, *5*(5), e10564.

Smeets, J. B. J., & Brenner, E. (1999). A new view on grasping. *Motor Control*, *3*(3), 237–271.

Smeets, J. B. J., van den Dobbelsteen, J. J., de Grave, D. D. J., van Beers, R. J., & Brenner, E. (2006). Sensory integration does not lead to sensory calibration. *Proceedings of the National Academy of Sciences of the United States of America*, *103*(49), 18781–18786.

Soto-Faraco, S., Sinnett, S., Alsius, A., & Kingstone, A. (2005). Spatial orienting of tactile attention induced by social cues. *Psychonomic Bulletin & Review*, *12*(6), 1024–1031.

Spence, C., Lloyd, D., McGlone, F., Nicholls, M. E., & Driver, J. (2000). Inhibition of return is supramodal: A demonstration between all possible pairings of vision, touch, and audition. *Experimental Brain Research*, *134*(1), 42–48.

Spence, C., Pavani, F., & Driver, J. (2000). Crossmodal links between vision and touch in covert endogenous spatial attention. *Journal of Experimental Psychology: Human Perception and Performance*, *26*(4), 1298–1319.

Taffou, M., & Viaud-Delmon, I. (2014). Cynophobic fear adaptively extends peripersonal space. *Frontiers in Psychiatry, 5*(September), 3–9.

Taylor-Clarke, M., Jacobsen, P., & Haggard, P. (2004). Keeping the world a constant size: Object constancy in human touch. *Nature Neuroscience*, 7(3), 219–220.

Teneggi, C., Canzoneri, E., Pellegrino, G., Serino, A., Giuridiche, S., Cicu, A., ... Paris, I. (2013). Report social modulation of peripersonal space boundaries. *Current Biology, 23*(5), 406–411.

Thakkar, K. N., Brugger, P., & Park, S. (2009). Exploring empathic space: Correlates of perspective transformation ability and biases in spatial attention. *PLoS One, 4*(6), e5864.

Tinazzi, M., Ferrari, G., Zampini, M., & Aglioti, S. M. (2000). Neuropsychological evidence that somatic stimuli are spatially coded according to multiple frames of reference in a stroke patient with tactile extinction. *Neuroscience Letters, 287*(2), 133–136.

Trenner, M. U., Heekeren, H. R., Bauer, M., Rossner, K., Wenzel, R., Villringer, A., & Fahle, M. (2008). What happens in between? Human oscillatory brain activity related to crossmodal spatial cueing. *PLoS One, 3*(1), e1467.

Tresilian, J. R. (1998). Attention in action or obstruction of movement? A kinematic analysis of avoidance behavior in prehension. *Experimental Brain Research, 120*(3), 352–368.

Tsakiris, M., & Haggard, P. (2005). The rubber hand illusion revisited: Visuotactile integration and self-attribution. *Journal of Experimental Psychology: Human Perception and Performance, 31*(1), 80–91.

Tsakiris, M., Prabhu, G., & Haggard, P. (2006). Having a body versus moving your body: How agency structures body-ownership. *Consciousness and Cognition, 15*(2), 423–432.

Valenza, N., Ptak, R., Zimine, I., Badan, M., Lazeyras, F., & Schnider, A. (2001). Dissociated active and passive tactile shape recognition: A case study of pure tactile apraxia. *Brain, 124*(Pt 11), 2287–2298.

Vallar, G. (1997). Spatial frames of reference and somatosensory processing: A neuropsychological perspective. *Philosophical Transactions of the Royal Society of London. Series B, Biological Sciences, 352*(1360), 1401–1409.

van Beers, R. J., Wolpert, D. M., & Haggard, P. (2002). When feeling is more important than seeing in sensorimotor adaptation. *Current Biology, 12*(10), 834–837.

van Stralen, H. E., & Dijkerman, H. C. (2011). Central touch disorders. *Scholarpedia, 6*(10), 8243.

van Stralen, H. E., van Zandvoort, M. J. E., Vissers, L. M. G., Hoppenbrouwers, S. S., Kappelle, L. J., & Dijkerman, H. C. (2014). Affective touch modulates the rubber hand illusion. *Cognition, 131* (1), 147–158.

Verhagen, L., Dijkerman, H. C., Grol, M. J., & Toni, I. (2008). Perceptuo-motor interactions during prehension movements. *The Journal of Neuroscience : The Official Journal of the Society for Neuroscience, 28*(18), 4726–4735.

Verhagen, L., Dijkerman, H. C., Medendorp, W. P., & Toni, I. (2012). Cortical dynamics of sensorimotor integration during grasp planning. *The Journal of Neuroscience: The Official Journal of the Society for Neuroscience, 32*(13), 4508–4519.

Verhagen, L., Dijkerman, H. C., Medendorp, W. P., & Toni, I. (2013). Hierarchical organization of parietofrontal circuits during goal-directed action. *The Journal of Neuroscience: The Official Journal of the Society for Neuroscience, 33*(15), 6492–6503.

Veronelli, L., Ginex, V., Dinacci, D., Cappa, S. F., & Corbo, M. (2014). Pure associative tactile agnosia for the left hand: Clinical and anatomo-functional correlations. *Cortex, 58*, 206–216.

Vesia, M., & Crawford, J. D. (2012). Specialization of reach function in human posterior parietal cortex. *Experimental Brain Research, 221*(1), 1–18.

von Hofsten, C., & Rösblad, B. (1988). The integration of sensory information in the development of precise manual pointing. *Neuropsychologia, 26*(6), 805–821.

Wann, J. P., & Ibrahim, S. F. (1992). Does limb proprioception drift? *Experimental Brain Research, 91*(1), 162–166.

Ward, J., Mensah, A., Jünemann, K., Ward, J., Mensah, A., & Jünemann, K. (2015). The rubber hand illusion depends on the tactile congruency of the observed and felt touch. *Journal of Experimental Psychology: Human Perception and Performance, 41*(5), 1203–1208.

Weber, E. H. (1834). In H. E. Ross, & D. J. Murray (Eds.), *The sense of touch*. London: Academic.

Weijers, N. R., Rietveld, A., Meijer, F. J. A., & de Leeuw, F. E. (2013). Macrosomatognosia in frontal lobe infarct-a case report. *Journal of Neurology, 260*(3), 925–926.

Weinstein, S. (1968). Intensive and extensive aspects of tactile sensitivity as a function of body part, sex, and laterality. In D. R. Kenskalo (Ed.), *The skin senses* (pp. 195–222). Sprinfield, IL: Charles C. Thomas.

Westwood, D. A., & Goodale, M. A. (2003). A haptic size-contrast illusion affects size perception but not grasping. *Experimental Brain Research, 153*, 253–259.

Whitwell, R. L., David Milner, A., Cavina-Pratesi, C., Byrne, C. M., & Goodale, M. A. (2014). DF's visual brain in action: The role of tactile cues. *Neuropsychologia, 55*, 41–50.

Wolpert, D. M., Goodbody, S. J., & Husain, M. (1998). Maintaining internal representations: The role of the human superior parietal lobe. *Nature Neuroscience, 1*(6), 529–533.

Yamamoto, S., & Kitazawa, S. (2001). Reversal of subjective temporal order due to arm crossing. *Nature Neuroscience, 4*(7), 759–765.

Zuidhoek, S., Kappers, A. M., Van Der Lubbe, R. H., & Postma, A. (2003). Delay improves performance on a haptic spatial matching task. *Experimental Brain Research, 149*(3), 320–330.

CHAPTER 4

Multisensory Perception and the Coding of Space

Nathan van der Stoep[1], Albert Postma[1,2,3] and Tanja C.W. Nijboer[1,4,5]
[1]Experimental Psychology, Helmholtz Institute, Utrecht University, Utrecht, The Netherlands
[2]Department of Neurology, University Medical Center, Utrecht, The Netherlands
[3]Korsakov Center Slingedael, Rotterdam, The Netherlands
[4]Rudolf Magnus Institute of Neuroscience and Center of Excellence for Rehabilitation Medicine, University Medical Center Utrecht and Rehabilitation Center De Hoogstraat, Utrecht, The Netherlands
[5]Department of Rehabilitation Medicine, University Medical Center, Utrecht, The Netherlands

Vision, audition, and touch all code the space around us, or rather the things that are located in the space around us, in a different way. Yet, together our senses form a coherent spatial representation of our environment. In this chapter we will discuss how space is coded through vision, audition, and touch, and how spatial information from these senses is combined or integrated. We will continue by discussing neuropsychological impairments that affect spatial perception and multisensory integration, and finally how multisensory stimulation may help reduce or overcome some of these impairments.

4.1 HOW VISION, TOUCH, AND AUDITION CODE SPACE

Our everyday experiences with the world are dependent on what we see, hear, feel, smell, and taste. In fact, living without any sensory organs seems useless, as we cannot interact with the world around us. Even losing a single sense can have a great impact on our daily lives (also see Boxes 4.1 and 4.2). The following situation demonstrates how nicely the senses get along (Fig. 4.1):

> *Imagine that it is your turn to hit a piñata at one of your friends' birthday parties. You are blindfolded, disorientated, and given a baseball bat. The piñata is dangling just above you, unaware of its fate. As you are blindfolded you will have to trust on auditory and tactile feedback to know whether you have actually hit the thing, much to the entertainment of your friends. You swing the bat randomly, and at your third attempt you suddenly feel some resistance and hear a crackling sound. You take off your blindfold, look up, and victoriously behold the cracked piñata exactly where you knew it was located once you hit it.*

Neuropsychology of Space.
DOI: http://dx.doi.org/10.1016/B978-0-12-801638-1.00004-5

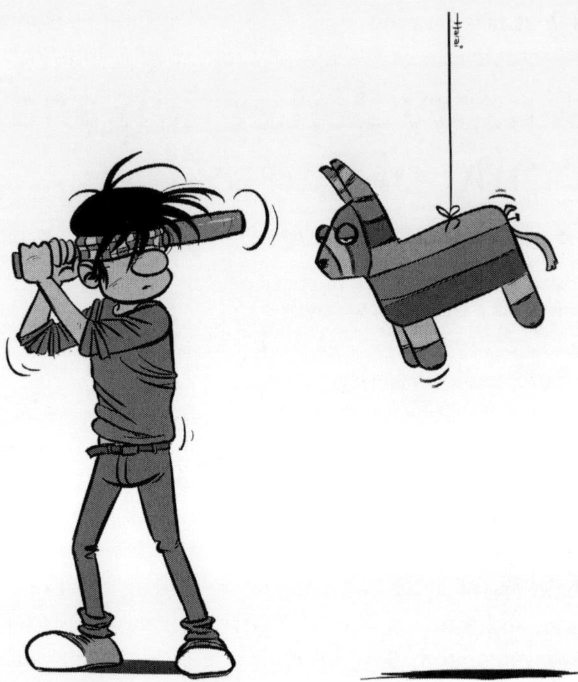

Figure 4.1 Knowing when and where you've hit a piñata requires close communication between the senses *(Illustration by N. van der Stoep).*

Although there does not seem to be anything special about this situation, a closer look at the piñata encounter reveals to us that something special has just happened. You were not aware of it, but your senses coded the space around you in very different ways, and yet, they all indicated the same location of the piñata in three-dimensional (3-D) space. Whereas you temporarily lost your sight you directly knew where to look after the blindfold was removed. This raises the question of how the remaining senses of audition, touch, and proprioception give input to the visual system. Before addressing multisensory integration let us first briefly discuss the basics of spatial localization through vision, audition, and somatosensation.

4.1.1 Vision

We can only see what we can see in the world around us because of our eyes. As obvious as this may sound, it determines the very nature of what is often considered to be the main exteroceptive system of the human brain: vision. Our sense of vision has several unique properties that help us interact efficiently with the world around us. With our eyes we perceive the light that is (or is not) reflected off things in the region of space in front of the body. As this light falls on the retina, the world around us is initially always coded in a retinotopic reference frame in the case of vision. This means that everything that we see is coded based on where the light reflections of an object in space fall on the retina. This way of representing the visual world can be seen throughout the visual pathway, from subcortical structures like the superior colliculi to the cortical structures like V1 (Grill-Spector & Malach, 2004; Sparks & Nelson, 1987; see also Chapter 2). The retinotopic mapping of visual information means that the region of space that we can see is directly spatially tuned. It allows us to accurately estimate the location of information in 3-D space, and provides size, shape, and texture information. Furthermore, it allows us to see and integrate many things in our visual field (ie, the part of space that we can see) and has many unique qualities such as the ability to differentiate between different colors, intensities, contrasts, textures, and shapes that help us to group and filter visual information (see Chapter 5 for a further discussion of filtering by spatial attention).

BOX 4.1 Lessons From the Blind: How Vision Loss Affects Spatial Cognition

Unfortunately, loss of vision is still a common ailment in the modern world. Estimates are that about 286 million individuals are severely visually impaired, with about 39 million to be considered blind (World Health Organization (WHO) fact sheet August 2014, http://www.who.int/mediacentre/factsheets/fs282/en/, see also Cattaneo & Vecchi, 2011; chapter 1: A Sense of Space). Within this population the condition of congenital blindness is rare, but in absolute numbers still makes a considerable amount. Gilbert and Foster (2001) estimated at about 1.4 million blind children in 2001 worldwide.

A central question is how blindness—especially early in life—affects cognition and in particular spatial thinking and behavior. Losing one sense could have various impacts on task performance by the remaining senses and on crossmodal integration in particular. Pavani and Röder (2012) discuss three possibilities for performance changes in the blind (see also Röder & Rosler, 2004).

First there is the option of hypercompensation. Due to higher reliance on the remaining senses these could become enhanced and start to function on a higher level. We may think here of increased tactile acuity in the blind as an example (Wong, Gnanakumaran, & Goldreich, 2011). At a neural level hypercompensation may be achieved by intramodal plasticity, by changes in multisensory brain areas, and by crossmodal plasticity (Pavani & Röder, 2012). In particular the latter has been demonstrated in studies in which the visual cortex of blind individuals becomes engaged in auditory or tactile tasks (Hamilton & Pascual-Leone, 1998; Sadato et al., 1996; Theoret, Merabet, & Pascual-Leone, 2004; Van der Lubbe, Van Mierlo, & Postma, 2010).

(*Continued*)

BOX 4.1 Lessons From the Blind: How Vision Loss Affects Spatial Cognition—cont'd

A second possibility is that performance on a certain task in the remaining sensory modalities stays at about the same level, suggesting independence between the lost modality and the remaining ones for the task at hand. Renier et al. (2010) showed that the right middle occipital gyrus in early blind participants was more tuned to auditory and tactile spatial stimuli than to nonspatial ones (the tuning to auditory and tactile inputs by this visual area again a sign of crossmodal plasticity). A similar preference in the right middle occipital gyrus was observed for visual spatial stimuli compared to nonspatial stimuli in sighted participants. Hence the spatial specialization of the extrastriate cortex remains unchanged even though it is driven in the blind by other modalities (Striem-Amit et al., 2015). The compensation explanation might also include another variant. Namely the lost sense does have some impact on task performance but this decrease in performance is masked or compensated for by changes in the contributions of other sensory modalities. There are several aids specifically designed to help the blind orient in the world that make use of this compensation possibility. A classic example is the white cane to support mobility (Maidenbaum et al., 2014; Maidenbaum, Levy-Tzedek, Chebat, Namer-Furstenberg & Amedi, 2014; Proulx, Ptito, & Amedi, 2014). In their book *Blind Vision: The Neuroscience of Visual Impairment* Cattaneo and Vecchi partly appear to adhere the compensation hypothesis: "... we think that shapes and space are represented in an analog format in the blind ..." (Cattaneo & Vecchi, 2011, p. 2). At the same time though, the authors acknowledge that intrinsic differences between blind and sighted individuals also exist.

A third consequence of losing a sense could be that it actually causes deficiencies in various cognitive domains, other than just the affected sensory modality. Some of these deficiencies might even be perceptual. Zwiers, Van Opstal, and Cruysberg (2001) found that blind participants performed more poorly in auditory localization in the vertical plane. Apparently vision is needed to calibrate the spectral sound cues in the pinnae in order to distinguish higher from lower in the vertical dimension. This again illustrates the importance of multisensory integration. Our senses tend to work together. If one sense becomes defective, performance in the other sensory modalities may drop as well.

Blindness may not only affect perceptual functioning of the remaining senses, it could have an impact at higher cognitive levels in particular. Of special interest here are higher forms of cognition such as mental imagery, spatial reasoning, and spatial memory. Can we really understand space if we cannot see (and never have done so)? Optimal sensory integration theories assume that weights are assigned to different sensory inputs in order to explain behavioral interactions (Millar, 1994). The weights depend on the precision and salience of an input for the task at hand. Vision as such is typically quite useful for spatial processing because it provides external, distal reference frame cues, often in a parallel, configurational manner, and with high acuity. However, Millar and Al-Attar (2005) demonstrated that

(*Continued*)

BOX 4.1 Lessons From the Blind: How Vision Loss Affects Spatial Cognition—cont'd

when concurrent visual information was experimentally manipulated to contain no spatial cues at all, blindfolded participants did not profit from it in a haptic spatial memory task. Hence vision per se is not enough for spatial memory. Its importance lays in the fact that under normal circumstances it offers an abundance of spatial cues. Moreover, offering external spatial haptic cues helped blindfolded participants to memorize irregular sequences of haptic spatial locations (Millar & Al-Attar, 2004). Thus, other modalities can also provide a large repertoire of spatial cues that can be used to remember space.

The last two findings suggest that vision per se is not sufficient nor necessary for building complex spatial representations. This again seems to support the option of compensation. Cattaneo et al. (2008) argue that in spatial reasoning and mental imagery, blind individuals often use different mental strategies. These strategies can still be rather effective even though they differ qualitatively from the cognitive solutions employed by sighted persons. At a neural level this may include functional reorganization of visual brain areas as well as the recruitment of supramodal or multisensory brain regions (Cattaneo et al., 2008).

How fixed are the idiosyncratic strategic biases of blind individuals? In their monumental paper *Vision as a Spatial Sense*, Thinus-Blanc and Gaunet (1997) emphasize that performance levels in spatial tasks depend on the particular strategies employed. Because of visual deprivation early on in life and its accompanying exploration behaviors, blind individuals either may have developed notable preferences to employ certain strategies and avoid others, or alternatively may become limited to just a few strategies (perhaps also implying the existence of a critical period to master spatial strategies). The former option is interesting because it may inspire education and training programs for the blind focusing on learning more optimal strategies to deal with spatial tasks.

Is vision a *sine qua non* for spatial cognition (see also Box 1.4)? Is compensation effective enough? Without doubt, vision is very important for understanding, representing, and acting in the spatial world. Congenitally blind clearly do worse on many spatial tests (see Cattaneo et al., 2008, Pasqualotto & Proulx, 2012, for recent overviews). However, at the same time it is also clear that they are not without spatial ability at all and quite often and perhaps surprisingly perform at high levels. Is the difference between blind and sighted individuals just quantitative or also reflecting a qualitative difference? Pasqualotto and Proulx (2012) argue that early visual inputs are essential for full development of multisensory integration abilities, which in turn are important for constructing allocentric spatial and survey representations. While blind do have certain allocentric reference skills (Tinti, Adenzato, Tamietto, & Cornoldi, 2006; Ungar, Blades, & Spencer, 1996), the difference with sighted persons' capacities makes it a large quantitative and even possibly quasiqualitative gap.

4.1.2 Touch

Our sense of touch is mediated by various receptors in the skin that allow us to perceive touch, heat, pressure, pain, etc. (see Chapter 3 for more on touch). As such, touch is always mapped to the body in space. Based on feedback from our muscles we know where in space a body part is located which enables us to know not only on which part of our body we have been touched, but also where in external space we have been touched. Think of, for example, being touched on your right hand both when holding your hand in front of your body and when placing it behind your back. You will be able to tell where on your body you have been touched (on the hand), but also where in external space your hand was when it was touched. When thinking of the region of space within which we can perceive touch, it becomes clear that it is limited in terms of the distance from the body at which we can perceive our environment as compared to, for example, vision and audition.

BOX 4.2 Lessons From the Deaf: How Hearing Loss Affects Spatial Cognition

According to the WHO (2015) around 360 million people worldwide these days suffer from disabling hearing loss (WHO fact sheet March 2015, http://www.who.int/mediacentre/factsheets/fs300/en/). The World Federation of the Deaf gives an estimate that about 70 million of these persons are considered deaf (http://wfdeaf.org/), that is, suffering a profound hearing loss (over 90 dB in their best ear), with about 32 million of them being children (http://www.deafchildworldwide.info/). Deafness in children is often accompanied by multiple other disabilities, either as a consequence of their deafness, or because of an underlying etiology that has several neurocognitive effects, deafness being one of them. The disabilities may include intellectual impairments, autism spectrum disorders, and concurrent perceptual deficits such as deafblindness (Van Dijk, Nelson, Postma, & Van Dijk, 2010). The group of deaf individuals without any comorbid symptoms and with normal intellectual development is particularly interesting. It allows investigating whether their visual abilities function at a superior level (see hypercompensation: Box 4.1) and whether this in turn leads to enhanced spatial abilities.

Deafness appears to incite selective improvements of visual skills, in particular peripheral vision and visual attention, whereas other dimensions remain unchanged (brightness, contrast, movement; Bavelier et al., 2000; Finney & Dobkins, 2001; Lomber, Meredith, & Kral, 2011). Pavani and Bottari (2012)

(Continued)

BOX 4.2 Lessons From the Deaf: How Hearing Loss Affects Spatial Cognition—cont'd

hypothesize that it is not the visual perception per se that is enhanced but rather visual attention and orienting (see also Bavelier, Dye, & Hauser, 2006). If visual orienting functions at a higher level in deaf individuals, the possibility emerges that spatial cognition at large is also boosted after hearing deprivation. There are several results suggesting that this is indeed the case (Emmorey & Kosslyn, 1996; Emmorey, Kosslyn, & Bellugi, 1993). It was reported that deaf individuals have enhanced mental imagery abilities. Importantly, this proficiency seems to depend on the fact that the deaf group used sign language. Emmorey et al. (1993) observed that hearing signers also showed a mental imagery advantage. Similarly, van Dijk, Kappers, and Postma (2013a) reported that both hearing and deaf signers performed better than hearing nonsigners on a haptic configuration learning task but to a similar extent. Sign language is an iconic type of language and has a large intrinsic spatial component (see also Box 6.3). When signing a story with different actors and when relaying a new bit of information about a particular actor, one might want to return to the area of manual action space where previously this actor was first introduced. This requires an implicit or explicit spatial memory. In line with this conjecture it was reported that spatial memory was increased on the basis of both auditory deprivation and (early) sign language experience (Cattani & Clibbens, 2005).

More research is needed to determine whether auditory deprivation (and subsequent visual attention proficiency) is more important for the development of spatial skills rather than sign language training. This might depend on the precise nature of the spatial task at stake. In contrast to the findings on haptic spatial configuration learning (van Dijk et al., 2013a), van Dijk, Kappers, & Postma (2013b) found that the same group of deaf participants outperformed both hearing signers and nonsigners on a bimanual haptic orientation matching of two bars that were 120 cm apart in space (see also Fig. 3.5). Hearing signers did not outperform the hearing nonsigners. This may suggest that auditory deprivation is responsible for the haptic orientation matching difference. However, as acknowledged by the authors, as all deaf participants also used sign language, we cannot rule out the possibility that profound sign language training early in life has made the difference. Cattani and Clibbens (2005) also point out the need to include nonsigning deaf participants as well in experimental studies.

It is not surprising that the growth in spatial efficiency with auditory deprivation is accompanied by changes at the brain level. As in the blind brain, major functional reorganization of the brain takes place in deaf individuals (Kral, 2007; Kral & Eggermont, 2007). Among others the deaf auditory cortex seems to adopt new visual functionality (Merabet & Pascual-Leone, 2010; Sharma, Nash, & Dorman, 2009). One of the most intriguing patterns of neural

(Continued)

BOX 4.2 Lessons From the Deaf: How Hearing Loss Affects Spatial Cognition—cont'd

plasticity is the observation of distinct hemispheric lateralization with prolonged auditory deprivation. It has been suggested that in the deaf the left hemisphere becomes more involved in visuospatial tasks that in hearing persons are typically associated with right hemisphere involvement (Bosworth, Petrich, & Dobkins, 2013; Cattaneo, Lega, Cecchetto, & Papagno, 2014). Cattaneo et al. (2014) point out that the default rightward tuning in space perception and representations might be absent in the deaf. Cattani and Clibbens (2005) even found a completely atypical lateralization in deaf participants in certain visuospatial memory conditions. Again, not just deafness itself may contribute to these changes in lateralization, also sign language usage seems to be a factor. Several researchers have claimed that (spatial) language processing by means of sign language causes larger right hemispheric activity (Emmorey et al., 2005; MacSweeney, Capek, Campbell, & Woll, 2008).

Based on the findings from Box 4.1 one might conclude that vision loss seems to depress spatial functioning. In contrast, the take home message from the current box would be that loss of audition strengthens spatial ability. It is remarkable that direct comparisons on spatial tasks between blind and deaf individuals are scarce. The obvious reason for this stems from the fact that the task designs have been adapted for the sense that is lost and thus often are greatly different with respect to input format. One of the few studies directly comparing deaf and blind participants was done by Berg and Worchel (1956). They had sex, age, and intelligence matched deaf, blind, and sighted-hearing children perform two haptic maze tasks. Perhaps surprisingly, deaf individuals performed more poorly than the blind, with sighted/hearing individuals performing better than the blind on one of the two mazes. The authors discussed that verbalization, motor imagery, and visual imagery strategies may all contribute to the performance differences in different extents. van Dijk et al. (2013a) tested deaf signers, hearing signers, and hearing nonsigners on a haptic spatial configuration learning test. They computed *Z*-scores for the former two groups relative to the performance levels of the third, control group. They also did this for the blind groups in an earlier study from their laboratory (Postma, Zuidhoek, Noordzij, & Kappers, 2007). Fig. 4.2 shows the results of their study. A negative *Z*-score means better haptic configuration learning relative to the matched controls. It can be seen from Fig. 4.2 that both blind and deaf individuals scored better than their controls (which are at the $Z = 0$ line, the horizontal line in Fig. 4.2). However, this effect was stronger in the blind.

The studies by Berg and Worchel (1956) and van Dijk et al. (2013a) seem to undermine the idea that deafness helps spatial cognition whereas blindness hampers it. However, it should be noted that these tasks were relatively complex and multiple factors play a role other than spatial efficiency. van Dijk et al. (2013a) point out that haptic fluency (handling the shapes by touch) also

(*Continued*)

BOX 4.2 Lessons From the Deaf: How Hearing Loss Affects Spatial Cognition—cont'd

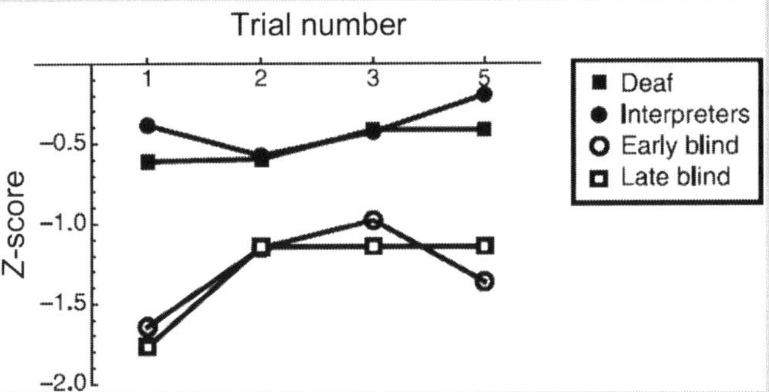

Figure 4.2 *Z*-scores on a haptic task where shapes have to be put in the corresponding slots on a board by touch. Raw scores over the subsequent trials would have shown any spatial learning effect but the *Z*-scores displayed here show the relative difference with respect to matched control groups over the various learning trials. It can be seen that the advantage of the blind and deaf groups is highest in the beginning of the experiment. *From van Dijk, R., Kappers, A. M., & Postma, A. (2013a). Haptic spatial configuration learning in deaf and hearing individuals.* PLoS One, *8(4), e61336, Figure 4.*

plays a role in their task and can speed up performance. Haptic fluency is clearly better trained in blind participants. Interestingly, a simpler test in which participants had to judge either duration or spatial length of a vibration stimulus on the index fingers revealed blind to be better in temporal judgment than the deaf, whereas the latter seemed to be better on the spatial task (but not significantly so; Papagno, Cecchetto, Pisoni, & Bolognini, 2016). Clearly further work on the comparison between blind and deaf individuals in spatial cognition is needed, controlling for task complexity, task familiarity, group matching, and the spatial process under scrutiny.

4.1.3 Audition

The localization of sound in space is very different from how we localize visual and tactile information. Whereas vision and somatosensation code space in a more or less direct way (visual space is coded in a retinotopic fashion, see Chapter 2, whereas somatosensation is coded in relation to different body parts, see Chapter 3), the auditory system needs to infer location in a more indirect manner. Two cues that help us localize sounds

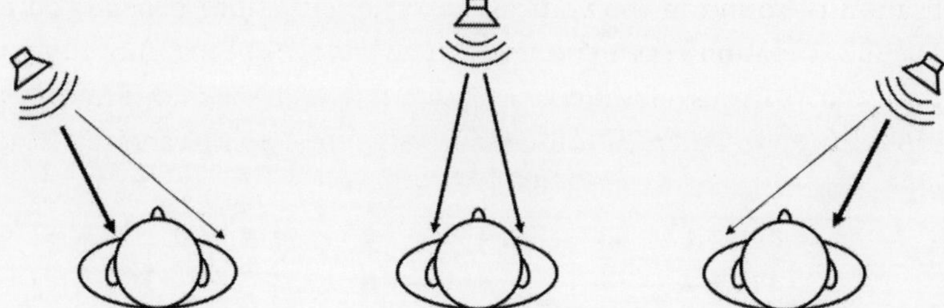

Figure 4.3 (Left) A sound that is presented from the left of the head arrives slightly earlier at the left than the right ear, and its intensity is higher for the left ear than for the right ear. (Center) A sound that is presented from right in front of the body midline arrives at both ears simultaneously at the same intensity. (Right) A sound that is presented from the right of the head arrives earlier to and has a higher intensity at the right relative to the left ear.

in horizontal space are interaural time and sound level differences (ITD and ILD; Middlebrooks & Green, 1991). The way our ears are positioned on our head causes a difference in arrival time of a sound at the left and the right ear depending on the position of a sound source relative to the head. Whenever a sound source is located on the right side of the head, a sound wave first arrives at the right ear, and a few microseconds later to the left ear. In contrast, when a sound source is located to the left of the head, a sound wave first arrives at the left ear, and a few milliseconds later to the right ear. Depending on the position of the sound source on the horizontal meridian, the ITD changes, allowing the brain to calculate the lateral position of a sound source in space (Fig. 4.3). Sounds located on the median plane will arrive at the same time at the left and right ear when no objects are in the way.

Another cue to a sound source's position in lateral space is the interaural level difference (ILD). When a sound is located to the right of the head, the sounds' intensity level will be slightly higher at the right ear as compared to the left ear, and vice versa for sounds located to the left of the head (Fig. 4.3).

Although we are generally less accurate in localizing sounds as compared to visual information, we are well able to do so when a sound contains many different frequencies (Frens, Van Opstal, & Van der Willigen, 1995; Middlebrooks & Green, 1991). When a sound consists of only a single frequency we are still able to tell from which horizontal spatial location the sound originated, but it is much harder to determine its elevation. This is because ITD and ILD cues mainly provide information about the location of a sound source in horizontal space. The localization of sound in the vertical plane (ie, elevation) depends on how the shape of the pinna (ie, the outer ear) affects the spectrum of the sound positioned at various elevations. These monaural spectral cues are also used to distinguish between sound coming from the front and rear space.

The distance of a sound source is estimated based on two types of cues: the intensity of a sound and the direct-to-reverberant ratio of a sound (Bronkhorst & Houtgast, 1999; Middlebrooks & Green, 1991). The intensity of a sound only provides a relative indication of distance when the intensity of a sound source is known. For example, when someone is speaking to you at a regular conversational level (~70 dB(A)) it is possible to determine whether someone is close by or further away from you. When we are in enclosed environments such as rooms, sounds not only are arriving directly at our ears, but also arrive in an indirect way because of sound reflections from the walls. It has been shown that we can estimate the absolute distance of a sound based on the ratio between the amplitude of the direct sound and the delay and amplitude of the reflections (Bronkhorst & Houtgast, 1999; see Kolarik, Moore, Zahorik, Cirstea, & Pardhan, 2015, for a review).

4.1.4 Spatial Reference Frames and Their Transformations

As we already mentioned above, vision, audition, and touch are initially all coded in different reference frames. Visual information is processed in a retinotopic reference frame, auditory information in a head-centered reference frame, and touch is coded in a body(-part) centered reference frame. However, to be able to compare spatial information between the senses, sensory information needs to get together at some point during sensory processing and be coded into a common reference frame (Cohen & Andersen, 2002). For example, head-related auditory spatial information needs to be coded into a retinotopic reference frame to make an eye-movement to a sound. Indeed, spatially aligned auditory and visual spatial maps have been found in the super colliculus, a midbrain structure that is heavily involved in generating eye movements (Stein & Meredith, 1993; also see Chapter 5: Spatial Attention and Eye Movements). The parietal cortex also seems to be involved in reference frame transformations for visual, auditory, and tactile information into eye-centered coordinates (ie, a reference frame that takes the orientation of the eyes in the head into account; Cohen & Andersen, 2002). Spatial information from one sense is transformed into the dominant frame of reference of a specific brain region

(Avillac, Deneve, Olivier, Pouget & Duhamel, 2005). These reference frame transformations also allow for comparison of spatial information from different senses regardless of movements of the eyes, head, and the body.

4.2 MULTISENSORY INTEGRATION

Neurophysiological observations of neurons that responded to the stimulation of more than one sense have played an important role in the formulation of various principles of multisensory integration. We will first discuss the neurophysiological principles of multisensory integration. Next, we will discuss behavioral evidence for multisensory integration in humans and its effect on spatial perception.

4.2.1 Principles Underlying Multisensory Integration

Much of the research on multisensory integration has been inspired by neurophysiological studies of the properties of multisensory neurons in monkeys, cats, and rodents (King & Palmer, 1985; Meredith, Nemitz, & Stein, 1987; Stein & Meredith, 1990, 1993). Typically, these studies report that a certain type of multisensory neurons responds to stimuli presented in different modalities. These neurons can be bimodal (eg, responsive to vision and audition) or trimodal (eg, responsive to vision, audition, and touch). Several rules or principles have emerged from these studies, which describe the circumstances under which these multisensory neurons show the largest activity during multisensory stimulation as compared to unimodal stimulation (ie, stimulation of a single sense).

First, multisensory response integration appears most pronounced when the components of a multisensory stimulus (eg, a sound and a light) are presented from the same spatial location (Kadunce, Vaughan, Wallace, & Stein, 2001; Stein & Meredith, 1990; Stein & Stanford, 2008). The influence of spatial alignment on multisensory integration has typically been studied by varying the stimuli in horizontal space (azimuth). However, at least for visual-tactile neurons, it has been shown that the response of multisensory neurons is modulated by the distance between visual and tactile stimuli in depth (Fogassi et al. 1996; Graziano & Gross, 1994). That is, certain multisensory neurons that responded to touch on the face only responded to visual stimuli that were presented within a limited distance from the face. The spatial region within which visual and tactile stimulation both trigger a response in a multisensory neuron is often referred to as peripersonal space (Fogassi et al., 1996; Graziano & Gross,

1994; Holmes & Spence, 2004; Serino, Canzoneri, & Avenanti, 2011; Van der Stoep et al., 2015; Van der Stoep, Serino, Farnè, Di Luca, & Spence, 2016; see also Chapter 1: A Sense of Space).

A second principle that appears to be important is the temporal proximity of the unisensory component stimuli (Meredith et al., 1987). The closer in time, for example, a sound and light flash are presented, the stronger is the response of multisensory cells. The temporal window within which unisensory stimuli from different senses are still integrated is called *the temporal binding window.* However, not all multisensory neurons follow these principles, as sometimes, multisensory integration can be observed in multisensory neurons, even with quite large spatial and temporal misalignment of the component unimodal stimuli (King & Palmer, 1985).

A third principle is called the principle of inverse effectiveness, which states that the relative increase in the activity of multisensory neurons due to multisensory stimulation is much larger when the unisensory component stimuli only evoke a weak response in the neuron (compare Fig. 4.4A–C, eg, a dim light and a soft sound) as compared to stronger stimuli (eg, a bright light and loud sound; Holmes, 2007, 2009; Meredith & Stein, 1983; Stein & Stanford, 2008). Due to inverse effectiveness weak signals are boosted more due to integration and have a higher probability of being perceived (Frassinetti, Pavani, & Ladavas, 2002, 2005; Lovelace, Stein, & Wallace, 2003). The absolute amount of activity in multisensory neurons will, however, be higher when the unisensory component stimuli produce a strong response in the neuron (see Fig. 4.4A).

4.2.2 Principles of Multisensory Integration in Human Behavior

The three main principles of multisensory integration that have been mentioned above have also been studied in humans. There is substantial support for each principle in human multisensory perception. For example, the principle of temporal alignment comes from studies of temporal order judgment (TOJ) and simultaneity perception (Vroomen & Keetels, 2010). When participants have to indicate which of two sequentially presented stimuli appeared first, the sound or the light signal, they generally cannot tell which came first when the sound and light are presented in close temporal proximity. Thus, stimuli that are presented within a temporal binding window are perceived as simultaneous, which could be taken as evidence of a temporal window of integration. The temporal binding window allows for some asynchrony between stimuli

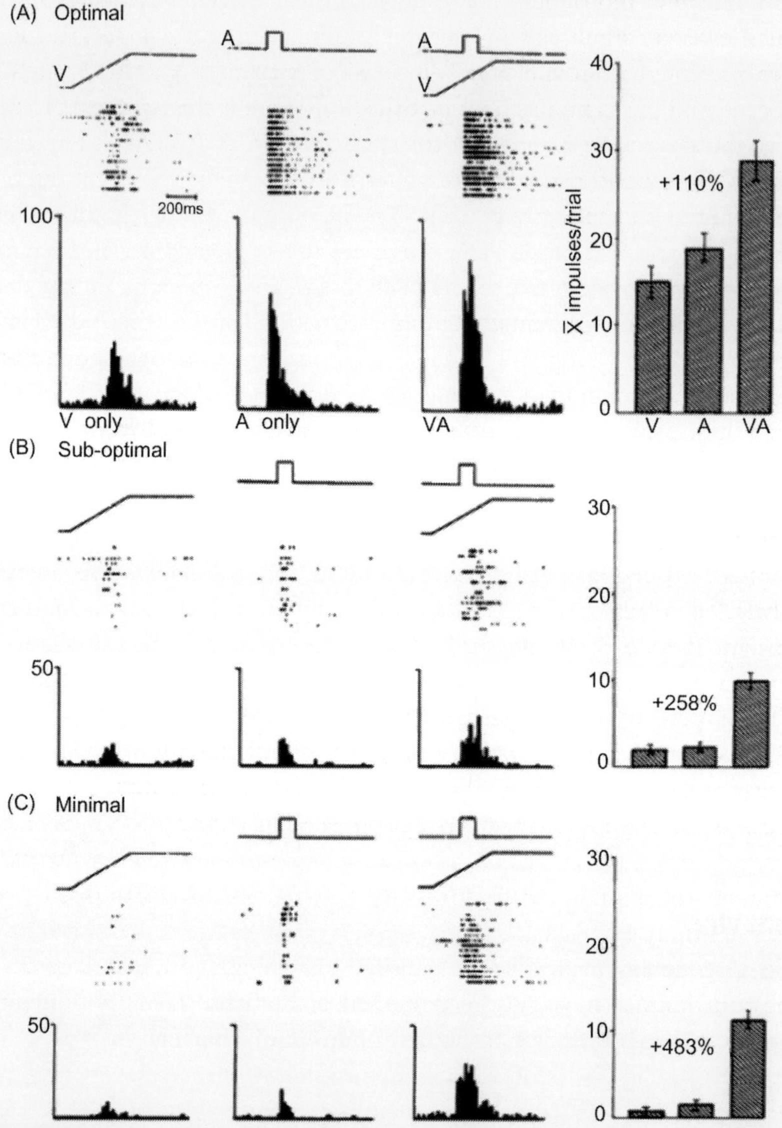

Figure 4.4 The principle of inverse effectiveness: The relative increase in spike rate in a multisensory neuron is greater when the unisensory component stimuli evoke a weak response in the neuron (B and C) as compared to when they evoke a strong response. *(A) From Meredith, M. A., & Stein, B. E. (1983). Interactions among converging sensory inputs in the superior colliculus. Science, 221(4608), 389–391, Figure 8.*

from different modalities. Interestingly, how accurate we are in telling which of two stimuli came first depends on whether the sound and light were presented from the same or a different spatial location (Keetels & Vroomen, 2005). This indicates that the temporal binding window is larger when stimuli are presented from the same rather than different spatial locations. When sound and light are presented from the same spatial location the brain tends to integrate the sound and light, making it more difficult to tell them apart. One could also argue that the brain simply has more information from which to tell apart the sound and light when they not only differ in terms of their temporal onset, but also differ in terms of the spatial location. Additional support for the principles of spatial and temporal alignment comes from studies of multisensory response enhancement (MRE). When participants have to respond as quickly as possible to the onset of a sound, a light, or their combination, response times (RTs) are generally much faster in the combined condition relative to the unisensory condition (Colonius & Diederich, 2004; Gondan & Minakata, 2015; Miller, 1982, 1986; Stevenson, Fister, Barnett, Nidiffer & Wallace, 2012). The amount of MRE depends on the spatial and temporal alignment of the sound and the light (Leone & McCourt, 2013; Van der Stoep, Spence, Nijboer, & Van der Stigchel, 2015). The closer in time and space the sound and the light are presented, the larger the facilitation.

Although the results mentioned above, as well as many other findings in humans, are in line with the principles of spatial and temporal alignment, there are also various circumstances in which human behavior diverges from these principles. For example, the importance of the spatial alignment of stimuli for multisensory integration has most often been observed in tasks in which space was somehow task-relevant, but not in tasks in which space was task-irrelevant (see Spence, 2013, for a review). The principles of multisensory integration thus seem to be more flexible in human behavior and can sometimes be task-dependent.

4.2.3 Multisensory Spatial Conflict

In certain circumstances the brain can receive conflicting spatial information from different senses. A typical example is when external loudspeakers of a television set are placed at a large distance from the screen. How does the brain deal with this conflicting information? Although vision is generally dominant in the spatial domain, audition seems to be more accurate in the temporal domain (Chen & Vroomen, 2013; Welch, DuttonHurt & Warren, 1986). The "modality appropriateness hypothesis" states that a

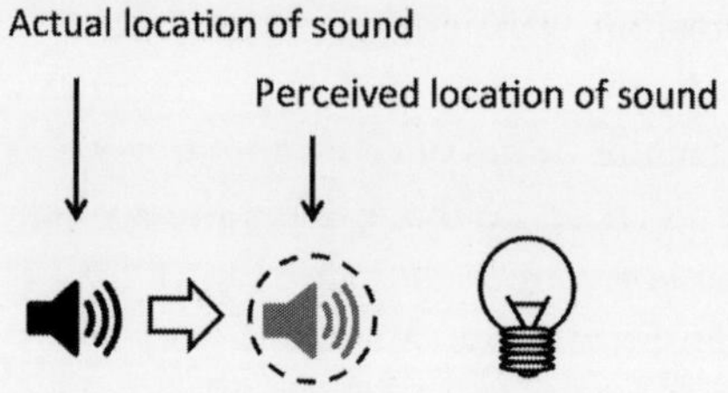

Figure 4.5 In the spatial ventriloquist effect, the perceived location of a sound source is shifted toward a visual source.

sense can dominate perception when it is best suited for a certain task (Spence & Squire, 2003; Welch & Warren, 1980). As a result, visual information can attract the perceived location of a sound that is presented at a slightly different location. This is called the spatial ventriloquist effect (Fig. 4.5). In the case of your television set, you localize sounds next to the screen to a location on the television screen.

In 2002, Marc Ernst and Martin Banks proposed a general principle that determines the degree with which each sense dominates perception. They showed that the contribution of each sense to perception depends on the reliability of sensory information (Alais & Burr, 2004; Battaglia, Jacobs, & Aslin, 2003; Ernst & Banks, 2002). For example, when visual information is more reliable than auditory information, vision mainly determines the perceived spatial location when sound and light are presented at slightly different spatial locations. In contrast, when auditory information is more reliable than visual spatial information, sound mainly determines the perceived spatial location. These findings can be explained by a simple model of optimal combination of visual and auditory spatial information in which the brain weighs auditory and visual information based on the reliability of sensory input. This has also been shown to occur in the depth dimension. When sound and light are presented from slightly different distances from the observer but from the same direction, the location of sounds in depth is perceived at a distance that is closer to the depth at which visual information was presented (Agganis, Muday, & Schirillo, 2010; Bowen, Ramachandran, Muday, & Schirillo, 2011).

4.3 CROSSMODAL EXOGENOUS SPATIAL ATTENTION

The previous section was concerned with how the integration of information from different senses into a unified whole affected spatial perception. However, information from one sense can also affect the perceptual processing of information from a different sense through crossmodal shifts of exogenous spatial attention (McDonald & Ward, 2000; Spence & Driver, 2004; see Chapter 5 for more information on the effects and different types of attention). For example, a sound (ie, an exogenous auditory cue) can attract attention to its spatial location and facilitate the processing of visual information that is presented a moment later at the same spatial location. Visual information that is presented at a different spatial location than that of the cue is not facilitated, demonstrating the spatial nature of the effects of crossmodal exogenous spatial attention.

By now, the benefits of crossmodal exogenous spatial attention shifts have been demonstrated between all combinations of auditory, visual, and tactile stimuli (Spence & McDonald, 2004). Whereas multisensory integration is typically most pronounced when stimuli from different modalities are presented within close temporal proximity, the beneficial effects of crossmodal shifts of exogenous spatial attention are often most pronounced when there is some time between the stimuli (eg, a ~200 ms stimulus onset asynchrony (SOA) between sound and light). Several researchers have suggested that the effects of crossmodal exogenous spatial attention and multisensory integration can be distinguished based on the time course of the facilitation effects of the two processes (McDonald, Teder-Sälejärvi, & Ward, 2001; Van der Stoep et al., 2015). It has been shown that at short SOAs (<50 ms), crossmodal facilitation is mainly the result of multisensory integration, whereas at intermediate SOAs (~50 ms) both crossmodal exogenous spatial attention and multisensory integration contribute to improvements in perception, and at longer SOAs (>100 ms) crossmodal exogenous spatial attention seems to be the main cause of perceptual benefits (Van der Stoep et al., 2015).

Given the benefits of multisensory integration, researchers wondered whether integrated (multisensory) cues are more effective in attracting spatial attention. This was investigated by comparing the effects of multisensory (audiovisual, audiotactile) and unisensory (auditory, visual, or tactile) exogenous spatial cues (Santangelo, Van der Lubbe, Belardinelli, & Postma, 2006, 2008). At first the effects of multisensory and unisensory cues did not seem to be very different in terms of the benefits of exogenous spatial attention. However, when participants were engaged in a secondary task (ie, doing multiple things at the same time; when the cognitive load was high), multisensory but not unisensory cues could still attract the participants' spatial attention (Santangelo & Spence, 2007; Santangelo, Ho, & Spence, 2008; see Spence & Santangelo, 2009, for a review). These results indicate a close relationship between multisensory integration and crossmodal exogenous spatial attention.

4.4 MULTISENSORY REGIONS OF SPACE

Although the field of multisensory research has grown rapidly over the last decades, most of the research has focused on multisensory interactions at a fixed distance from the body. Recently, however, researchers started to recognize the importance of the influence of variations in distance on multisensory integration. The brain seems to process information from various regions of space differently (see Fig. 4.6 for the different regions of space; see also Chapter 1: A Sense of Space). The different regions of space can be defined by: (1) the distance at which multisensory interactions between different sensory modalities take place (Occelli, Spence, & Zampini, 2011; Van der Stoep, Nijboer, Van der Stigchel, & Spence, 2015); (2) the behavioral functions that are associated with different regions of space (Previc, 1998; Van der Stoep et al., 2016); and (3) distance-specific impairments in spatial perception (Aimola, Schindler, Simone & Venneri, 2012; Halligan & Marshall, 1991; Van der Stoep et al., 2013).

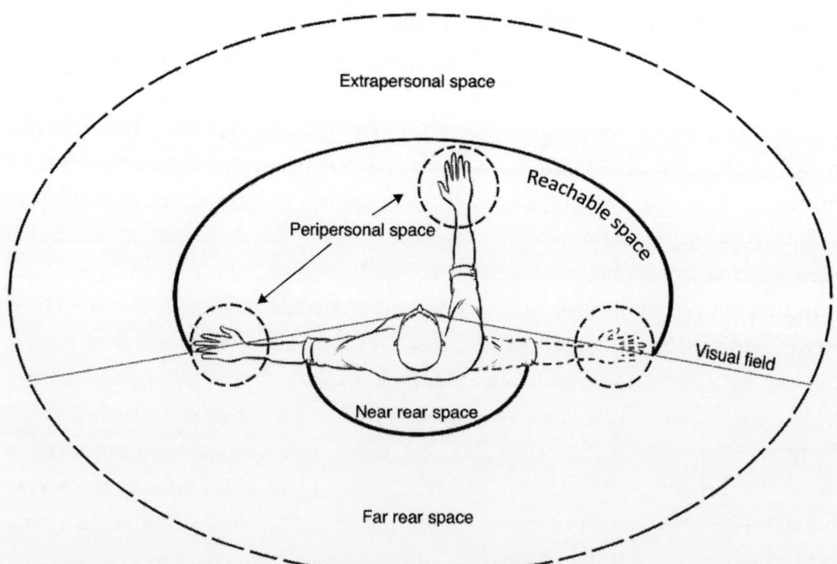

Figure 4.6 A schematic bird's-eye view of the different regions of multisensory space. *From Van der Stoep, N., Serino, A., Farnè, A., Di Luca, M., & Spence, C. (2016). Depth: The forgotten dimension in multisensory research.* Multisensory Research, *Figure 1.*

4.4.1 Peripersonal Space

About 20 years ago, neurophysiologists observed neurons in the premotor cortex of the macaque monkey that respond to both visual and tactile stimulation (Fogassi et al., 1996; Graziano & Gross, 1994; Graziano, Hu, & Gross, 1997). For example, a neuron could respond to tactile stimulation of the hand and visual stimulation near or on the hand. Importantly, some of these multisensory neurons did not respond to visual stimuli that were presented further away from the hand. The spatial region around the hand within which visual and tactile stimuli evoke a response in multisensory neurons is now commonly termed peripersonal (hand) space. Similar multisensory spatial regions have been observed around the face, shoulders, trunk, and the back of the head (Fogassi et al., 1996; Graziano et al., 1997; Graziano, Reiss, & Gross, 1999; see Graziano & Cooke, 2006, for a review).

There is increasing support for the idea that a peripersonal space around different body parts exists also in humans (see Makin, Holmes, & Ehrsson, 2008; Occelli et al., 2011; Van der Stoep et al., 2015; Van der Stoep et al., 2016, for reviews). For example, sounds that are close to, rather than far away from, the hand make responses to touch on the hand faster (Canzoneri, Magosso & Serino, 2012; Canzoneri, Ubaldi et al., 2013; Canzoneri, Marzolla, Amoresano, Verni & Serino, 2013). Multisensory interactions in human peripersonal hand space seem to crucially depend on ventral premotor and posterior parietal areas (Serino et al., 2011).

The peripersonal space seems to be flexible in that its size can change depending on the circumstances (Fig. 4.7). For example, tool-use allows interactions between the body and information in extrapersonal space. This novel distance at which interactions with the body can take place seems to trigger a change in the size of peripersonal space to now also incorporate the region of space that was coded as extrapersonal space before tool-use (Berti & Frassinetti, 2000; Farnè, Bonifazi, & Ládavas, 2005; Holmes & Spence, 2004; Van der Stoep et al., 2016). Action preparation (Brozzoli, Ehrsson, & Farnè, 2014), moving through the environment (Galli, Noel, Canzoneri, Blanke, & Serino, 2015; Noel et al., 2015), social interactions (Teneggi, Canzoneri, Di Pellegrino, & Serino, 2013), and anxiety (Lourenco, Longo, & Pathman, 2011; Sambo & Iannetti, 2013; Taffou & Viaud-Delmon, 2014) all seem to be able to change the size or the extent of peripersonal space.

The brain thus seems to flexibly update the space around different body parts within which visual or auditory information can interact with touch on the body. This flexible updating makes sense in that it not only

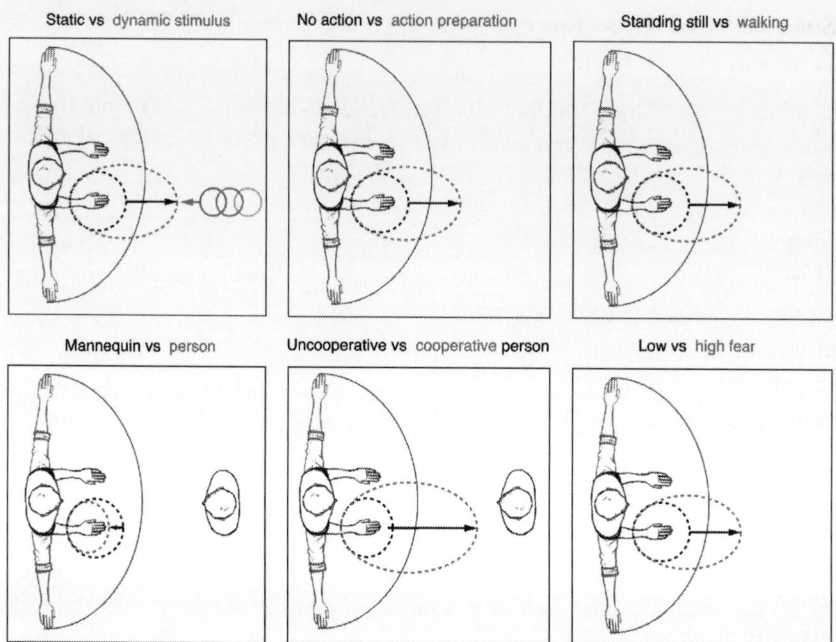

Figure 4.7 A bird's-eye view of how the extent of peripersonal space can change depending on the circumstances. The solid black line represents the reachable space, the dashed black and red circles represent peripersonal hand space in different situations. *Taken from Van der Stoep, N., Serino, A., Farnè, A., Di Luca, M., & Spence, C. (2016). Depth: The forgotten dimension in multisensory research.* Multisensory Research, *Figure 3.*

allows efficiently responding to and predicting of possible interactions with the environment, but also allows defending the body against potentially harmful interactions with the world.

4.4.2 Extrapersonal Space

Whereas it has become quite clear that multisensory interactions involving touch and vision/audition shape the peripersonal space around different body parts, much less is known about how audiovisual interactions progress in extrapersonal space. Recently, it has been shown that audiovisual interactions are modulated by the distance from which information is presented in extrapersonal space. For example, it was shown that the principle of inverse effectiveness is especially pronounced when decreases in stimulus intensity co-occur with increases in the distance between the stimuli and the observer (Van der Stoep, Van der

Stigchel, Nijboer, & Van der Smagt, 2015). In everyday life, when we view an object from a large distance the retinal image is smaller relative to when we view the object from a smaller distance. Similarly, sounds that we perceive from a closer distance arrive with a higher intensity at our ears than sounds that we perceive from afar. In the study by Van der Stoep, Van der Stigchel, Nijboer, & Van der Smagt, (2015), audiovisual integration was more enhanced when audiovisual stimuli were presented at ~2 m as compared to when the exact same stimuli were presented at 80 cm. This could not be explained solely by the principle of inverse effectiveness because presenting stimuli in near space with the same retinal size and auditory/visual intensity did not boost audiovisual integration. Interestingly, a situation in which stimulus size and intensity decrease with distance is quite common in everyday life. Yet, it is not entirely clear as to why audiovisual integration increases in far space. The authors proposed that spatial localization might generally be less reliable in far space, and that the brain therefore benefits more from integrating spatial information from vision and audition in far as compared to near space.

Further support for the idea that the distance from which information is presented in extrapersonal space modulates audiovisual interactions comes from a study of crossmodal exogenous spatial attention (Van der Stoep, Nijboer, & Van der Stigchel, 2014). If sounds can attract spatial attention to a specific location in depth it should only enhance visual information that is presented at that specific location in depth, but not at different distance. This was indeed observed. Sounds that were presented far away facilitated the processing of visual information that was presented at the same depth, but not at a closer distance and vice versa. These results indicate that the distance from which information is presented is taken into account in crossmodal interactions.

4.4.3 Front Versus Rear Space

A region of space that has not been discussed yet is the space behind the body. Audition and touch are dominant in rear space given the lack of visual input. Several studies have shown that sounds that are presented close to the back of the head interact strongly with tactile stimulation of the head. When sounds are presented at a larger distance from the head, the interaction between auditory and tactile information is not as strong (Farnè & Làdavas, 2002). The region of space around the head within which auditory and tactile information interacts is called the near rear space or rear peripersonal head space. Others have shown that sounds that are presented from behind the body are slightly more effective in attracting a driver's attention to rear space (the rear viewing mirror) than sounds that are presented from front space and vice versa (Ho & Spence, 2005). However, this does not mean that auditory information from rear space cannot affect visual information processing in front space. When participants only had to respond to visual information in front space, auditory cues that were presented in rear space were as effective as the same cues that were presented from front space (Lee & Spence, 2015).

4.5 IMPAIRMENTS IN MULTISENSORY INTEGRATION

As described above, the brain has a large capacity for automatic simultaneous processing and integration of sensory information. Combining information from different sensory modalities can facilitate primary as well as higher order cortical operations such as detection, discrimination, and recognition of sensory stimuli (Ghazanfar & Schroeder, 2006). Multisensory integration helps to create a stable and organized percept of the world and allows for efficient perception of and interaction with the environment. Given the benefits of multisensory integration, an impaired ability to integrate information from different senses may have quite severe consequences for perception and cognitive abilities at large (eg, attention, memory; see Dionne-Dostie, Paquette, Lassonde, & Gallagher, 2015, for a review). For example, recent studies indicate that multisensory integration is impaired in individuals with autism spectrum disorder beyond what would be expected based on already present changes in unisensory processing (Baum, Stevenson, & Wallace, 2015). Difficulties with integrating sensory information may increase distractibility and a general feeling of being quickly overwhelmed by stimuli from the environment. In contrast, multisensory conditions rather than being a problem might also work as a tool to enhance unisensory perception and attention (see Tinga et al., 2015, for a review). Below, we will focus on how multisensory stimulation may or may not improve perception in *sensory* and *attention* disorders such as hemianopia, neglect, and extinction (Heilman, Watson, & Valenstein, 1993).

Losing or being born without one of our senses impairs integrating sensory information from that sense and other, intact, senses because there is no sensory input from the absent sense. For example, in the blind and the deaf, there is no visual or auditory input, respectively. Interestingly, in these situations the brain can recruit brain regions that are traditionally considered visual or auditory in nature to improve processing of the intact senses (see Boxes 4.1 and 4.2 for more on this topic). However, there are also cases in which vision and/or audition is impaired, but not fully lost. In such cases there may be some residual sensory information processing from the impaired sense, which may still allow the integration of information from the impaired and intact senses. First, we will discuss multisensory processing in a condition that is called hemianopia, or cortical blindness. Next, we will discuss multisensory integration in a condition that is called neglect in which attentional processing is affected. Patients with neglect are typically unaware of visual information in a certain region of space while visual pathways are typically unaffected.

4.5.1 Hemianopia

As a result of lesions in the early visual pathways, patients may fail to adequately respond or report contralesional visual stimuli. This condition is known as hemianopia. Hemianopia has a strong negative impact on several functions and/or activities of daily living, such as reading, scanning a scene or the environment, obstacle avoidance, crossing streets. A few studies have looked into the direct, short-term, as well as longer lasting effects of multisensory stimulation on the performance of patients with subacute and chronic hemianopia. For example, Frassinetti et al. (2005) and Leo et al. (2008) demonstrated that the simultaneous presentation of a sound and light could enhance the detection of a visual target in the blind field of hemianopia patients. In a very recent study, however, no influence of visual stimuli on aurally guided saccades (ie, eye movements to sounds) was observed in patients with hemianopia (Ten Brink, Nijboer, Bergsma, Barton & Van der Stigchel, 2015). In this study, eight patients with hemianopia had to make eye movements to an auditory target that was either presented in isolation (unisensory condition) or accompanied by a visual stimulus (multisensory condition). The visual stimulus could be presented either at the same or at a different location as the auditory target. Saccade landing points were compared between conditions for each patient. In seven of the eight patients with hemianopia saccade accuracy to the auditory target was influenced by the visual stimulus in the intact field, but not in the blind field. Only one patient, a patient with quadrantanopia, showed a facilitation effect in the blind quadrant.

Apart from these direct and short-term improvements, longer lasting effects have also been studied. For example, Bolognini, Rasi, and Làdavas (2005) investigated whether auditory localization could be improved using multisensory stimulation in patients with hemianopia. In multisensory trials the sound and light were presented either spatially congruent (ie, same spatial location) or spatially incongruent (ie, different spatial location). Auditory localization improved at all four tested locations (7.5 and 20 degrees in both hemifields). Importantly, the improvement was dependent on the spatial congruency of sound and light signals. These findings are in line with the principle of spatial alignment. Effects were restricted to the contralesional (impaired) visual field.

Bolognini, Rasi, Coccia, and Làdavas (2005) trained patients with hemianopia with audiovisual stimulation, in daily sessions of about 4 h for nearly 2 weeks. During these training sessions, patients had to shift their gaze toward the visual stimulus in the blind hemifield. This visual stimulus was either presented in isolation or accompanied by an auditory stimulus. Patients improved in visual detection, visual exploration, and in different tasks of daily life. Importantly, these improvements were still visible 1 month after the training. Since patients were instructed to make eye movements, multisensory stimulation might have enhanced the responsiveness of the oculomotor system, reinforcing orientation toward the blind hemifield and oculomotor visual exploration, resulting in improved visual detection. This study, however, did not look at the effects of the unimodal versus multisensory conditions. Similar improvement might be obtained by only using unimodal (visual) stimulation, given that each training session contained both unisensory and multisensory stimulation. To investigate the potential benefits of multisensory stimulation over unisensory stimulation, Passamonti et al. (2009) incorporated a unisensory visual control training and compared this to the effects of an audiovisual training. The results indicated that only audiovisual training improved visual detection and exploration, oculomotor scanning and on activities of daily life. These effects remained stable at a 3-month follow-up and a 1-year follow-up. Patients' oculomotor scanning was more similar to the healthy control subjects after audiovisual training, whereas the group of patients receiving the control (visual only) training showed no significant change. These findings indicate a long-term persistence of audiovisual treatment effects on the oculomotor system, which might encourage a more organized pattern of visual exploration.

In a similar study by Keller and Lefin-Rank (2010) the effects of audiovisual stimulation in patients in the subacute phase after brain damage was studied. Either an audiovisual training or a visual training was given to patients with hemianopia. Patients were instructed to detect visual targets as fast as possible. The audiovisual training resulted in a larger improvement in visual exploration compared to the visual training. Additionally, only patients that received audiovisual training showed near normal daily living activities after training.

Interestingly, proprioceptive stimulation may also help to improve visual detection (Schendel & Robertson, 2004) or target size processing (Brown, Kroliczak, Demonet, & Goodale, 2008). Schendel and Robertson showed that visual detection in the blind field of a single patient improved when the contralesional arm was extended into the blind field, but only when the hand was placed near the visual targets, not when the hand was placed further away. These results could not be replicated, however, in a very similar study by Smith et al. (2008), in which five patients were tested. As for object size estimations, it was shown that performance was significantly improved when the patients' contralesional hand was placed near the objects (Brown et al., 2008). Although some of these results look promising, it should be noted that only very small samples of patients were included in these studies and variation in effect or effect sizes appears to be large.

Although the results of the above mentioned studies look promising with respect to the benefits of multisensory stimulation or training, it is still unclear which patients will benefit from this. Given that some patients have shown no improvements during multisensory stimulation (Ten Brink et al., 2015), isolating the factors that determine whether a patient will benefit from such a multisensory training may help improve and individualize treatment.

4.5.2 Neglect

Neglect is a common disorder that affects approximately 50% of stroke patients in (sub)acute stage after stroke, in which patients are impaired in detecting stimuli or orienting attention toward the contralesional side of space (Bisiach & Luzzatti, 1978; Halligan, Fink, Marshall, & Vallar, 2003; Heilman & Valenstein, 1979; Heilman et al., 1993; Nijboer, Kollen, &

Kwakkel, 2013). Neglect is an important negative prognostic factor for (motor) recovery (Cherney, Halper, Kwasnica, Harvey, & Zhang, 2001; Nijboer, Kollen, & Kwakkel, 2014) and independence in activities of daily living (Nijboer, Van de Port, Schepers, Post, & Visser-Meily, 2013). The current theory is that neglect is better explained by dysfunction of distributed cortical attention networks than by structural damage to specific brain areas (Corbetta & Shulman, 2011; Karnath & Rorden, 2012; Urbanski et al, 2011; see also Chapter 5). The aim of many treatments for neglect is to reduce the imbalance between the two hemispheres. Multisensory stimulation could be such a treatment.

Frassinetti et al. (2005) showed that the combination of visual and auditory stimulation could improve visual detection accuracy in neglect. Seven patients with neglect took place in a setup where four visual stimuli could be presented on the left, and four on the right with respect to body midline of the patients. At the exact same locations as the visual stimuli, auditory stimuli could be presented. Patients were asked to detect the location of the visual stimuli. On average only approximately 18% of the visual stimuli were detected, a percentage that increased to approximately 49% when an auditory stimulus was presented at the same time, at the exact same location. When the auditory stimulus was presented at the same time, but from a different location as the visual stimulus, detection accuracy was approximately 35%. In an earlier study, Frassinetti et al. (2002) showed that the detection accuracy heavily relied on the spatial distance between visual and auditory stimuli. With a comparable setup, seven patients with neglect were asked to indicate the location of a visual stimulus and the accuracy was best when the visual and auditory stimuli were located at the exact same position. When the auditory stimulus was presented from the location directly adjacent to the location of the visual stimulus, performance decreased but was still significantly better compared to no auditory stimulus. With increasing distance from the location of the visual stimuli, the beneficial effect of the auditory stimulus diminished.

Sambo et al. (2011) investigated whether the combination of visual and tactile stimuli could enhance processing of tactile stimuli in patients with visual neglect and tactile extinction. Extinction is related to neglect, but not the same. Patients with extinction will detect stimuli on the left and on the right side, but will ignore stimuli on one side when the left and the right side are presented simultaneously. Extinction can occur in different sensory modalities: visual, auditory, and tactile extinction frequently occur after stroke. In the study by Sambo et al. (2011), patients fixated on a fixation cross and had to indicate as quickly and accurately as possible when they detected a tactile stimulus. Detection of a tactile stimulus to the left hand was significantly faster when the left hand was placed in the right (ie, intact) visual field compared to the left (ie, neglect) visual field.

Visuo-somatosensory combinations have also been studied in a patient with visual extinction (Di Pellegrino and Frassinetti, 2000). When patients with visual extinction had to report digits on a monitor they reported the digit on the right almost every trial, whereas the stimulus on the left was often ignored. Only when the patient was allowed to place their own hands near the visual stimuli did performance increase significantly. No changes in performance were found when the hands were further away from the stimuli, or when images of hands were presented near the stimuli.

4.6 CONCLUSION

Space is a feature of the world that is shared by our senses: we can see, hear, and feel where things are. Moreover, though not well developed in all humans (and ignored in this book), we also have a coarse sense of smell for direction. In this chapter we started with a brief discussion of how the senses code space. More importantly we have paid attention to the question of how they work together in multisensory integration and crossmodal interactions. We wish to emphasize here that in clinical patient work a very promising approach lies in applying multisensory interventions. Patients with sensory impairments (deaf, blind; see Boxes 4.1 and 4.2) could particularly benefit from applying combinations of stimuli from the remaining senses (see also the use of sensory substitution devices; Maidenbaum et al., 2014; Proulx et al., 2014). Similarly treatment of neurological disorders might entertain multisensory stimulation techniques. Several patient studies have already indicated that multisensory stimulation can enhance performance on several different tasks (eg, detection, localization, search, exploration, some activities of daily living) in which a response is required to sensory stimuli.[1]

[1] It should be kept in mind, though, that the studies described here used very small groups of patients and none of the studies were proper randomized controlled trials (RCTs). In this design, usually larger groups of patients are randomly assigned to either the experimental condition or a control or placebo condition. In this case, a placebo condition could be care as usual, where the optimal design would incorporate two experimental conditions: one in which only unisensory stimulation would take place and one in which multisensory stimulation would be given.

Impairments due to stroke may be reduced during multisensory stimulation because multisensory brain regions still function and enhance perceptual processing. In the case of hemianopia, when a patient's visual cortex has been affected by stroke, there may still be some subcortical processing of visual information. In subcortical multisensory brain regions, such as the superior colliculus, multisensory integration can still enhance the analysis of visual input and improve spatial orienting. Given that multiple brain regions are involved in multisensory integration, damage to one unisensory or multisensory brain area may not necessarily lead to an overall impairment in multisensory integration or perception in general. This makes multisensory stimulation a highly interesting candidate for diagnostics and rehabilitation of motor, sensory, or attention deficits (ie, neglect) after stroke.

REFERENCES

Agganis, B. T., Muday, J. A., & Schirillo, J. A. (2010). Visual biasing of auditory localization in azimuth and depth. *Perceptual and Motor Skills*, *111*(3), 872–892.

Aimola, L., Schindler, I., Simone, A. M., & Venneri, A. (2012). Near and far space neglect: Task sensitivity and anatomical substrates. *Neuropsychologia*, *50*(6), 1115–1123.

Alais, D., & Burr, D. (2004). The ventriloquist effect results from near-optimal bimodal integration. *Current Biology*, *14*(3), 257–262.

Avillac, M., Deneve, S., Olivier, E., Pouget, A., & Duhamel, J. R. (2005). Reference frames for representing visual and tactile locations in parietal cortex. *Nature Neuroscience*, *8*(7), 941–949.

Battaglia, P. W., Jacobs, R. A., & Aslin, R. N. (2003). Bayesian integration of visual and auditory signals for spatial localization. *Journal of the Optical Society of America A*, *20*(7), 1391–1397.

Baum, S. H., Stevenson, R. A., & Wallace, M. T. (2015). Behavioral, perceptual, and neural alterations in sensory and multisensory function in autism spectrum disorder. *Progress in Neurobiology*, *134*, 140–160.

Bavelier, D., Dye, M. W., & Hauser, P. C. (2006). Do deaf individuals see better? *Trends in Cognitive Sciences*, *10*(11), 512–518. wdoi:S1364-6613(06)00243-9.

Bavelier, D., Tomann, A., Hutton, C., Mitchell, T., Corina, D., Liu, G., & Neville, H. (2000). Visual attention to the periphery is enhanced in congenitally deaf individuals. *Journal of Neuroscience*, *20*(17), RC93.

Berg, J., & Worchel, P. (1956). Sensory contributions to human maze-learning—A comparison of matched blind, deaf, and normals. *Journal of General Psychology*, *54*(1), 81–93.

Berti, A., & Frassinetti, F. (2000). When far becomes near: Remapping of space by tool use. *Journal of Cognitive Neuroscience*, *12*(3), 415–420.

Bisiach, E., & Luzzatti, C. (1978). Unilateral neglect of representational space. *Cortex*, *14* (1), 129–133.

Bolognini, N., Rasi, F., Coccia, M., & Làdavas, E. (2005). Visual search improvement in hemianopic patients after audio-visual stimulation. *Brain*, *128*(12), 2830–2842.

Bolognini, N., Rasi, F., & Làdavas, E. (2005). Visual localization of sounds. *Neuropsychologia, 43*(11), 1655–1661.

Bosworth, R. G., Petrich, J. A., & Dobkins, K. R. (2013). Effects of attention and laterality on motion and orientation discrimination in deaf signers. *Brain and Cognition, 82*(1), 117–126. Available from http://dx.doi.org/10.1016/j.bandc.2013.01.006.

Bowen, A. L., Ramachandran, R., Muday, J. A., & Schirillo, J. A. (2011). Visual signals bias auditory targets in azimuth and depth. *Experimental Brain Research, 214*(3), 403–414.

Bronkhorst, A. W., & Houtgast, T. (1999). Auditory distance perception in rooms. *Nature, 397*(6719), 517–520.

Brown, L. E., Kroliczak, G., Demonet, J. F., & Goodale, M. A. (2008). A hand in blindsight: Hand placement near target improves size perception in the blind visual field. *Neuropsychologia, 46*(3), 786–802.

Brozzoli, C., Ehrsson, H. H., & Farnè, A. (2014). Multisensory representation of the space near the hand from perception to action and interindividual interactions. *The Neuroscientist, 20*, 122–135.

Canzoneri, E., Magosso, E., & Serino, A. (2012). Dynamic sounds capture the boundaries of peripersonal space representation in humans. *PLoS One, 7*, e44306. Available from http://dx.doi.org/10.1371/journal.pone.0044306.

Canzoneri, E., Marzolla, M., Amoresano, A., Verni, G., & Serino, A. (2013). Amputation and prosthesis implantation shape body and peripersonal space representations. *Scientific Reports, 3*, 2844. Available from http://dx.doi.org/10.1038/srep02844.

Canzoneri, E., Ubaldi, S., Rastelli, V., Finisguerra, A., Bassolino, M., & Serino, A. (2013). Tool-use reshapes the boundaries of body and peripersonal space representations. *Experimental Brain Research, 228*, 25–42.

Cattaneo, Z., Lega, C., Cecchetto, C., & Papagno, C. (2014). Auditory deprivation affects biases of visuospatial attention as measured by line bisection. *Experimental Brain Research, 232*(9), 2767–2773. Available from http://dx.doi.org/10.1007/s00221-014-3960-7.

Cattaneo, Z., & Vecchi, T. (2011). *Blind vision: The neuroscience of visual impairment*. Cambridge, MA, London: MIT Press.

Cattaneo, Z., Vecchi, T., Cornoldi, C., Mammarella, I., Bonino, D., Ricciardi, E., & Pietrini, P. (2008). Imagery and spatial processes in blindness and visual impairment. *Neuroscience & Biobehavioral Reviews, 32*(8), 1346–1360. Available from http://dx.doi.org/10.1016/j.neubiorev.2008.05.002.

Cattani, A., & Clibbens, J. (2005). Atypical lateralization of memory for location: Effects of deafness and sign language use. *Brain and Cognition, 58*(2), 226–239. Available from http://dx.doi.org/10.1016/j.bandc.2004.12.001.

Chen, L., & Vroomen, J. (2013). Intersensory binding across space and time: A tutorial review. *Attention, Perception, & Psychophysics, 75*(5), 790–811.

Cherney, L. R., Halper, A. S., Kwasnica, C. M., Harvey, R. L., & Zhang, M. (2001). Recovery of functional status after right hemisphere stroke: Relationship with unilateral neglect. *Archives of Physical Medicine and Rehabilitation, 82*(3), 322–328.

Cohen, Y. E., & Andersen, R. A. (2002). A common reference frame for movement plans in the posterior parietal cortex. *Nature Reviews Neuroscience, 3*(7), 553–562.

Colonius, H., & Diederich, A. (2004). Multisensory interaction in saccadic reaction time: a time-window-of-integration model. *Journal of Cognitive Neuroscience, 16*(6), 1000–1009.

Corbetta, M., & Shulman, G. L. (2011). Spatial neglect and attention networks. *Annual Review of Neuroscience, 34*, 569.

di Pellegrino, G., & Frassinetti, F. (2000). Direct evidence from parietal extinction of enhancement of visual attention near a visible hand. *Current Biology, 10*(22), 1475–1477.

Dionne-Dostie, E., Paquette, N., Lassonde, M., & Gallagher, A. (2015). Multisensory integration and child neurodevelopment. *Brain Sciences*, *5*(1), 32–57.

Emmorey, K., Grabowski, T., McCullough, S., Ponto, L. L., Hichwa, R. D., & Damasio, H. (2005). The neural correlates of spatial language in English and American Sign Language: A PET study with hearing bilinguals. *Neuroimage*, *24*(3), 832–840. Available from http://dx.doi.org/10.1016/j.neuroimage.2004.10.008.

Emmorey, K., & Kosslyn, S. M. (1996). Enhanced image generation abilities in deaf signers: A right hemisphere effect. *Brain and Cognition*, *32*(1), 28–44. doi:S0278-2626(96)90056-1.

Emmorey, K., Kosslyn, S. M., & Bellugi, U. (1993). Visual imagery and visual–spatial language: Enhanced imagery abilities in deaf and hearing ASL signers. *Cognition*, *46*(2), 139–181. doi:0010-0277(93)90017-P.

Ernst, M. O., & Banks, M. S. (2002). Humans integrate visual and haptic information in a statistically optimal fashion. *Nature*, *415*(6870), 429–433.

Farnè, A., Bonifazi, S., & Làdavas, E. (2005). The role played by tool-use and tool-length on the plastic elongation of peri-hand space: A single case study. *Cognitive Neuropsychology*, *22*(3–4), 408–418.

Farnè, A., & Làdavas, E. (2002). Auditory peripersonal space in humans. *Journal of Cognitive Neuroscience*, *14*(7), 1030–1043.

Finney, E. M., & Dobkins, K. R. (2001). Visual contrast sensitivity in deaf versus hearing populations: exploring the perceptual consequences of auditory deprivation and experience with a visual language. *Cognitive Brain Research*, *11*(1), 171–183.

Fogassi, L., Gallese, V., Fadiga, L., Luppino, G., Matelli, M., & Rizzolatti, G. (1996). Coding of peripersonal space in inferior premotor cortex (area F4). *Journal of Neurophysiology*, *76*(1), 141–157.

Frassinetti, F., Bolognini, N., Bottari, D., Bonora, A., & Làdavas, E. (2005). Audiovisual integration in patients with visual deficit. *Journal of Cognitive Neuroscience*, *17*(9), 1442–1452.

Frassinetti, F., Pavani, F., & Ladavas, E. (2002). Acoustical vision of neglected stimuli: Interaction among spatially converging audiovisual inputs in neglect patients. *Journal of Cognitive Neuroscience*, *14*(1), 62–69.

Frens, M. A., Van Opstal, A. J., & Van der Willigen, R. F. (1995). Spatial and temporal factors determine auditory–visual interactions in human saccadic eye movements. *Perception & Psychophysics*, *57*(6), 802–816.

Galli, G., Noel, J. P., Canzoneri, E., Blanke, O., & Serino, A. (2015). The wheelchair as a full-body tool extending the peripersonal space. *Frontiers in Psychology*, *6*, 639.

Ghazanfar, A. A., & Schroeder, C. E. (2006). Is neocortex essentially multisensory? *Trends in Cognitive Sciences*, *10*(6), 278–285.

Gilbert, C., & Foster, A. (2001). Childhood blindness in the context of VISION 2020—the right to sight. *Bulletin World Health Organ*, *79*(3), 227–232.

Gondan, M., & Minakata, K. (2015). A tutorial on testing the race model inequality. *Attention, Perception, & Psychophysics*, 1–13.

Graziano, M. S., & Cooke, D. F. (2006). Parieto-frontal interactions, personal space, and defensive behavior. *Neuropsychologia*, *44*(6), 845–859.

Graziano, M. S., & Gross, C. G. (1994). The representation of extrapersonal space: A possible role for bimodal, visual-tactile neurons. In M. S. Gazzaniga (Ed.), *The cognitive neurosciences* (pp. 1021–1034). Cambridge, MA: MIT Press.

Graziano, M. S., Hu, X. T., & Gross, C. G. (1997). Visuospatial properties of ventral premotor cortex. *Journal of Neurophysiology*, 77(5), 2268–2292.

Graziano, M. S., Reiss, L. A., & Gross, C. G. (1999). A neuronal representation of the location of nearby sounds. *Nature*, *397*(6718), 428–430.

Grill-Spector, K., & Malach, R. (2004). The human visual cortex. *Annual Reviews in Neuroscience, 27*, 649–677.

Halligan, P. W., Fink, G. R., Marshall, J. C., & Vallar, G. (2003). Spatial cognition: Evidence from visual neglect. *Trends in Cognitive Sciences*, 7(3), 125–133.

Halligan, P. W., & Marshall, J. C. (1991). Left neglect for near but not far space in man. *Nature, 350*(6318), 498–500.

Hamilton, R. H., & Pascual-Leone, A. (1998). Cortical plasticity associated with Braille learning. *Trends in Cognitive Sciences, 2*(5), 168–174.

Heilman, K. M., & Valenstein, E. (1979). Mechanisms underlying hemispatial neglect. *Annals of Neurology, 5*(2), 166–170.

Heilman, K. M., Watson, R. T., & Valenstein, E. (1993). Neglect and related disorders. In K. M. Heilman, & E. Valenstein (Eds.), *Clinical Neuropsychology* (pp. 243–294). New York, NY: Oxford University Press.

Ho, C., & Spence, C. (2005). Assessing the effectiveness of various auditory cues in capturing a driver's visual attention. *Journal of Experimental Psychology: Applied, 11*(3), 157.

Holmes, N. P. (2007). The law of inverse effectiveness in neurons and behaviour: Multisensory integration versus normal variability. *Neuropsychologia, 45*(14), 3340–3345.

Holmes, N. P. (2009). The principle of inverse effectiveness in multisensory integration: Some statistical considerations. *Brain Topography, 21*(3–4), 168–176.

Holmes, N. P., & Spence, C. (2004). The body schema and multisensory representation(s) of peripersonal space. *Cognitive Processing, 5*(2), 94–105.

Kadunce, D. C., Vaughan, W. J., Wallace, M. T., & Stein, B. E. (2001). The influence of visual and auditory receptive field organization on multisensory integration in the superior colliculus. *Experimental Brain Research, 139*(3), 303–310.

Karnath, H. O., & Rorden, C. (2012). The anatomy of spatial neglect. *Neuropsychologia, 50*(6), 1010–1017.

Keetels, M., & Vroomen, J. (2005). The role of spatial disparity and hemifields in audio-visual temporal order judgments. *Experimental Brain Research, 167*(4), 635–640.

Keller, I., & Lefin-Rank, G. (2010). Improvement of visual search after audiovisual exploration training in hemianopic patients. *Neurorehabilitation and Neural Repair, 24*(7), 666–673.

King, A. J., & Palmer, A. R. (1985). Integration of visual and auditory information in bimodal neurones in the guinea-pig superior colliculus. *Experimental Brain Research, 60*(3), 492–500.

Kolarik, A. J., Moore, B. C., Zahorik, P., Cirstea, S., & Pardhan, S. (2015). Auditory distance perception in humans: A review of cues, development, neuronal bases, and effects of sensory loss. *Attention, Perception, & Psychophysics*, 1–23.

Kral, A. (2007). Unimodal and cross-modal plasticity in the "deaf" auditory cortex. *International Journal of Audiology, 46*(9), 479–493. Available from http://dx.doi.org/10.1080/14992020701383027.

Kral, A., & Eggermont, J. J. (2007). What's to lose and what's to learn: Development under auditory deprivation, cochlear implants and limits of cortical plasticity. *Brain Research Reviews, 56*(1), 259–269. Available from http://dx.doi.org/10.1016/j.brainresrev.2007.07.021.

Lee, J., & Spence, C. (2015). Audiovisual crossmodal cuing effects in front and rear space. *Frontiers in Psychology*, 6.

Leone, L. M., & McCourt, M. E. (2013). The roles of physical and physiological simultaneity in audiovisual multisensory facilitation. *i-Perception, 4*(4), 213–228.

Leo, F., Bolognini, N., Passamonti, C., Stein, B. E., & Làdavas, E. (2008). Cross-modal localization in hemianopia: New insights on multisensory integration. *Brain, 131*(3), 855–865.

Lomber, S. G., Meredith, M. A., & Kral, A. (2011). Adaptive crossmodal plasticity in deaf auditory cortex: Areal and laminar contributions to supranormal vision in the deaf. *Progress in Brain Research, 191*, 251–270. Available from http://dx.doi.org/10.1016/B978-0-444-53752-2.00001-1.

Lourenco, S. F., Longo, M. R., & Pathman, T. (2011). Near space and its relation to claustrophobic fear. *Cognition, 119*(3), 448–453.

Lovelace, C. T., Stein, B. E., & Wallace, M. T. (2003). An irrelevant light enhances auditory detection in humans: A psychophysical analysis of multisensory integration in stimulus detection. *Cognitive Brain Research, 17*(2), 447–453.

MacSweeney, M., Capek, C. M., Campbell, R., & Woll, B. (2008). The signing brain: The neurobiology of sign language. *Trends in Cognitive Sciences, 12*(11), 432–440. Available from http://dx.doi.org/10.1016/j.tics.2008.07.010.

Maidenbaum, S., Hanassy, S., Abboud, S., Buchs, G., Chebat, D. R., Levy-Tzedek, S., & Amedi, A. (2014). The "EyeCane", a new electronic travel aid for the blind: Technology, behavior & swift learning. *Restorative Neurology and Neuroscience, 32*(6), 813–824. Available from http://dx.doi.org/10.3233/RNN-130351.

Maidenbaum, S., Levy-Tzedek, S., Chebat, D. R., Namer-Furstenberg, R., & Amedi, A. (2014). The effect of extended sensory range via the EyeCane sensory substitution device on the characteristics of visionless virtual navigation. *Multisensory Research, 27* (5-6), 379–397.

Makin, T. R., Holmes, N. P., & Ehrsson, H. H. (2008). On the other hand: Dummy hands and peripersonal space. *Behavioural Brain Research, 191*(1), 1–10.

McDonald, J. J., Teder-Sälejärvi, W. A., & Ward, L. M. (2001). Multisensory integration and crossmodal attention effects in the human brain. *Science, 292*(5523), 1791.

McDonald, J. J., & Ward, L. M. (2000). Involuntary listening aids seeing: Evidence from human electrophysiology. *Psychological Science, 11*(2), 167–171.

Merabet, L. B., & Pascual-Leone, A. (2010). Neural reorganization following sensory loss: The opportunity of change. *Nature Reviews Neuroscience, 11*(1), 44–52. Available from http://dx.doi.org/10.1038/nrn2758.

Meredith, M. A., Nemitz, J. W., & Stein, B. E. (1987). Determinants of multisensory integration in superior colliculus neurons. I. Temporal factors. *The Journal of Neuroscience*, 7(10), 3215–3229.

Meredith, M. A., & Stein, B. E. (1983). Interactions among converging sensory inputs in the superior colliculus. *Science, 221*(4608), 389–391.

Middlebrooks, J. C., & Green, D. M. (1991). Sound localization by human listeners. *Annual Review of Psychology, 42*(1), 135–159.

Millar, S. (1994). *Understanding and representing space: Theory and evidence from studies with blind and sighted children*. Oxford: Oxford University Press, Clarendon Press.

Millar, S., & Al-Attar, Z. (2004). External and body-centered frames of reference in spatial memory: Evidence from touch. *Perception & Psychophysics, 66*(1), 51–59.

Millar, S., & Al-Attar, Z. (2005). What aspects of vision facilitate haptic processing? *Brain and Cognition, 59*(3), 258–268. Available from http://dx.doi.org/10.1016/j.bandc.2005.07.005.

Miller, J. (1982). Divided attention: Evidence for coactivation with redundant signals. *Cognitive Psychology, 14*(2), 247–279.

Miller, J. (1986). Timecourse of coactivation in bimodal divided attention. *Perception & Psychophysics, 40*(5), 331–343.

Nijboer, T. C., Kollen, B. J., & Kwakkel, G. (2013). Time course of visuospatial neglect early after stroke: A longitudinal cohort study. *Cortex, 49*(8), 2021–2027.

Nijboer, T. C., Kollen, B. J., & Kwakkel, G. (2014). The impact of recovery of visuospatial neglect on motor recovery of the upper paretic limb after stroke. *PLoS One, 9*(6), e100584.

Nijboer, T., Van de Port, I., Schepers, V., Post, M., & Visser-Meily, A. (2013). Predicting functional outcome after stroke: The influence of neglect on basic activities in daily living. *Frontier in Human Neuroscience*, 7(182), 1–6. Available from http://dx.doi.org/10.3389/fnhum.2013.00182.

Noel, J. P., Grivaz, P., Marmaroli, P., Lissek, H., Blanke, O., & Serino, A. (2015). Full body action remapping of peripersonal space: The case of walking. *Neuropsychologia*, *70*, 375–384.

Occelli, V., Spence, C., & Zampini, M. (2011). Audiotactile interactions in front and rear space. *Neuroscience & Biobehavioral Reviews*, *35*(3), 589–598.

Papagno, C., Cecchetto, C., Pisoni, A., & Bolognini, N. (2016). Deaf, blind or deaf-blind: Is touch enhanced? *Experimental Brain Research*, *234*(2), 627–636. Available from http://dx.doi.org/10.1007/s00221-015-4488-1.

Pasqualotto, A., & Proulx, M. J. (2012). The role of visual experience for the neural basis of spatial cognition. *Neuroscience Biobehavioral Reviews*, *36*(4), 1179–1187. Available from http://dx.doi.org/10.1016/j.neubiorev.2012.01.008.

Passamonti, C., Bertini, C., & Làdavas, E. (2009). Audio-visual stimulation improves oculomotor patterns in patients with hemianopia. *Neuropsychologia*, *47*(2), 546–555.

Pavani, F., & Bottari, D. (2012). Visual abilities in individuals with profound deafness: A critical review. In M. M. Murray, & M. T. Wallace (Eds.), *The neural bases of multi-sensory processes*. Boca Raton, FL: CRC Press/Taylor & Francis.

Pavani, F., & Röder, B. (2012). Crossmodal plasticity as a consequence of sensory loss: Insights from blindness and deafness. In B. E. Stein (Ed.), *The new handbook of multi-sensory processes* (pp. 737–760). Cambridge, MA: MIT Press.

Postma, A., Zuidhoek, S., Noordzij, M. L., & Kappers, A. M. (2007). Differences between early-blind, late-blind, and blindfolded-sighted people in haptic spatial-configuration learning and resulting memory traces. *Perception*, *36*(8), 1253–1265.

Previc, F. H. (1998). The neuropsychology of 3-D space. *Psychological Bulletin*, *124*(2), 123–164.

Proulx, M. J., Ptito, M., & Amedi, A. (2014). Multisensory integration, sensory substitution and visual rehabilitation. *Neuroscience and Biobehavioral Reviews*, *41*, 1–2.

Renier, L. A., Anurova, I., De Volder, A. G., Carlson, S., VanMeter, J., & Rauschecker, J. P. (2010). Preserved functional specialization for spatial processing in the middle occipital gyrus of the early blind. *Neuron*, *68*(1), 138–148. Available from http://dx.doi.org/10.1016/j.neuron.2010.09.021.

Röder, B., & Rosler, F. (2004). Compensatory plasticity as a consequence of sensory loss. In G. Calvert, C. Spence, & B. E. Stein (Eds.), *The handbook of multisensory processes* (pp. 719–747). Cambridge, MA: MIT Press.

Sadato, N., Pascual-Leone, A., Grafman, J., Ibanez, V., Deiber, M. P., Dold, G., & Hallett, M. (1996). Activation of the primary visual cortex by Braille reading in blind subjects. *Nature*, *380*(6574), 526–528. Available from http://dx.doi.org/10.1038/380526a0.

Sambo, C. F., & Iannetti, G. D. (2013). Better safe than sorry? The safety margin surrounding the body is increased by anxiety. *The Journal of Neuroscience*, *33*(35), 14225–14230.

Sambo, C. F., Vallar, G., Fortis, P., Ronchi, R., Posteraro, L., Forster, B., & Maravita, A. (2011). Visual and spatial modulation of tactile extinction: Behavioural and electrophysiological evidence. *Frontiers in Human Neuroscience*, *6*(217). Available from http://dx.doi.org/10.3389/fnhum.2012.00217.

Santangelo, V., & Spence, C. (2007). Multisensory cues capture spatial attention regardless of perceptual load. *Journal of Experimental Psychology: Human Perception and Performance*, *33*(6), 1311.

Santangelo, V., Van der Lubbe, R. H., Belardinelli, M. O., & Postma, A. (2006). Spatial attention triggered by unimodal, crossmodal, and bimodal exogenous cues: A comparison of reflexive orienting mechanisms. *Experimental Brain Research, 173*(1), 40–48.

Santangelo, V., Van der Lubbe, R. H., Belardinelli, M. O., & Postma, A. (2008). Multisensory integration affects ERP components elicited by exogenous cues. *Experimental Brain Research, 185*(2), 269–277.

Schendel, K., & Robertson, L. C. (2004). Reaching out to see: Arm position can attenuate human visual loss. *Journal of Cognitive Neuroscience, 16*(6), 935–943.

Serino, A., Canzoneri, E., & Avenanti, A. (2011). Fronto-parietal areas necessary for a multisensory representation of peripersonal space in humans: An rTMS study. *Journal of Cognitive Neuroscience, 23*(10), 2956–2967.

Sharma, A., Nash, A. A., & Dorman, M. (2009). Cortical development, plasticity and re-organization in children with cochlear implants. *Journal of Communication Disorders, 42* (4), 272–279. Available from http://dx.doi.org/10.1016/j.jcomdis.2009.03.003.

Smith, D. T., Lane, A. R., & Schenk, T. (2008). Arm position does not attenuate visual loss in patients with homonymous field deficits. *Neuropsychologia, 46*(9), 2320–2325.

Sparks, D. L., & Nelson, I. S. (1987). Sensory and motor maps in the mammalian superior colliculus. *Trends in Neurosciences, 10*(8), 312–317.

Spence, C. (2013). Just how important is spatial coincidence to multisensory integration? Evaluating the spatial rule. *Annals of the New York Academy of Sciences, 1296*(1), 31–49.

Spence, C., & Santangelo, V. (2009). Capturing spatial attention with multisensory cues: A review. *Hearing Research, 258*(1), 134–142.

Spence, C., & McDonald, J. (2004). The cross-modal consequences of the exogenous spatial orienting of attention. In G. A. Calvert, C. Spence, & B. E. Stein (Eds.), *The handbook of multisensory processes* (pp. 3–26). Cambridge, MA: MIT Press.

Spence, C., & Driver, J. (Eds.). (2004). *Crossmodal space and crossmodal attention*. Oxford, UK: Oxford University Press.

Spence, C., & Squire, S. (2003). Multisensory integration: maintaining the perception of synchrony. *Current Biology, 13*(13), R519–R521.

Stein, B. E., & Stanford, T. R. (2008). Multisensory integration: Current issues from the perspective of the single neuron. *Nature Reviews Neuroscience, 9*(4), 255–266.

Stein, B. E., & Meredith, M. (1990). Multisensory integration. *Annals of the New York Academy of Sciences, 608*(1), 51–70.

Stein, B. E., & Meredith, M. A. (1993). *The merging of the senses*. Cambridge, MA: The MIT Press.

Stevenson, R. A., Fister, J. K., Barnett, Z. P., Nidiffer, A. R., & Wallace, M. T. (2012). Interactions between the spatial and temporal stimulus factors that influence multisensory integration in human performance. *Experimental Brain Research, 219*(1), 121–137.

Striem-Amit, E., Ovadia-Caro, S., Caramazza, A., Margulies, D. S., Villringer, A., & Amedi, A. (2015). Functional connectivity of visual cortex in the blind follows retinotopic organization principles. *Brain, 138*(6), 1679–1695.

Taffou, M., & Viaud-Delmon, I. (2014). Cynophobic fear adaptively extends peripersonal space. *Frontiers in Psychiatry, 5*, 122. Available from http://dx.doi.org/10.3389/fpsyt.2014.00122.

Ten Brink, A. F., Nijboer, T. C., Bergsma, D. P., Barton, J. J., & Van der Stigchel, S. (2015). Lack of multisensory integration in hemianopia: No influence of visual stimuli on aurally guided saccades to the blind hemifield. *PLoS One, 10*(4), e0122054.

Teneggi, C., Canzoneri, E., Di Pellegrino, G., & Serino, A. (2013). Social modulation of peripersonal space boundaries. *Current Biology, 23*(5), 406–411.

Theoret, H., Merabet, L., & Pascual-Leone, A. (2004). Behavioral and neuroplastic changes in the blind: Evidence for functionally relevant cross-modal interactions. *Journal of Physiology, 98*(1–3), 221–233. Available from http://dx.doi.org/10.1016/j.jphysparis.2004.03.009.

Thinus-Blanc, C., & Gaunet, F. (1997). Representation of space in blind persons: Vision as a spatial sense? *Psycholigical Bulletin, 121*(1), 20–42.

Tinga, A. M., Visser-Meily, J. M. A., van der Smagt, M. J., Van der Stigchel, S., van Ee, R., & Nijboer, T. C. W. (2015). Multisensory stimulation to improve low-and higher-level sensory deficits after stroke: A systematic review. *Neuropsychology Review, 26*(1), 73–91.

Tinti, C., Adenzato, M., Tamietto, M., & Cornoldi, C. (2006). Visual experience is not necessary for efficient survey spatial cognition: Evidence from blindness. *Quarterly Journal of Experimental Psychology, 59*(7), 1306–1328. Available from http://dx.doi.org/10.1080/17470210500214275.

Ungar, S., Blades, M., & Spencer, C. (1996). The ability of visually impaired children to locate themselves on a tactile map. *Journal of Visual Impairment & Blindness, 90*(6), 526–535.

Urbanski, M., De Schotten, M. T., Rodrigo, S., Oppenheim, C., Touzé, E., Méder, J. F., & Bartolomeo, P. (2011). DTI-MR tractography of white matter damage in stroke patients with neglect. *Experimental Brain Research, 208*(4), 491–505.

Van der Lubbe, R. H., Van Mierlo, C. M., & Postma, A. (2010). The involvement of occipital cortex in the early blind in auditory and tactile duration discrimination tasks. *Journal of Cognitive Neuroscience, 22*(7), 1541–1556.

Van der Stoep, N., Nijboer, T. C. W., & Van der Stigchel, S. (2014). Exogenous orienting of crossmodal attention in 3-D space: Support for a depth-aware crossmodal attentional system. *Psychonomic Bulletin & Review, 21*(3), 708–714.

Van der Stoep, N., Nijboer, T. C. W., Van der Stigchel, S., & Spence, C. (2015). Multisensory interactions in the depth plane in front and rear space: A review. *Neuropsychologia, 70*, 335–349.

Van der Stoep, N., Serino, A., Farnè, A., Di Luca, M., & Spence, C. (2016). Depth: The forgotten dimension in multisensory research. *Multisensory Research.* Available from http://dx.doi.org/10.1163/22134808-00002525.

Van der Stoep, N., Spence, C., Nijboer, T. C. W., & Van der Stigchel, S. (2015). On the relative contributions of multisensory integration and crossmodal exogenous spatial attention to multisensory response enhancement. *Acta Psychologica, 162*, 20–28.

Van der Stoep, N., Van der Stigchel, S., Nijboer, T. C. W., & Van der Smagt, M. J. (2015). Audiovisual integration in near and far space: effects of changes in distance and stimulus effectiveness. *Experimental Brain Research, 234*(5), 1175–1188.

Van der Stoep, N., Visser-Meily, J. M., Kappelle, L. J., de Kort, P. L., Huisman, K. D., Eijsackers, A. L., & Nijboer, T. C. (2013). Exploring near and far regions of space: distance-specific visuospatial neglect after stroke. *Journal of Clinical and Experimental Neuropsychology, 35*(8), 799–811.

van Dijk, R., Kappers, A. M., & Postma, A. (2013a). Haptic spatial configuration learning in deaf and hearing individuals. *PLoS One, 8*(4), e61336. Available from http://dx.doi.org/10.1371/journal.pone.0061336.

van Dijk, R., Kappers, A. M., & Postma, A. (2013b). Superior spatial touch: Improved haptic orientation processing in deaf individuals. *Experimental Brain Research, 230*(3), 283–289. Available from http://dx.doi.org/10.1007/s00221-013-3653-7.

Van Dijk, R., Nelson, C., Postma, A., & Van Dijk, J. (2010). Deaf children with severe multiple disabilities: Etiologies, intervention, and assessment. In M. Marschark, & P. E. Spencer (Eds.), *The Oxford handbook of deaf studies, language, and education volume 2* (Vol. 2) Oxford: Oxford University Press.

Vroomen, J., & Keetels, M. (2010). Perception of intersensory synchrony: A tutorial review. *Attention, Perception, & Psychophysics*, *72*(4), 871–884.

Welch, R. B., DuttonHurt, L. D., & Warren, D. H. (1986). Contributions of audition and vision to temporal rate perception. *Perception & Psychophysics*, *39*(4), 294–300.

Welch, R. B., & Warren, D. H. (1980). Immediate perceptual response to intersensory discrepancy. *Psychological Bulletin*, *88*(3), 638.

Wong, M., Gnanakumaran, V., & Goldreich, D. (2011). Tactile spatial acuity enhancement in blindness: Evidence for experience-dependent mechanisms. *Journal of Neuroscience*, *31*(19), 7028–7037. Available from http://dx.doi.org/10.1523/JNEUROSCI.6461-10.2011.

Zwiers, M. P., Van Opstal, A. J., & Cruysberg, J. R. (2001). A spatial hearing deficit in early-blind humans. *Journal of Neuroscience*, *21*(9), 141–145, RC142.

FURTHER READING

Làdavas, E., Di Pellegrino, G., Farnè, A., & Zeloni, G. (1998). Neuropsychological evidence of an integrated visuotactile representation of peripersonal space in humans. *Journal of Cognitive Neuroscience*, *10*(5), 581–589.

Meredith, M. A., & Stein, B. E. (1986). Visual, auditory, and somatosensory convergence on cells in superior colliculus results in multisensory integration. *Journal of Neurophysiology*, *56*(3), 640–662.

Nidiffer, A. R., Stevenson, R. A., Fister, J. K., Barnett, Z. P., & Wallace, M. T. (2016). Interactions between space and effectiveness in human multisensory performance. *Neuropsychologia*. Available from http://dx.doi.org/10.1016/j.neuropsychologia.2016.01.031.

Rizzolatti, G., Fadiga, L., Fogassi, L., & Gallese, V. (1997). The space around us. *Science*, *277*(5323), 190.

Ross, L. A., Saint-Amour, D., Leavitt, V. M., Javitt, D. C., & Foxe, J. J. (2007). Do you see what I am saying? Exploring visual enhancement of speech comprehension in noisy environments. *Cerebral Cortex*, *17*(5), 1147–1153.

Stevenson, R. A., & James, T. W. (2009). Audiovisual integration in human superior temporal sulcus: Inverse effectiveness and the neural processing of speech and object recognition. *Neuroimage*, *44*(3), 1210–1223.

Van Atteveldt, N. M., Formisano, E., Blomert, L., & Goebel, R. (2007). The effect of temporal asynchrony on the multisensory integration of letters and speech sounds. *Cerebral Cortex*, *17*(4), 962–974.

CHAPTER 5

Spatial Attention and Eye Movements

Stefan Van der Stigchel[1] and Tanja C.W. Nijboer[1,2,3]
[1]Experimental Psychology, Helmholtz Institute, Utrecht University, Utrecht, The Netherlands
[2]Rudolf Magnus Institute of Neuroscience and Center of Excellence for Rehabilitation Medicine, University Medical Center Utrecht and Rehabilitation Center De Hoogstraat, Utrecht, The Netherlands
[3]Department of Rehabilitation Medicine, University Medical Center, Utrecht, The Netherlands

The space around us is highly crowded: even when performing a simple task like making a cup of coffee, there are generally a huge number of distracting elements in our environment that could interfere with the performance of this particular task. Although very few people will be able to arrange their kitchen such that there are no distracting elements, even the most tidy people with clean kitchens will face a challenging task: making coffee involves multiple elements that are relevant during different moments in the process. To keep performance on track, information relevant to the current goal and intention needs to be selected, while irrelevant information needs to be filtered out. This selection of a spatial element in the face of competition for selection by other elements has been termed "spatial attention." As we will outline in this chapter, spatial attention is a multifaceted concept which involves various different components and functions. Although spatial attention is perhaps one of the most ill-defined terms in experimental psychology, the aim of the current chapter is to provide some understanding about what spatial attention entails and how deficits in spatial attention can inform us about its underlying mechanisms. The description of the consequences of deficits in spatial attention will illustrate how crucial spatial attention is for our daily functioning.

5.1 TOP-DOWN AND BOTTOM-UP ATTENTION

While making coffee, we have a clear goal and we will select the element that is important for achieving this goal. When information is selected according to the goals, intentions, and beliefs of the observer, spatial selection is said to be under "top-down" control. By definition, we have

Neuropsychology of Space.
DOI: http://dx.doi.org/10.1016/B978-0-12-801638-1.00005-7

full control of this type of selection, as we voluntarily decide to allocate our attention to a certain object. This is in sharp contrast to "bottom-up" control, which is determined in full by the physical properties of the environment, irrespective of the observer's goals or intentions. While making coffee, a door might unexpectedly open, which might constitute such a salient event, that attention will be captured in a bottom-up manner. Any element that is salient, because of its physical properties, might capture attention away from the current focus of attention. As will be clear from this description, there is a continuous competition for attentional selection: salient bottom-up information battles with the top-down settings for attentional priority. This is perhaps most evident from studies on eye movements, as will be discussed later in this chapter. Because we can only execute one eye movement at a time, there is a continuous competition between bottom-up and top-down information in determining the next fixation.

Theorists have long been debating to what extent top-down control is able to influence what we select. Although some theories claim that top-down control is dominant in determining what we select (Bacon & Egeth, 1994; Folk, Remington, & Johnston, 1992), others have argued that bottom-up control is more dominant (Itti & Koch, 2000; Nothdurft, 2000; Theeuwes, 1991), or argued for a combination of both (Wolfe, 1994, 1998). More recent views focus on the timescale of visual processing in determining when a certain type of control is most dominant. This view argues that visual selection is driven solely by bottom-up control during the first sweep of information processing, while top-down control progressively becomes stronger as information processing progresses: top-down control can influence selection only after the first initial sweep is completed (Van der Stigchel et al., 2009). This is, for instance, evident from eye movement studies, which have shown that the endpoints of saccades with a short reaction time are fully determined by the bottom-up information in a display (van Zoest, Donk, & Theeuwes, 2004; van Zoest, Donk, & Van der Stigchel, 2012).

When discussing the concept of attentional selection, attention has frequently been conceptualized as a "spotlight" as an analogy for an attentional window which travels through space and selects a certain element while ignoring the elements in the environment (Posner & Petersen, 1990) or as a "zoom-lens" which selects a certain element for further inspection (Eriksen & St James, 1986). The spotlight analogy also works for the interaction between top-down and bottom-up control: although we can guide the attentional spotlight voluntarily through a scene, any novel or salient element can disrupt this voluntary control and guide the spotlight automatically to the potent element. Besides the spatial location of the spotlight, observers can also adjust the size of the attentional spotlight given the requirements of a specific task at hand. For instance, when the task is to select the most salient item in the display, the spotlight is set such that the spotlight encompasses the full visual display. A more difficult task in which each individual item has to be inspected one by one will require a spotlight with a smaller size (Nakayama & Joseph, 1998). Metaphorically, the spotlight can therefore also be considered a zoom lens which can change size depending on the task at hand (Box 5.1).

BOX 5.1 Is Attention the Only Ill-defined Cognitive Domain?

Although William James wrote that "everyone knows what attention is" (James, 1890), there have been many claims that attention is ill-defined. For instance, Elisabeth Styles (1997) stated that attention is not a single concept and that is not possible to define attention as a unitary concept (see also, Duncan, 2006). Some have even argued that attention does not exist at all (Rubin, 1965/1925). In the domain of visual attention, the topic of the current chapter, already many different types of attention exist: bottom-up, top-down, covert, overt, etc. Attention might therefore be considered a multifaceted concept consisting of different components, all in need of their own definition. Although there is currently a lack of a common theory of attention, it might be questioned how unique attention is in this respect. How about memory? There are many different types of memory as well, each subcomponent having its own rules and characteristics. Executive control might even be worse: there are already so many different names for this domain (eg, cognitive control, executive functioning), that it is difficult to propose a common definition for this domain as well. So, although it might be true that attention is ill-defined, it begs the question whether attention is truly unique compared to other cognitive domains.

5.2 VISUAL SEARCH AND ATTENTIONAL CAPTURE

One of the hallmark tasks in the visual attention literature to understand the characteristics of the spotlight is the visual search task. In a visual search task, the participant has to search for a "target" element which is presented together with other nontarget elements, generally termed "distractors." The speed with which the target is identified with respect to the number of distractors in the visual display is

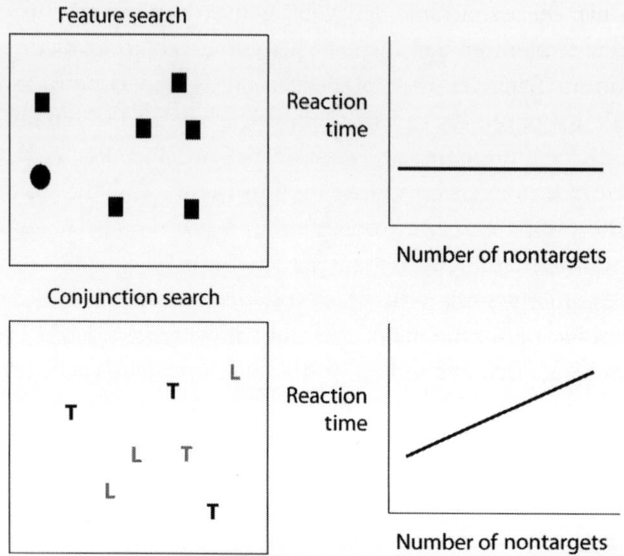

Figure 5.1 Examples of a search display for a feature and a conjunction search task. A feature search task will result in parallel search in which the reaction time is independent of the number of elements in the screen. In a conjunction search task, reaction time will increase with the number of items in the display, which is the signature of serial search.

indicative for the extent to which a target element is able to automatically attract attention (Treisman & Gelade, 1980). When the reaction time is largely independent of the number of distractors, search is claimed to be "parallel," indicating that the target automatically attracted attention and could be identified immediately. Parallel search is generally observed during feature search in which the target has a feature which is not shared by any of the distractors (eg, a green target among red distractors). Because of the unique aspect of the target, attention will be guided to the target before any of the distractors is selected. Parallel search is contrasted with "serial search," which is observed when the reaction time increases with the number of distractors (see Fig. 5.1). Serial search is generally associated with conjunction search in which the target does not have a unique feature but is defined by a conjunction of features (eg, a green T presented among green Ls and red Ts as distractors). In this case, each individual element in the display needs to be selected until the target is identified, as there is not a unique feature which can guide attention. Reaction times then increase linearly as a function of the number of elements in the display.

In the parallel search task described above, the bottom-up capture of attention due to the unique feature of the target is helpful, as it allows for a rapid response during the task. There is therefore no reason for the attentional system to ignore this information. This makes the attentional capture task particularly interesting as it entails a task in which observers have to ignore irrelevant bottom-up information (Theeuwes, 1992, 1994). In the attentional capture paradigm, the target has a unique feature compared to the other elements and the task is to identify the orientation of a line segment inside the target. On a subset of trials, a salient distractor is also present which is unique in a different dimension. One example would be a green diamond-shaped target presented among green circle-shaped nontargets, with the salient distractor being a red circle. Although the distractor should be ignored by the observer, as it is incongruent with the current top-down goal, numerous studies have now shown that reaction times are increased when the salient distractor is present (for an overview, see Theeuwes, 2010). This increase in reaction time indicates that the salient distractor captured attention before attention could be allocated to the target, irrespective of the top-down goal. Recent studies measuring event-related potentials (ERPs) have provided additional converging evidence for the capture of attention by measuring an ERP component named the "N2pc" which is considered an index of the allocation of spatial attention (Luck, Girelli, McDermott, & Ford, 1997). The N2pc is a larger negative voltage at electrodes contralateral to the attended stimulus. When ERPs were recorded during the traditional attentional capture task in which the target was presented at the vertical meridian and the salient distractor in the left or right visual field, Hickey, McDonald, and Theeuwes (2006) revealed a clear N2pc contralateral to the distractor, indicating that attention had shifted to the location of the distractor.

Variations of the attentional capture paradigm have convincingly shown that not every salient feature is capable of attracting attention in a bottom-up manner (Jonides & Yantis, 1988; Yantis & Hillstrom, 1994). This discrepancy in results might be caused by different sizes of the attentional window (Belopolsky, Zwaan, Theeuwes, & Kramer, 2007; Theeuwes, Kramer, & Belopolsky, 2004): when the task requires a small attentional window, salient elements outside of this window might not capture attention, whereas any salient element inside the attentional window will capture attention. Attentional capture by a salient element is then always observed with an easy task in which the attentional window spreads over the entire visual display, but might be absent in tasks in which there is a need for serial search, requiring a small attentional window.

5.3 ATTENTIONAL CUEING

Additional distinctions between bottom-up and top-down attentional control can be revealed by investigating how these types of attention can be directed in space. A task which is well suited to study the orienting of spatial attention is the attentional cueing paradigm, developed by Michael Posner (1980). In this paradigm, subjects have to respond as quickly as possible to the presentation of a target element which may appear either to the left or to the right of a central fixation point. Before the target is presented, a cue appears in the periphery. A distinction is made between informative and noninformative cues: an informative cue provides information about the likely location of the subsequent target, whereas a noninformative cue has no predictive value. For instance, an informative cue with a validity of 80% will appear at the location of the target at 80% of the trials, whereas it will appear at the nontarget location in the remaining trials. For both types of cues, response times are decreased on valid trials, in which the cue is presented at the same location as the target, compared to invalid trials, in which the cued location is not the location of the subsequently presented target. This can be explained by the attention-grabbing nature of the cue: the presentation of the cue results in a shift of attention to the location of the target which is then presented at an attended location. Because attention speeds up the processing of elements presented at an attended location, reaction times will be faster.

Because of its abrupt appearance in the periphery, the cue constitutes a salient event and will therefore automatically attract attention. Therefore an informative peripheral cue does not solely tap into top-down control, because the presentation of the peripheral cue will also elicit a bottom-up shift of attention. One way to solve this problem and elicit a fully voluntary shift of attention is to present an arrow at fixation point, pointing either to the location of the target or to the nontarget location. Although later studies have shown that also the presentation of a nonpredictive central arrow cue results in a small automatic shift of attention in the direction of the cue (Hommel, Pratt, Colzato, & Godijn, 2001), these cues are often used to study more voluntary shifts of attention. It might not be easy to develop a fully voluntary cue in the center of the screen, as research has revealed that symbols like numbers (Fischer, Castel, Dodd, & Pratt, 2003) and gaze cues (Friesen & Kingstone, 1998) can also elicit a reflexive voluntary shift of attention. Not every word or symbol elicits a reflexive shift of attention, however, as letters of the alphabet, days of the week, and months of the year do not have these abilities (Dodd, Van der Stigchel, Leghari, Fung, & Kingstone, 2008).

When examining the timing between the presentation of the cue and the presentation of a peripheral noninformative cue, a striking phenomenon becomes apparent. As expected, when the cue-target interval is short, reaction times to the target are faster when the cue is valid compared to the invalid condition. However, when the interval between cue onset and target onset is more than 300 ms, detection times are slower at the cued location than at the uncued location. This phenomenon is known as inhibition of return (IOR) and has shown to be one of the most reliable effects in attention research (R. M. Klein & Taylor, 1994; Posner & Cohen, 1984). IOR even occurs for up to five cued locations before a target is presented, showing that IOR can be observed at multiple locations when attention is rapidly shifting between locations (Dodd, Castel, & Pratt, 2003). IOR has been explained by the fact that the relatively long interval between cue and target allows the attentional spotlight sufficient time to return to the central fixation point in the absence of the presentation of a target. Because there is presumably a bias to not return to a previously attended location in order to prevent perseverative types of errors in behavior, an inhibitory tag is placed at the previously attended location, resulting in a delay in the shift of attention back to the cued location for long cue-target intervals. Some have even argued that IOR has evolved to allow for an effective search routine while searching for essential elements, like food (R. M. Klein & MacInnes, 1999); IOR then allows for covering a maximum amount of territory in as little time as possible because previously searched locations will have a small chance of being revisited due to the inhibitory tag associated with these locations. Importantly, IOR only occurs for peripheral noninformative cues and is not observed for central informative cues. For these cues, the attentional benefits at the cued location last and no reversal of these benefits is observed. This has led many to believe that voluntary and involuntary shifts of attention reflect two different components (Jonides, 1981) (Box 5.2).

5.4 ATTENTION AND EYE MOVEMENT PREPARATION

Although visual attention is responsible for the selection of a certain area in the visual space for further selection, the initial visual processing depends first and foremost on the position of the eye and the head. Given

BOX 5.2 Visual Attention and Working Memory

There are many different ways in which visual attention and working memory are related. In this chapter, we explain that IOR is a mechanism which inhibits previously attended locations. In this way, IOR functions as a memory for locations where you have already searched. But this is not the only link between visual attention and working memory. For instance, spatial working memory (remembering a location during a delay period in which no visual input is presented) is known to be mediated by visual attention in that the spotlight of attention is allocated to the location in spatial working memory (Awh & Jonides, 2001). Presenting an attention-grabbing onset in the delay period indeed modulates the memory representation (Van der Stigchel, Merten, Meeter, & Theeuwes, 2007). There is also neural overlap between the areas responsible for attention and spatial working memory (Postle, Awh, Jonides, Smith, & D'Esposito, 1999). Similar to *spatial* working memory, visual attention and *visual* working memory are also intimately related in that visual attention is reflexively captured by a stimulus in visual working memory (Olivers, Meijer, & Theeuwes, 2006). Furthermore, eye movements are automatically guided to a stimulus matching the content of visual working memory (Silvis & Van der Stigchel, 2014).

the high acuity of the fovea, the most effective way to process an element is by executing a saccade to its location. It is therefore not surprising that many researchers have been interested in the question whether the attentional and oculomotor system are related. Although we generally assume that a person is attending the location to which his or her eyes are pointing, it is definitely possible to shift our attentional spotlight without moving our eyes. This comes in handy during a party in which you might be looking at your colleague, while your attention is scanning the room for other, perhaps more interesting, attendees.

Although it is clear that there is no one-to-one mapping between the locus of attention and the position of the eyes, it could still be possible that the shifting of attention and the programming of an eye movement are part of a common integrated system. Although the eyes do not move, but attention does, it could be the case that an eye movement is programmed to the attended location, but not executed. This concept has been the foundation of the premotor theory of attention, which has been the dominant view in the last decades regarding the relation between the attentional and the oculomotor system. According to this view, the mechanisms involved in both the programming of an eye movement and the shift of spatial attention are basically the same (Rizzolatti, Riggio, Dascola, & Umilta, 1987; Rizzolatti, Riggio, & Sheliga, 1994). Two strong predictions follow from this idea: first, the execution of an eye movement should be accompanied by a shift of attention to the saccade target location. Second, any shift of attention should result in an activation of the oculomotor system.

Evidence for the first prediction comes from dual-task studies in which participants have to prepare and execute a saccade while performing an identification task (Deubel & Schneider, 1996; Van der Stigchel & Theeuwes, 2005). Performance on the identification task can then be used as a proxy of the locus of attention during the preparation of the eye movement. In a typical paradigm, the primary task for the observer is to execute an eye movement to a peripheral saccade goal as indicated by a central cue, like an arrow pointing to the left or right of the visual field. While preparing the eye movement, a probe stimulus is presented, either at the location of the saccade goal or at a different location in the visual field. Observers are required to report the identification of the probe stimulus (eg, a letter). The rationale for this type of paradigm is that the accuracy on the identification task should be dependent on where visual attention is allocated during the preparation of the saccade. If attention and eye movements are indeed tightly coupled, performance on the identification task should be best at the location of the saccade goal shortly before the execution of the eye movement and should be impaired at any other location in the display. This is indeed what is observed in many different variations of this paradigm (Hoffman & Subramaniam, 1995a, 1995b; Kowler, Anderson, Dosher, & Blaser, 1995; Van der Stigchel & Theeuwes, 2005). For instance, Deubel and Schneider (1996) observed that the identification of a letter stimulus, which was presented shortly just before the execution of a saccade, was at chance level when presented at any location different from the saccade target location, while performance was best at the saccade target location. Additional experiments showed that this finding could not be attributed to any strategic effect, as these same results were obtained when prior knowledge was provided regarding the location of the to-be-identified letter: it was simply not possible to shift attention to any other location in space than to the goal of the programmed eye movement (see also, Deubel, 2008; Deubel & Schneider, 2003). Although the dual-task paradigms discussed until now have mainly focused on voluntary executed saccades, similar results have been obtained for more reflexive involuntary saccades in which a saccade was triggered by the presentation of an abrupt onset (Peterson, Kramer, & Irwin, 2004). Results of dual-task experiments therefore provide clear evidence for the first prediction of the premotor theory: any execution of a saccade, voluntary or involuntary, is accompanied by a shift of attention to the saccade goal location.

5.5 ATTENTION AND SACCADE TRAJECTORIES

A second prediction of the premotor theory of attention is that any shift of attention should result in an activation of the oculomotor system. Evidence for this prediction comes from studies in which shifts of attention resulted in a modulation of the oculomotor program. More specifically, these studies have examined the trajectory between the start and the end of the eye movement. This trajectory is not straight but generally is slightly curved, as already noted by Yarbus (1967) in his now classic eye movement recordings. Interestingly, this baseline curvature can be influenced by various internal and environmental factors, like the allocation of attention in space (for reviews, see Van der Stigchel, 2010; Van der Stigchel, Meeter, & Theeuwes, 2006). The first reports of these modulations of the saccade trajectory by the allocation of attention were described by Sheliga, Riggio, and Rizzolatti (1994). In their experiments, participants made a vertical saccade to a target above or below the central fixation point. A peripheral cue, presented in one of four possible boxes to the left or right of the fixation point, determined the direction of the required eye movement. In order to successfully perform the task, participants therefore had to attend to this cue without the execution of an eye movement. When the subsequent eye movement to the target was examined in detail, it was observed that the trajectory of this eye movement deviated away from the cued location. This indicates that directing attention in space results in an activation of the oculomotor system.

Deviations in saccade trajectories have generally been explained in terms of population coding (Tipper, Howard, & Houghton, 2000; Tipper, Howard, & Jackson, 1997). This explanation is based on the idea that each neuron in a motor map codes an individual vector that encodes the movement toward the corresponding location. The direction of the average of these vectors then determines the direction in which the eye movement is initiated. Crucial for this idea is that a movement program results in activation of a broad population of vectors. When two elements are presented in relatively close proximity, the average vector will therefore point to an intermediate location. According to this view, this average vector can be influenced by inhibiting one of the two active populations. This way, eye movements do not generally land in between two elements, but can be successfully biased toward one specific element. As a by-product of the distributed nature of the population code, the inhibition of this one population will also inhibit a subset of the vectors coding for the other population. Because of this, the resulting vector will point slightly away from the target location, because part of the vectors coding for the desired movement will also be inhibited. With respect to the results of Sheliga, Riggio, and Rizzolatti (1995), this explanation indicates that the shift of attention to a location different from the desired target location evoked a movement vector to the attended location. Because this vector needed to be inhibited in order to execute a saccade to the desired target location, the saccade trajectory deviated away from the location of the cue. This provides strong evidence for the second prediction of the premotor theory of attention, as a shift of attention resulted in an activation of the oculomotor system.

These findings were later extended in a study that showed that the strength of the trajectory deviation is a measure of the amount of attention allocated to any particular location in space (Van der Stigchel & Theeuwes, 2007). Observers were endogenously cued to attend to a peripheral location without making an eye movement. As expected, when a letter was presented at the cued location, performance on the letter identification task was superior compared to the condition in which the letter was presented at an uncued location. On a subset of trials, however, observers had to execute a saccade to a location above or below the central fixation (as indicated by a specific letter, the "go-letter"). When this go-letter was presented at the cued location, saccade trajectories deviated away from the cued location, in line with the premotor theory of attention. Saccades also deviated away from the uncued location, but less strongly compared to when the go-letter was presented at the cued location. These differences in the strength of the deviation are therefore related to the amount of attention allocated to the cued and the uncued locations, showing that these deviations reflect the amount of attention allocated in space. It was concluded that the activation in the oculomotor system elegantly travels along with the spotlight of attention: wherever attention is allocated, the oculomotor system is activated. Interestingly, this also seems to hold for reflexive shifts of visual attention as obtained by central symbolic cues: when a gaze cue was presented at central fixation, saccade trajectories deviated away from the direction toward which the gaze was oriented (Nummenmaa & Hietanen, 2006), similar to implicitly learned symbolic central cues (Van der Stigchel, Mills, & Dodd, 2010).

5.6 HOW OBLIGATORY IS THE LINK BETWEEN ATTENTION AND EYE MOVEMENTS?

Not only behavioral studies have provided evidence for the overlap between the attentional and the oculomotor system, but both functional neuro-imaging studies (Corbetta et al., 1998; Nobre, Gitelman, Dias, & Mesulam, 2000) and microstimulation in the monkey brain (Moore & Fallah, 2004) have provided converging evidence for such an overlap. There is, for instance, strongly overlapping neural activation in both parietal and frontal lobes when participants either shift their eyes or shift attention (Corbetta et al., 1998). Although these results are clearly in line with a strong relation between the two systems, it does raise the question of whether motor preparation is both necessary and sufficient for a shift of spatial attention to occur (Smith & Schenk, 2012). There have now been numerous studies showing a dissociation between attention and saccade preparation (Belopolsky & Theeuwes, 2009; Hunt & Kingstone, 2003).

One interesting manipulation to explore this question is by creating a situation in which the capacity to perform a saccade is restricted. This situation can be created by rotating the eyes of the observer such that there is inability to make an eye movement further toward the temporal side (Craighero, Carta, & Fadiga, 2001). By placing the stimulus display off to one side, a stimulus can be presented at a location which cannot be reached by a saccade. Because visual acuity is not influenced by the rotation of the eyes, any possible differences in attentional deployment cannot be attributed to any low-level effect, but is caused by the restricted capacity to perform a saccade. When performing a voluntary and an involuntary attentional cueing task, Smith, Rorden, and Schenk (2012) observed a difference between both types of attention with respect to the ability to perform an eye movement. Eye abduction did not have an effect on voluntary attention, since cueing effects were similar across the abducted and nonabducted hemifields. A difference between both hemifields was observed for involuntary attention, however, in that a nonpredictive cue did not result in a standard cueing effect when presented in the abducted hemifield, whereas the cue did capture attention in the nonabducted hemifield. These results suggest that eye abduction does not produce a deficit in voluntary attention, which seems to implicate that, in contrast to involuntary attention, there is a strong independence between voluntary attention and the oculomotor system. Although one might argue that this is a rather "abnormal" situation which might not generalize to other situations, it does implicate that there is not a strict obligatory coupling between attention and eye movements, at least for voluntary attention.

This lack of a strict coupling between voluntary attention and eye movements also becomes evident from studies on patients with oculomotor deficits. When performing attentional cueing tasks, a patient with a complete paralysis of both eyes still showed normal voluntary cueing, whereas involuntary attention was clearly impaired (Smith, Rorden, & Jackson, 2004). Similar results were observed in patients suffering from Duane's retraction syndrome, a chronic condition which impairs mobility of one of the eyes (Gabay, Henik, & Gradstein, 2010). Although the findings on involuntary attention in these patients are nicely in line with the idea that any deficit in oculomotor control should result in problems in spatial attention, observations of an intact voluntary attention are clearly not in line with the premotor theory of attention. Does this mean that eye movements are not a good proxy of the locus of attention? No, it does not. In the vast majority of the situations, attention and eye movements will be highly correlated, although a dissociation can be observed under certain circumstances.

5.7 THE DYNAMICS OF SELECTION IN OCULOMOTOR CONTROL

Because attention and eye movement are so strongly coupled, eye movement paradigms can be used to study the dynamics of attentional selection. With standard reaction time experiments, the locus of attention at a certain moment in time is difficult to determine. With the rise of affordable and easy-to-use eye trackers, there has been a great increase in studies on the dynamics of oculomotor control. These studies have the advantage of revealing the outcome of the competition between different elements in the display. Similar to attention, the endpoint of an eye movement is the result of a continuous competition between bottom-up and top-down factors. The dynamics of top-down and bottom-up control can therefore be studied by measuring eye movements in situations in which there is strong competition in a given visual display.

When eye movements are measured in visual search displays, eye movements can reveal which locations were foveated before the target was selected. In an oculomotor version of the attentional capture paradigm, Theeuwes and colleagues (Godijn & Theeuwes, 2002; Theeuwes, Kramer, Hahn, & Irwin, 1998) observed that eye movements can be captured by a salient stimulus, similar to attention. Observers were presented with a display containing a number of gray circles positioned on an imaginary circle around a central fixation point. After a short interval, all elements changed color, expect one. This color singleton was the target location to which an eye movement should be executed as fast and accurately as possible. In a subset of trials, an onset distractor was presented simultaneously with the target at an empty location. Because this element is new, it is a salient element and will therefore grab attention. In line with this, a reflexive eye movement was executed to the distractor on 30–40% of the trials: the eye was "captured" by the distractor before landing on the target location (hence the term "oculomotor capture") (Fig. 5.2). Interestingly, this capture was most prominent for saccades with a short latency, consistent with the idea that bottom-up factors strongly influence the initial phase of the selection process. Because of the short latency, capture saccades are generally characterized as "reflexive." These results were later extended by van Zoest and colleagues who showed that eye movements with short latencies are completely stimulus-driven, as the initial direction was determined by the relative salience of target and distractor (van Zoest & Donk, 2005; van Zoest et al., 2004). The effects of saliency were absent for eye movements with a longer latency.

In terms of the vector theory, this oculomotor capture is caused by the competition between multiple vectors in the oculomotor system. One vector is evoked by the presentation of the target. Because of the task instructions, this vector will be mainly evoked on the basis of top-down influences; it does not constitute a salient element and the vector will therefore not be very strong early on during the selection process, in contrast to the vector associated with the onset distractor. Because of the salience of this element, its corresponding vector will be strong early on in the selection process. When a saccade is initiated with a short latency, the strongest vector in the system will therefore be the distractor vector. If the observer wants to perform this task successfully, it therefore has to inhibit the distractor vector and activate the target vector. This process involves top-down inhibition, based on task demands, and will therefore take time to develop. The high percentage of capture trials in a typical oculomotor capture paradigm indicates that oculomotor inhibition of a salient distractor is only successful in a subset of trials.

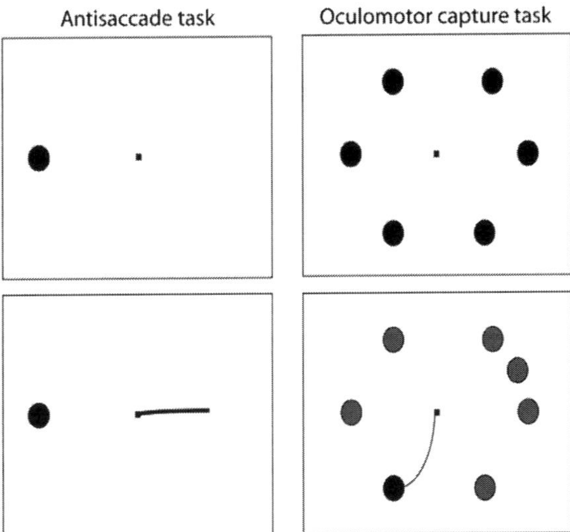

Figure 5.2 Examples of an antisaccade and oculomotor capture trial. In the antisaccade task, observers have to execute an eye movement in the opposite direction of an onset, while observers in the oculomotor capture task have to execute an eye movement to the target while ignoring the onset distractor.

5.8 THE CHARACTERISTICS OF OCULOMOTOR INHIBITION

The advantage of the oculomotor capture paradigm is that the erroneous eye movement is fully based on bottom-up information. The subsequent oculomotor inhibition therefore has to be applied to a reflexive oculomotor program. This is in contrast to the antisaccade task. In this task, the observer has to execute an eye movement in the opposite direction from an onset element, termed an "antisaccade." Because the onset is the only element in the visual display, it is highly salient and will therefore attract a high amount of attention. Because of this, observers generally execute a high number of erroneous "prosaccades" toward the onset before correcting and making an eye movement to the mirrored location. Although a correct antisaccade is fully voluntary, given the empty location toward which it should be executed, the erroneous prosaccade is not fully involuntary. In contrast to the oculomotor capture paradigm, the onset in the antisaccade task is relevant for the execution of the task. Without being aware of its presence and location, it is not possible to correctly perform the task, since the location of the onset distractor should be coded in order to know where the antisaccade should be initiated toward. In the oculomotor capture paradigm, this is not the case as the location of the target is independent of the location of the distractor. Observers in this task are frequently even unaware of the presence of the onset distractor (Kramer, Hahn, Irwin, & Theeuwes, 2000). Differences in inhibition between these two types of tasks have been observed in various populations. For instance, younger children generally perform worse on the antisaccade task compared to older children, whereas no such differences exist on the oculomotor capture task (Kramer, Gonzalez de Sather, & Cassavaugh, 2005). The same holds for elderly, in which older adults show deficits on the antisaccade task compared to younger adults, although no such difference exists on the oculomotor capture task (Kramer et al., 2000). Lastly, children with attention-deficit hyperactivity disorder (ADHD) are impaired on the antisaccade task (C. Klein, Raschke, & Brandenbusch, 2003), whereas they perform normal on the oculomotor capture task, when strictly looking at the percentage oculomotor capture (Van der Stigchel et al., 2007). These results led Kramer et al. (2000) to suggest that there are two types of oculomotor inhibition: an intentional/effortful inhibition, associated with the inhibition of task-relevant information as in the antisaccade task, and automatic/implicit inhibition, observed in the oculomotor capture paradigm associated with the inhibition of task-irrelevant information. According to this view, intentional inhibition is dependent on working memory functioning, explaining the age differences and the deficits in intentional inhibition observed in children with ADHD. Indeed, performance on the antisaccade task is impaired when healthy controls perform a working memory task simultaneously (Mitchell, Macrea, & Gilchrist, 2002).

The dynamics of oculomotor inhibition become evident from studies measuring saccade trajectory deviations. As explained earlier, these deviations in saccade trajectories are generally explained by the inhibition of an unwanted saccade program, resulting in a shift of the initial vector pointing away from the target location. These deviations therefore also reflect the competition between top-down and bottom-up factors. When measured during visual search task in which there is competition between a target and a distractor, two directions of deviations are observed: for saccades with a short latency, saccade trajectories deviate *toward* the distractor (Mulckhuyse, Van der Stigchel, & Theeuwes, 2009; R. Walker, McSorley, & Haggard, 2006). This deviation toward has been claimed to be caused by the unresolved competition between the vector coding for the target and the vector coding for the distractor. Early during the selection process, top-down inhibition did not have the time yet to resolve this competition, because of which the resulting saccade is the average of the two vectors. Later in time, top-down inhibition has inhibited the vector associated with the distractor, resulting in saccade trajectories that deviate *away* from the distractor (Doyle & Walker, 2001; Van der Stigchel, Meeter, & Theeuwes, 2007).

The strength of the deviation away from a distractor is modulated by the strength of the inhibition applied to the distractor vector. For instance, if observers were cued in advance where the target would appear, saccades deviated consistently away from the distractor (R. Walker et al., 2006). The prior knowledge of the target location results in a strong contribution of top-down processes, because the competition can already be partly resolved before the target and distractor are actually presented. These deviations were much smaller, and even in the opposite direction for short latencies, when the target location was unpredictable. These results were extended by findings that cueing the distractor location in advance results in deviation away from the distractor, even in trials in which the distractor location was cued, but the distractor was not presented (Van der Stigchel & Theeuwes, 2006). This result indicates that the observer use such a distractor cue to already inhibit the vector coding for the distractor location, even though this location is empty at the time the cue is presented. Deviations away were even stronger when the distractor was also presented, indicating that additional inhibition was applied based on the physical presence of the distractor, summing up with the inhibition applied on the basis of the distractor cue.

5.9 TOP-DOWN INFLUENCES IN SACCADE AVERAGING

In the studies described above, the distance between the target and the distractor was relatively large. When the target and distractor are presented in close proximity, typically within 30 degrees of angular distance, eye movements to the target generally land on an intermediate location between the target and the distractor (Coren & Hoenig, 1972). This phenomenon has been termed "the global effect" and is claimed to be the result of the averaging of the two saccade vectors (for a review, see Van der Stigchel & Nijboer, 2011). Because the two elements are presented so closely aligned, the application of a large amount of inhibition to the distractor vector would also strongly inhibit the target vector (for a computational model, see Meeter, Van der Stigchel, & Theeuwes, 2010). Therefore, inhibitory processes do not play a large role in the global effect and results are generally explained in terms of the strength of the saccade averaging.

Interestingly, the global effect is more frequent for short saccade latencies (Findlay, 1982). This is in line with the idea that bottom-up information influence the selection process early on, while top-down information becomes dominant for saccades with a longer latency. In the case where a target and distractor are presented, the corresponding vectors will have the same strength as in the case where no top-down influence is present yet. Indeed, the only way to avoid a global effect is to wait 300 ms to initiate a saccade (Ottes, Van Gisbergen, & Eggermont, 1985). When the latency was shorter, the task instruction to fixate the target hardly influenced the saccade endpoint and the saccade was predominantly executed to a location in between the target and the distractor. The relation between the strength of top-down influence and saccade latency has been shown to be linear, with a clear decrease of the global effect with increasing latencies (Heeman, Theeuwes, & Van der Stigchel, 2014). The effect of saccade latency on the global effect is only observed when there is a clear instruction to foveate the target and ignore the distractor and there is a need for selection. In conditions in which no instructions are given, the global effect is observed across the whole latency range (Heeman et al., 2014). In monkeys, the global effect is associated with express saccades, which are saccades with an extremely short latency of less than 100 ms (Chou, Sommer, & Schiller, 1999). Express saccades have been proposed to be purely reflexive movements and are thought to occur within the fastest time possible for a visual stimulus to be translated into a saccade target (Dorris, Pare, & Munoz, 1997).

The strength of the global effect is known to reflect the strength of the various vectors in the oculomotor system. A detailed analysis of the saccade endpoint can therefore unravel the strength of the competition evoked by a certain element. For instance, when two elements are presented, the saccade endpoint will deviate in the direction of the largest stimulus (Findlay, Brogan, & Wenban-Smith, 1993) and the stimulus with the strongest intensity (Deubel, Wolf, & Hauske, 1984). These results indicate that measuring eye movements allow for a more detailed analysis of the dynamics of the selection process compared to simple reaction time experiments, as the temporal and spatial properties of this process can be revealed by examining metrics like the saccade endpoint and the saccade trajectory.

Until now, we have discussed the mechanisms of an intact attentional system. In such a system, the link between attention and eye movements is strong, and there is much control over the programming of eye movements. Although attention might be considered an ill-defined term, studies on patients with deficits in spatial attention have contributed much to a better understanding of the functioning of spatial attention. Most importantly, the consequences of deficits in spatial attention have illustrated how crucial spatial attention is for our daily functioning.

5.10 SPATIAL NEGLECT

Deficits in attention can occur after stroke in that some patients might suffer from a disorder called "hemispatial neglect" which occurs frequently after especially right-hemisphere damage (Stone, Patel, & Greenwood, 1993). Patients with neglect fail to orient to, look at, and/or respond to people or objects approaching from one side of space. Neglect is clinically assessed using varieties of neuropsychological tests (Fig. 5.3), ranging from primarily perceptual-attentional tests (eg, visual search), tests for internal representation (eg, drawing from memory) up to motor-intentional tests (eg, balance, posture) (Barrett, Goedert, & Basso, 2012).

Next to the so-called "spatial bias," patients with neglect often have difficulties in maintaining alertness and vigilance and detecting *nonlateralized* stimuli, probably as a result of deficits in attentional capacity (Husain & Rorden, 2003; Robertson, Mattingley, Rorden, & Driver, 1998). The most common sites of damage are the right inferior parietal up to the ventral frontal cortex (Mort et al., 2003; Vallar & Perani, 1986), superior temporal cortex (Karnath, Fruhmann Berger, Küker, & Rorden, 2004),

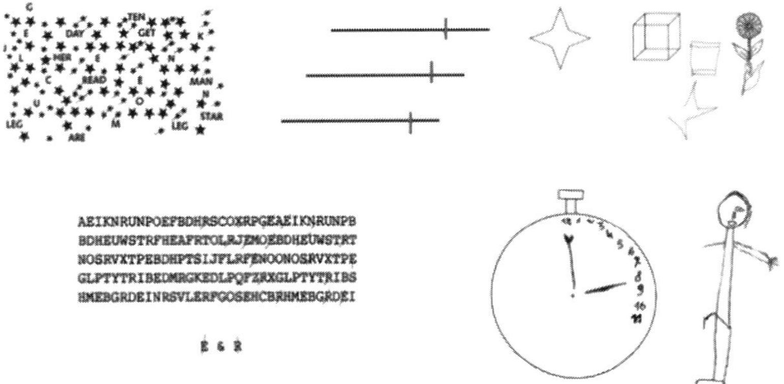

Figure 5.3 Examples of typical neglect tests and typical performance of individuals with neglect.

along with subcortical nuclei (Karnath et al., 2004; Vallar & Perani, 1986). All these regions have been assumed to serve as specialized nodes of one of the two frontoparietal networks that mediates spatial attention, eye-hand coordination (visuomotor behavior) and vigilance (Corbetta, Kincade, Lewis, Snyder, & Sapir, 2005; Heilman, Bowers, Valenstein, & Watson, 1987; Mesulam, 1999). As such, neglect might result from dysfunction of two frontoparietal networks involved in control of attention (Corbetta & Shulman, 2002; He et al., 2007): the *dorsal attention network* that controls allocation of spatial attention to extrapersonal space and selection of stimuli and responses in contralesional space as well as the *ventral attention network* that controls for target detection and reorienting toward salient unexpected events in either hemifield. There appears to be an important asymmetry between ventral and dorsal parietal areas (Abdullaev & Posner, 2005; Corbetta et al., 2005), as damage to the ventral areas also produces dysfunction of the dorsal attention network, causing neglect, whereas more dorsal lesions do not cause malfunctions of the ventral attention network (Friedrich, Egly, Rafal, & Beck, 1998).

5.11 NEGLECT AND CAPTURE

Broadly speaking there are two theories about neglect. Kinsbourne (1987) stressed the inability to direct attention to the contralesional hemispace, either in perception or in representations from memory and imagery. In contrast Marshall and Halligan (1989) emphasized extreme capture of information in the ipsilesional hemispace as the primary cause of neglect. Recording eye movements in neglect patients has given great insight in the underlying mechanisms of spatial attention and especially the abilities and impairments related to neglect. Walker and Findlay (1996), for example, presented neglect patients with two bilateral and simultaneous visual stimuli. Neglect patients predominantly made eye movements to the ipsilesional stimulus. Van der Stigchel and Nijboer (2010) recorded eye movements in a single patient during an oculomotor distractor paradigm. The most important difference between such a paradigm and the paradigm of Walker and Findlay is that the distractor has to be ignored in order to be able to perform the task correctly. The patient in the study by Van der Stigchel and Nijboer was able to make eye movements to targets in both the contralesional and ipsilesional hemifields, suggesting that, at least in that patient, it was not an inability to direct attention to the contralesional hemispace. Yet when the distractor was

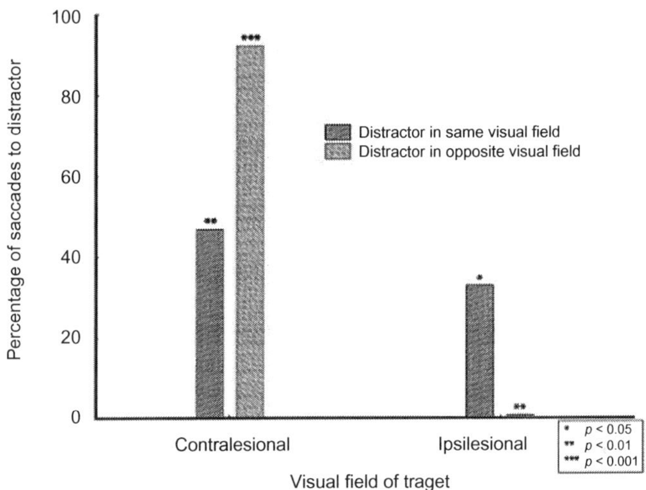

Figure 5.4 Percentage capture when the distractor was presented in the same or opposite field as the target in a single patient with chronic neglect.

presented in the ipsilesional (ie, nonneglected) hemispace, hardly any eye movements were made toward the contralesional target. When the distractor was presented in the contralesional (ie, neglected) hemispace, almost no eye movements were made toward this distractor (see Fig. 5.4). These results were taken to conclude that visual neglect is associated with an imbalance in the saccadic system, with extreme capture by ipsilesional information.

5.12 NEGLECT AND CUEING

The Posner cueing paradigm has been widely used to study spatial attention in neglect. In healthy controls but also stroke patients without neglect, there are no differences between the left and right sided targets. Yet in neglect patients, contralesional target preceded by ipsilesional (invalid) cues result in extremely large reaction times. This is called the extinction like pattern (Posner, 1980) and is often interpreted as a "disengage deficit" (Losier & Klein, 2001; Morrow & Ratcliff, 1988; Olk, Hildebrandt, & Kingstone, 2010; Schindler et al., 2009). Recently, Ten Brink et al. (in revision) investigated whether neglect patients have more difficulties disengaging attention from an object in space compared to a spatial location only. Stroke patients with ($n = 14$) or without ($n = 69$) neglect performed a cueing task. In one version of the task, the informative peripheral cue remained onscreen (object-in-space-condition), whereas in the other version, the cue disappeared (spatial-location-condition). In both versions, neglect patients had difficulties disengaging their attention from ipsilesional invalid cues and this disengage deficit was positively correlated with neglect severity, especially in the object-in-space-condition. Importantly, neglect patients were even slower to respond to contralesional targets when the cue remained on screen compared to when the cue disappeared, showing engage deficits as well. These patterns differed between patients and it is very likely that engage and disengage deficits have a different underlying mechanism, which is likely to be related to a spatial bias.

5.13 RECOVERY OF NEGLECT

Spontaneous neurobiological recovery of neglect occurs within the first 10–12 weeks poststroke onset (Nijboer, Kollen, & Kwakkel, 2013). The presence of neglect has been associated with poor and more attenuated motor recovery (Nijboer, Kollen, & Kwakkel, 2014) and higher disability and lesser independence in activities of daily living compared to patients without neglect (Buxbaum et al., 2004; Cherney, Halper, Kwasnica, Harvey, & Zhang, 2001; Katz, Hartman-Maeir, Ring, & Soroker, 1999; Nijboer, Van de Port, Schepers, Post, & Visser-Meily, 2013). As a result, many studies aim at alleviating neglect with different treatments, such as visual scanning training, limb activation training, sensory stimulation, mental imagery training, and prism adaptation (Kerkhoff & Schenk, 2012; Luaute, Halligan, Rode, Jacquin-Courtois, & Boisson, 2006).

Especially prism adaptation appears to be a promising treatment (Kerkhoff & Schenk, 2012; Luaute et al., 2006). It was first described by Rossetti et al. (1998) and has been widely studied since. Exposure to prisms produces a lateral shift of the visual field so that targets appear displaced (Fig. 5.5A). Usually 10 degrees rightward displacing prisms are

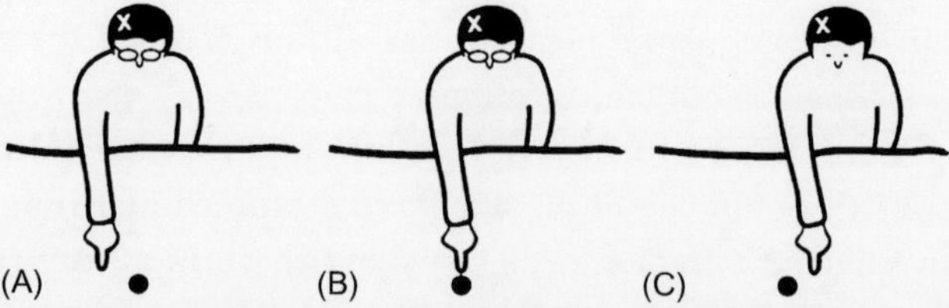

Figure 5.5 Schematic overview of the prism adaptation procedure. *From: Ten Brink, A. F., Visser-Meily, J. M. A. , & Nijboer, T. C. W. , (2014). Effectiviteit van prisma-adaptatie als behandeling voor hemispatieel neglect. Tijdschrift voor Neuropsychologie, 9(1), 2–15. Reproduced with permission from Boom Uitgevers.*

used, so all visual stimuli are perceived to be 10 degrees to the right of their true location. Now when a pointing movement has to be made, the felt position of the arm and hand is not displaced and the pointing movement toward the seen (displaced) position will result in a pointing error. Adaptation to this optical shift requires a set of successive visuomotor pointing movements (Fig. 5.5B). Two important factors contribute to this adaptation: *strategic recalibration* and *spatial realignment* (Newport & Schenk, 2012). Strategic recalibration is the act of consciously perceiving the errors in pointing endpoints, whereas spatial realignment is the more unconscious process of gradually realigning the visual and proprioceptive maps in order to slowly and gradually reduce the errors in pointing endpoints. Especially spatial realignment is considered as the key component of prism adaptation. When the prisms are removed after the adaptation phase, the magnitude of the observed after-effects reflect the amount of realignment between visual and proprioceptive information (Fig. 5.5C).

Rossetti et al. (1998) demonstrated a significant reduction of spatial neglect following a brief period of prism adaptation with rightward prisms. Effects of prism adaptation have been reported across clinical tests of neglect, but also in more daily situations, such as wheelchair navigation (Jacquin-Courtois, Rode, Pisella, Boisson, & Rossetti, 2008), mental imagery (Rode, Rossetti, & Boisson, 1998), and balance (Nijboer, Olthoff, Van der Stigchel, & Visser-Meily, 2014). The beneficial effects of prism adaptation have been reported to last two hours (Rossetti et al., 1998) up to 1 week (Dijkerman, Webeling, ter Wal, Groet, & van Zandvoort, 2004; Pisella, Rode, Farne, Boisson, & Rossetti, 2002) after a single session, and even up to 6 weeks following repetitive prism adaptation (McIntosh, Rossetti, & Milner, 2002; Nys, Seurinck, & Dijkerman, 2008; Shiraishi, Yamakawa, Itou, Muraki, & Asada, 2008). Additionally, long-term prism training has been reported to show long-lasting beneficial effects, from weeks (Frassinetti, Angeli, Meneghello, Avanzi, & Làdavas, 2002; Serino, Barbiani, Rinaldesi, & Làdavas, 2009; Serino, Bonifazi, Pierfederici, & Làdavas, 2007) up to 2 years (Nijboer, Nys, Van der Smagt, Van der Stigchel, & Dijkerman, 2011) after ending prism adaptation.

Prism adaptation seems to alleviate many, yet not all aspects of neglect. Even though this might be frustrating for implementation in a rehabilitation setting, it does create a unique opportunity to investigate the neuroanatomical systems and disentangle various subcategories of the neglect syndrome.

The neuroanatomical systems supporting prism adaptation effects are currently still largely unknown. Both the cerebellum as well as several areas in the parietal cortex have been associated with effects of prism adaptation. Imaging studies have suggested that the right cerebellum is active during both early (Fig. 5.5A) and later (Fig. 5.5B) stages of adaptation and a positive relation was found between activity in the cerebellum during adaptation and prolonged error reduction (Chapman et al., 2010; Luauté et al., 2006). Within the parietal cortex, the inferior and superior parietal lobules and the intraparietal sulcus have been associated with early and late stages of prism adaptation: with improving pointing accuracy, activity in the intraparietal sulcus was reduced and activity in the parieto-occipital sulcus increased (Chapman et al., 2010). It was concluded that error detection involved more inferior regions, while error correction activated more superior regions of the parietal cortex.

Emergent research suggests that prism adaptation might primarily and specifically ameliorate the more motor-intentional deficits and not the perceptual-attentional deficits (Barrett et al., 2012; Nijboer, McIntosh, Nys, Dijkerman, & Milner, 2008; Nijboer, Vree, Dijkerman, & Van der Stigchel, 2010). An additional distinction can be made between vision-for-action and vision-for-perception (Milner & Goodale, 2006; Striemer & Danckert, 2010). Distinct pathways have been described: the ventral pathway (occipito-temporal areas) is largely involved in vision-for-perception, whereas the dorsal pathway (occipito-parietal areas) is largely involved in vision-for-action. As such, Striemer and Danckert (2010) suggested that prism adaptation affects primarily the visuomotor aspects of neglect. This suggestion, however, cannot explain all evidence of the effects of prism adaptation on neglect, such as mental imagery (Rode et al., 1998), visual search performance (Saevarsson, Kristjánsson, Hildebrandt, & Halsband, 2009), but also improvement on the line-bisection task when this task is viewed in the traditional perception-action model distinction (ie, perceptual task). Attention is likely to play an important role here, but its exact role is largely unknown. Interesting dissociations have been reported.

First, there appears to be a dissociation between implicit versus explicit perceptual tasks (Newport & Schenk, 2012): deficits in performance on explicit perceptual tasks seem to benefit more from prism adaptation compared to implicit perceptual tasks. Three different perceptual tasks were used; two in which patients had to judge either emotional expression in chimeric faces or brightness of gray-scale images in which brightness was increased from left to right or from right to left. Importantly, in both these tasks, no right or wrong answer could be given. In the third task, patients had to indicate whether images of faces were normal or chimeric. Here, the given answer could be right or wrong. Performance of neglect patients only improved on the latter task.

Second, prism adaptation seems to improve voluntary attentional shifts but not reflexive ones. In the study of Nijboer et al. (2008) two neglect patients were tested with an adapted version of the Posner cueing paradigm and both patients showed the typical pattern of longer reaction times to left-sided targets, especially when they were preceded by an invalid, right ward cue (Fig. 5.6). After prism adaptation, only the reaction times on the endogenous variant of the cueing task were significantly reduced, especially for the left targets preceded by an arrow pointing toward the right.

Importantly, these dissociations have only been investigated in a few studies with small numbers of patients. It remains to be seen if such dissociations account for larger populations of neglect patients and how prism adaptation influences perception, attention, and/or intention at a neuronal level.

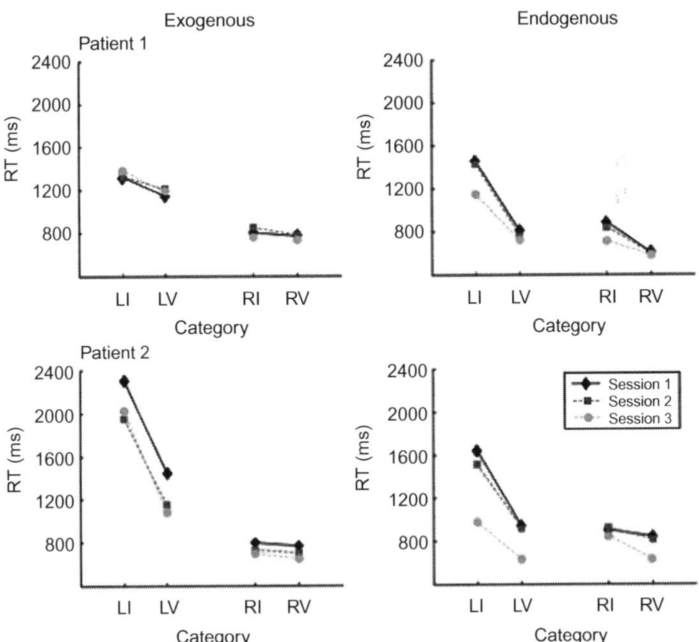

Figure 5.6 Reaction times of the two patients (top vs bottom row). The left panels illustrate the reaction times on the exogenous cueing task, the right panels illustrate the reaction times on the endogenous cueing task. *LV*, left valid; *LI*, left invalid; *RV*, right valid; *RI*, right invalid.

5.14 PROBLEMS WITH THE ATTENTIONAL EXPLANATION OF SPATIAL NEGLECT: A NEW THEORY

Although spatial neglect has been generally explained as an attentional deficit (Kinsbourne, 1987; Mesulam, 1999), it is becoming increasingly evident that the concept of attention is not sufficient to explain all of the problems observed in patients with neglect. This is partly due to the fact that attention is so ill-defined. Until now, this chapter has not provided a clear definition of what attention is. The reason for this is quite simple: nobody knows what attention is. The description of neglect is helpful to support this claim: although neglect is considered an attentional problem, it is questionable what this attentional problem exactly is. If you realize that normal observers without neglect only have a very limited attentional capacity and ignore a large portion of their environment, one might argue that everyone has an attentional deficit to some extent. Still, there is something special about neglect which results in ignoring a large portion of their visual worlds. Although we are not going to solve this puzzle in this chapter, we will highlight one aspect of the neglect syndrome that might contribute to their problems in daily life. In order to do this, we will first introduce a concept known as "spatial remapping."

The image projected on our retina changes rapidly with each saccade. With each new fixation our brain therefore has to integrate the old and new retinal images with information about the current eye position and the magnitude and direction in which gaze was displaced by the most recent saccade. The saving, updating, and relocalization of the different parts of a visual scene, referred to as "spatial remapping," allow us to accurately determine the location of external targets and generate eye or limb movements to these targets. So, imagine that after each eye movement ("saccade") you make, you would lose all information about the position of all objects in your environment. You would have no idea which shelves you have already searched when looking for that one jazz record, simply because that information is not maintained after a saccade (see Fig. 5.7). This will likely result in very inefficient search in which you revisit previously searched shelves. Although hard to imagine, it may be one of the problems you encounter when you do not have the capacity to remap and update spatial information.

Neurons with spatial remapping properties have been identified in a region within the posterior parietal cortex, the lateral intraparietal area (Duhamel, Colby, & Goldberg, 1992). Using single cell recording in

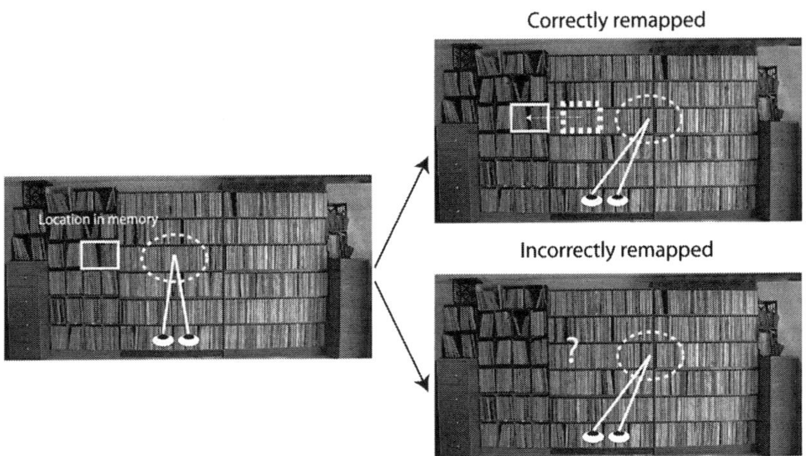

Figure 5.7 After each saccade, the brain has to remap the location of objects in memory to maintain a representation of their correct location in space. When remapping is successful, the true world coordinates of objects will still be available after the saccade. In this example, this would mean that the remembered location of where you had previously searched would be updated with respect to new fixation location. When remapping fails, however, the location of the previously searched shelves relative to the current one will be wrong or completely lost.

monkeys, Duhamel and colleagues observed neurons that responded when a saccade brought the location of a target into their receptive field, even when the target was extinguished before the saccade. Furthermore, other cells responded to targets outside their current receptive field, but only if the target would be brought into the receptive field by an imminent saccade, suggesting predictive shifts in the representations of visual stimuli (Colby, Duhamel, & Goldberg, 1996; Gnadt & Andersen, 1988). This updating in the posterior parietal cortex occurs in concert with other areas with spatial remapping properties: the superior colliculus (M. F. Walker, Fitzgibbon, & Goldberg, 1995), frontal eye fields (Umeno & Goldberg, 1997), and striate and extrastriate cortex (Nakamura & Colby, 2002). These remapping properties are often thought to underlie our perception of a stable visual world, by compensating for the shifts in retinal image that accompany each saccade (Burr & Morrone, 2011; Melcher, 2007; Sommer & Wurtz, 2006).

Although we have the perception of a fully stable world, experimental studies have shown that this stability only reflects a surprisingly limited number of objects. For instance, it is possible to make remarkably large changes to a visual scene during a saccade without the viewer becoming aware of them (Henderson & Hollingworth, 1999). Furthermore, it has been estimated that at most three or four objects can be retained across a saccade (Irwin, 1992) and that only the most salient or behaviorally relevant objects (ie, attended objects) are actually remapped (Cavanagh, Hunt, Afraz, & Rolfs, 2010; Gottlieb, Kusunoki, & Goldberg, 1998). As a result, the perception of a stable visual world only reflects the few objects that are remapped after a saccade. Spatial remapping is therefore a selective mechanism that allows retention of relevant spatial information across saccades. Because we execute multiple saccades per second, any attended location has to be remapped almost continuously. Any information about an attended object might be lost after a saccade if spatial remapping is inadequate. Successful spatial attention therefore crucially depends on reliable remapping.

Deficits in spatial remapping might be one of the factors contributing to the neglect syndrome (Pisella & Mattingley, 2004). As mentioned, there are numerous problems with the explanation of neglect as a disorder of spatial attention. For instance, why would a neglect patient frequently revisit targets in the ipsilesional visual field during a search task (Malhotra, Mannan, Driver, & Husain, 2004; Mannan et al., 2005; Nys, Stuart, & Dijkerman, 2010; Rusconi, Maravita, Bottini, & Vallar, 2002) or have difficulty determining whether he or she has already looked at an element (Behrmann, Watt, Black, & Barton, 1997; Husain et al., 2001; Wojciulik, Husain, Clarke, & Driver, 2001)? If their deficit were merely one of a reduced attentional field, then the patient would simply stop searching once they had explored all of ipsilateral space. It may be that due to failures in remapping, memory for previously visited locations is impaired, resulting in frequent revisits. Furthermore, patients copy only half a picture, but in doing so sometimes transport visual information from the contralesional side to the ipsilesional side (*allochiria*) (Di Pellegrino, 1995; Halligan, Marshall, & Wade, 1992). By viewing neglect as a problem in spatial remapping, allochiria can be explained by deficits in remapping: information is wrongly remapped and is therefore transported to the wrong location in a visual scene (Pisella & Mattingley, 2004). There is indeed some evidence that neglect patients have problems with remapping information (Denis, Beschin, Logie, & Della Sala, 2002; Pisella, Berberovic, & Mattingley, 2004; Pisella & Mattingley, 2004; Vuilleumier et al., 2007). For instance, Vuilleumier and colleagues showed in a visual working memory task that when neglect patients had to remember the location of a stimulus, memory of the spatial location was diminished after a saccade had been made, indicating that the location of the to be remembered stimulus was not remapped correctly (Vuilleumier et al., 2007).

Although we do not claim that deficits in spatial remapping can explain all deficits in spatial neglect, it might be that any attentional imbalance between the two visual fields is modulated by a deficit in spatial remapping. As neglect is a syndrome with a large number of different brain areas involved, it is very likely that not every neglect patient will have remapping deficit. Depending on the location of the lesion, one neglect patient might show deficits in remapping, whereas another patient with neglect will perform normally on experiments tapping into spatial remapping.

5.15 CONCLUSION

In this chapter, our aim was to provide an overview of what spatial attention entails. As we already warned in the introduction, spatial attention consists of multiple components, varying from bottom-up and top-down attention to subcomponents like spatial remapping and spatial working memory. Perhaps the most simple definition is one in which the limited processing capacity is not explained as a limitation, but as a way to select one specific spatial location and successfully ignore information presented at other locations. For efficient behavior, the key is to know which information is relevant and to keep focus on that information. Imagine a situation in which one can process all information: entering a supermarket will cause an overflow of completely irrelevant information, resulting in a problem for systems governing our memory and reasoning. Selection of relevant information allows these other cognitive systems to work effectively.

With the rise of affordable eye-trackers, eye movement recording systems will soon be integrated in many communication systems, like tablets and smartphones. These systems will therefore be able to know what is relevant for the user at a given moment in time, given the close link between attention and eye movements. This will allow companies to know where we are looking and will give advertisers control about where to present an advertisement such that the user will foveate it.

Perhaps these new technologies will aid also patients suffering from deficits in spatial attention. Although many rehabilitation techniques, like prism adaptation, are promising, there is still little transition between the experimental studies on these techniques and actual neural rehabilitation treatments. The gap between experimental psychology, neuropsychology, and neural rehabilitation will hopefully be filled in the coming years. One crucial factor in this transition will be a better diagnosis of which aspect of spatial attention is impaired in a given patient. Different techniques might improve different aspects of spatial attention, whereas not all patients might be impaired in all aspects of spatial attention. It is therefore very unlikely that one rehabilitation technique will be effective for all patients, given the wide variety in possible underlying disorders.

REFERENCES

Abdullaev, Y., & Posner, M. I. (2005). How the brain recovers following damage. *Nature Neuroscience*, *8*(11), 1424–1425.

Awh, E., & Jonides, J. (2001). Overlapping mechanisms of attention and spatial working memory. *Trends in Cognitive Sciences*, *5*(3), 119–126.

Bacon, W. F., & Egeth, H. E. (1994). Overriding stimulus-driven attentional capture. *Perception & Psychophysics*, *55*, 485–496.

Barrett, A. M., Goedert, K. M., & Basso, J. C. (2012). Prism adaptation for spatial neglect after stroke: Translational practice gaps. *Nature Reviews Neurology*, *8*, 567–577.

Behrmann, M., Watt, S., Black, S. E., & Barton, J. J. S. (1997). Impaired visual search in patients with unilateral neglect: An oculographic analysis. *Neuropsychologia*, *35*(11), 1445–1458.

Belopolsky, A. V., & Theeuwes, J. (2009). When are attention and saccade preparation dissociated? *Psychological Science*, *29*, 1340–1347.

Belopolsky, A. V., Zwaan, L., Theeuwes, J., & Kramer, A. F. (2007). The size of an attentional window modulates attentional capture by color singletons. *Psychonomic Bulletin & Review*, *14*(5), 934–938.

Burr, D., & Morrone, M. C. (2011). Spatiotopic coding and remapping in humans. *Philosophical Transactions of the Royal Society: B*, *366*, 504–515.

Buxbaum, L. J., Ferraro, M. K., Veramonti, T., Farne, A., Whyte, J., Ladavas, E., et al. (2004). Hemispatial neglect: Subtypes, neuroanatomy, and disability. *Neurology*, *9*(62), 749–756.

Cavanagh, P., Hunt, A. R., Afraz, A., & Rolfs, M. (2010). Visual stability based on remapping of attention pointers. *Trends in Cognitive Sciences*, *14*(4), 147–153.

Chapman, H. L., Eramudugolla, R., Gavrilescu, M., Strudwick, M. W., Loftus, A., Cunnington, R., et al. (2010). Neural mechanisms underlying spatial realignment during adaptation to optical wedge prisms. *Neuropsychologia*, *48*(9), 2595–2601.

Cherney, L. R., Halper, A. S., Kwasnica, C. M., Harvey, R. L., & Zhang, M. (2001). Recovery of functional status after right hemisphere stroke: Relationship with unilateral neglect. *Archives of Physical Medicine and Rehabilitation*, *82*(3), 322–328.

Chou, I., Sommer, M. A., & Schiller, P. H. (1999). Express averaging saccades in monkeys. *Vision Research*, *39*, 4200–4216.

Colby, C. L., Duhamel, J.-R., & Goldberg, M. E. (1996). Visual, motor and cognitive activation in the monkey lateral intraparietal area. *Journal of Neurophysiology*, *76*, 2841–2852.

Corbetta, M., Akbudak, E., Conturo, T., Snyder, A. Z., Ollinger, J. M., Drury, H. A., et al. (1998). A common network of functional areas for attention and eye movements. *Neuron*, *21*(4), 761–773.

Corbetta, M., Kincade, M. J., Lewis, C., Snyder, A. Z., & Sapir, A. (2005). Neural basis and recovery of spatial attention deficits in spatial neglect. *Nature Neuroscience*, *8*(11), 1603–1610.

Corbetta, M., & Shulman, G. L. (2002). Control of goal-directed and stimulus-driven attention in the brain. *Nature Neuroscience*, *3*, 201–215.

Coren, S., & Hoenig, P. (1972). Effect of non-target stimuli on the length of voluntary saccades. *Perceptual and Motor Skills*, *34*, 499–508.

Craighero, L., Carta, A., & Fadiga, L. (2001). Peripheral oculomotor palsy affects orienting of visuospatial attention. *Neuroreport*, *12*, 3283–3286.

Denis, M., Beschin, N., Logie, R. H., & Della Sala, S. (2002). Visual perception and verbal descriptions as sources for generating mental representations: Evidence from representational neglect. *Cognitive Neuropsychology*, *19*(2), 97–112.

Deubel, H. (2008). The time course of presaccadic attention shifts. *Psychological Research*, *72*(6), 630–640.

Deubel, H., & Schneider, W. X. (1996). Saccade target selection and object recognition: Evidence for a common attentional mechanism. *Vision Research*, *36*(12), 1827–1837.

Deubel, H., & Schneider, W. X. (2003). Delayed saccades, but not delayed manual aiming movements, require visual attention shifts. *Annals of the New York Academy of Sciences*, *1004*, 289–296.

Deubel, H., Wolf, W., & Hauske, M. (1984). The evaluation of the oculomotor error signal. In A. G. Gale, & F. W. Johnson (Eds.), *Theoretical and applied aspects of oculomotor research* (pp. 55–62). Amsterdam: Elsevier.

Di Pellegrino, G. (1995). Clock-drawing in a case of left visuo-spatial neglect: A deficit of disengagement. *Neuropsychologia*, *33*(3), 353–358.

Dijkerman, H. C., Webeling, M., ter Wal, J. M., Groet, E., & van Zandvoort, M. J. (2004). A long-lasting improvement of somatosensory function after prism adaptation, a case study. *Neuropsychologia*, *42*(12), 1697–1702.

Dodd, M. D., Castel, A. D., & Pratt, J. (2003). Inhibition of return with rapid serial shifts of attention: Implications for memory and visual search. *Perception & Psychophysics*, *65*(7), 1126–1135.

Dodd, M. D., Van der Stigchel, S., Leghari, M. A., Fung, G., & Kingstone, A. (2008). Attentional SNARC: There's something special about numbers (let us count the ways). *Cognition*, *108*(3), 810–818.

Dorris, M. C., Pare, M., & Munoz, D. P. (1997). Neuronal activity in monkey superior colliculus related to the initiation of saccadic eye movements. *Journal of Neuroscience*, *17*, 8566–8579.

Doyle, M. C., & Walker, R. (2001). Curved saccade trajectories: Voluntary and reflexive saccades curve away from irrelevant distractors. *Experimental Brain Research*, *139*, 333–344.

Duhamel, J.-R., Colby, C. L., & Goldberg, M. E. (1992). The updating of the representation of visual space in parietal cortex by intended eye movements. *Science*, *255*, 90–92.

Duncan, J. (2006). Brain mechanisms of attention. *The Quarterly Journal of Experimental Psychology*, *59*(1), 2–27.

Eriksen, C. W., & St James, J. (1986). Visual attention within and around the field of focal attention: A zoom lens model. *Perception & Psychophysics*, *40*, 225–240.

Findlay, J. M. (1982). Global visual processing for saccadic eye movements. *Vision Research*, *22*, 1033–1045.

Findlay, J. M., Brogan, D., & Wenban-Smith, M. G. (1993). The spatial signal for saccadic eye movements emphasizes visual boundaries. *Perception & Psychophysics*, *53*(6), 633–641.

Fischer, M. H., Castel, A. D., Dodd, M. D., & Pratt, J. (2003). Perceiving numbers causes spatial shifts of attention. *Nature Neuroscience*, *6*, 555–556.

Folk, C. L., Remington, R. W., & Johnston, J. C. (1992). Involuntary covert orienting is contingent on attentional control settings. *Journal of Experimental Psychology: Human Perception and Performance*, *18*(4), 1030–1044.

Frassinetti, F., Angeli, V., Meneghello, F., Avanzi, S., & Làdavas, E. (2002). Long-lasting amelioration of visuospatial neglect by prism adaptation. *Brain*, *125*(3), 608–623.

Friedrich, F. J., Egly, R., Rafal, R. D., & Beck, D. (1998). Spatial attention deficits in humans: A comparison of superior parietal and temporal-parietal junction lesions. *Neuropsychology*, *12*(2), 193–207.

Friesen, C. K., & Kingstone, A. (1998). The eyes have it! Reflexive orienting is triggered by nonpredictive gaze. *Psychonomic Bulletin & Review*, *5*(3), 490–495.

Gabay, S., Henik, A., & Gradstein, L. (2010). Ocular motor ability and covert attention in patients with Duane Retraction Syndrome. *Neuropsychologia*, *48*(10), 3102–3109.

Gnadt, J. W., & Andersen, R. A. (1988). Memory related motor planning activity in posterior parietal cortex of macaque. *Experimental Brain Research*, *70*(1), 216–220.

Godijn, R., & Theeuwes, J. (2002). Programming of endogenous and exogenous saccades: Evidence for a competitive integration model. *Journal of Experimental Psychology: Human Perception and Performance*, *28*(5), 1039–1054.

Gottlieb, J. P., Kusunoki, M., & Goldberg, M. E. (1998). The representation of visual salience in monkey parietal cortex. *Nature*, *391*, 481–484.

Halligan, P. W., Marshall, J. C., & Wade, D. T. (1992). Left on the right: Allochiria in a case of left visuo-spatial neglect. *Journal of Neurology, Neurosurgery & Psychiatry*, *55*, 717–719.

He, B. J., Snyder, A. Z., Vincent, J. L., Epstein, A., Shulman, G. L., & Corbetta, M. (2007). Breakdown of functional connectivity in frontoparietal networks underlies behavioral deficits in spatial neglect. *Neuron*, *53*(6), 905–918.

Heeman, J., Theeuwes, J., & Van der Stigchel, S. (2014). The time course of top-down control on saccade averaging. *Vision Research*, *100*, 29–37.

Heilman, K. M., Bowers, D., Valenstein, E., & Watson, R. T. (1987). Hemispace and hemispatial neglect. In M. Jeannerod (Ed.), *Neurophysiological and neuropsychological aspects of spatial neglect* (pp. 115–150). Amsterdam: North-Holland.

Henderson, J. M., & Hollingworth, A. (1999). High-level scene perception. *Annual Review of Psychology*, *50*, 243–271.

Hickey, C., McDonald, J. J., & Theeuwes, J. (2006). Electrophysiological evidence of the capture of visual attention. *Journal of Cognitive Neuroscience*, *18*(4), 604–613.

Hoffman, J. E., & Subramaniam, B. (1995a). The role of visual attention in saccadic eye movements. *Perception & Psychophysics*, *37*(6), 787–795.

Hoffman, J. E., & Subramaniam, B. (1995b). Saccadic eye movements and visual selective attention. *Perception & Psychophysics*, *57*, 787–795.

Hommel, B., Pratt, J., Colzato, L., & Godijn, R. (2001). Symbolic control of visual attention. *Psychological Science*, *12*(5), 360–365.

Hunt, A. R., & Kingstone, A. (2003). Covert and overt voluntary attention: Linked or independent? *Cognitive Brain Research*, *18*, 102–105.

Husain, M., Mannan, S., Hodgson, T. L., Wojciulik, E., Driver, J., & Kennard, C. (2001). Impaired spatial working memory across saccades contributes to abnormal search in parietal neglect. *Brain*, *124*(5), 941–952.

Husain, M., & Rorden, C. (2003). Non-spatially lateralized mechanisms in hemispatial neglect. *Nature Reviews Neuroscience*, *4*, 26–36.

Irwin, D. E. (1992). Memory for position and identity across eye movements. *Journal of Experimental Psychology: Learning, Memory and Cognition*, *18*(2), 307–317.

Itti, L., & Koch, C. (2000). A saliency-based search mechanism for overt and covert shifts of visual attention. *Vision Research*, *40*, 1489–1506.

Jacquin-Courtois, S., Rode, G., Pisella, L., Boisson, D., & Rossetti, Y. (2008). Wheel-chair driving improvement following visuo-manual prism adaptation. *Cortex*, *44*(1), 90–96.

James, W. (1890). *The principles of psychology*. London: MacMillan.
Jonides, J. (1981). Voluntary versus automatic control over the mind's eye's movement. *Attention and performance* (Vol. IX, pp. 187–203). Hillsdale, NJ: Erlbaum.
Jonides, J., & Yantis, S. (1988). Uniqueness of abrupt visual onset in capturing attention. *Perception & Psychophysics, 43*, 346–354.
Karnath, H. O., Fruhmann Berger, M., Küker, W., & Rorden, C. (2004). The anatomy of spatial neglect based on voxelwise statistical analysis: A study of 140 patients. *Cerebral Cortex, 14*(10), 1164–1172.
Katz, N., Hartman-Maeir, A., Ring, H., & Soroker, N. (1999). Functional disability and rehabilitation outcome in right hemisphere damaged patients with and without unilateral spatial neglect. *Archives of Physical Medicine and Rehabilitation, 80*(4), 379–384.
Kerkhoff, G., & Schenk, T. (2012). Rehabilitation of neglect: An update. *Neuropsychologia, 50*(6), 1072–1079.
Kinsbourne, M. (1987). Mechanisms of unilateral neglect. In M. Jeannerod (Ed.), *Neurophysiological and neuropsychological aspects of spatial neglect* (pp. 69–86). Amsterdam: Elsevier Science Publishers.
Klein, C., Raschke, A., & Brandenbusch, A. (2003). Development of pro- and antisaccades in children with attention-deficit hyperactivity disorder (ADHD) and healthy controls. *Psychophysiology, 40*, 17–28.
Klein, R. M., & MacInnes, W. J. (1999). Inhibition of return is a foraging facilitator in visual search. *Psychological Science, 10*, 346–352.
Klein, R. M., & Taylor, T. L. (1994). Categories of cognitive inhibition with reference to attention. In D. Dagenbach, & T. H. Carr (Eds.), *Inhibitory processes in attention, memory, and language* (pp. 113–150). San Diego, CA: Academic Press.
Kowler, E., Anderson, E., Dosher, B., & Blaser, E. (1995). The role of attention in the programming of saccades. *Vision Research, 35*(13), 1897–1916.
Kramer, A. F., Gonzalez de Sather, J. C. M., & Cassavaugh, N. D. (2005). Development of attentional and oculomotor control. *Developmental Psychology, 41*(5), 760–772.
Kramer, A. F., Hahn, S., Irwin, D. E., & Theeuwes, J. (2000). Age differences in the control of looking behavior: Do you know where your eyes have been? *Psychological Science, 11*(3), 210–217.
Losier, B. J., & Klein, R. M. (2001). A review of the evidence for a disengage deficit following parietal lobe damage. *Neuroscience and Biobehavioural Reviews, 25*(1), 1–13.
Luaute, J., Halligan, P., Rode, G., Jacquin-Courtois, S., & Boisson, D. (2006). Prism adaptation first among equals in alleviating left neglect: A review. *Restorative Neurology and Neuroscience, 24*, 409–418.
Luauté, J., Michel, C., Rode, G., Pisella, L., Jacquin-Courtois, S., Costes, N., et al. (2006). Functional anatomy of the therapeutic effects of prism adaptation on left neglect. *Neurology, 66*, 1859–1867.
Luck, S. J., Girelli, M., McDermott, M. T., & Ford, M. A. (1997). Bridging the gap between monkey neurophysiology and human perception: An ambiguity resolution theory of visual selective attention. *Cognitive Psychology, 33*, 64–87.
Malhotra, P., Mannan, S., Driver, J., & Husain, M. (2004). Impaired visual spatial memory: One component of the visual neglect syndrome? *Cortex, 40*, 667–676.
Mannan, S. K., Mort, D. J., Hodgson, T. L., Driver, J., Kennard, C., & Husain, M. (2005). Revisiting previously searched locations in visual neglect: Role of right parietal and frontal lesions in misjudging old locations as new. *Journal of Cognitive Neuroscience, 17*(2), 340–354.
Marshall, J. C., & Halligan, P. W. (1989). Does the midsagittal plane play any privileged role in "left" neglect? *Cognitive Neuropsychology, 6*(4), 403–422.
McIntosh, R. D., Rossetti, Y., & Milner, A. D. (2002). Prism adaptation improves chronic visual and haptic neglect: A single case study. *Cortex, 38*, 309–320.

Meeter, M., Van der Stigchel, S., & Theeuwes, J. (2010). A competitive integration model of exogenous and endogenous eye movements. *Biological Cybernetics*, *102*, 271–291.

Melcher, D. (2007). Predictive remapping of visual features precedes saccadic eye movements. *Nature Neuroscience*, *10*(7), 903–907.

Mesulam, M. M. (1999). Spatial attention and neglect: Parietal, frontal and cingulate contributions to the mental representation and attentional targeting of salient extrapersonal events. *Philosophical Transactions of the Royal Society: B*, *354*, 1325–1346.

Milner, A. D., & Goodale, M. A. (2006). *The visual brain in action* (2nd ed.). Oxford: Psychology Press.

Mitchell, J. P., Macrea, C. N., & Gilchrist, I. D. (2002). Working memory and the suppression of reflexive saccades. *Journal of Cognitive Neuroscience*, *14*(1), 95–103.

Moore, T., & Fallah, M. (2004). Microstimulation of the frontal eye field and its effects on covert spatial attention. *Journal of Neurophysiology*, *91*(1), 152–162.

Morrow, L. A., & Ratcliff, G. (1988). The disengagement of covert attention and the neglect syndrome. *Psychobiology*, *16*, 261–269.

Mort, D. J., Malhotra, P., Mannan, S. K., Rorden, C., Pambakian, A., Kennard, C., et al. (2003). The anatomy of visual neglect. *Brain*, *126*(9), 1986–1997.

Mulckhuyse, M., Van der Stigchel, S., & Theeuwes, J. (2009). Early and late modulation of saccade deviations by target distractor similarity. *Journal of Neurophysiology*, *102*(3), 1451–1458.

Nakamura, K., & Colby, C. L. (2002). Updating of the visual representation in monkey striate and extrastriate cortex during saccades. *Proceedings of the National Academy of Sciences*, *99*(6), 4026–4031.

Nakayama, K., & Joseph, J. S. (1998). Attention, pattern recognition, and pop-out in visual search. In R. Parasuraman (Ed.), *The attentive brain* (pp. 279–298). Cambridge: MIT Press.

Newport, R., & Schenk, T. (2012). Prisms and neglect: What have we learned? *Neuropsychologia*, *50*(6), 1080–1091.

Nijboer, T. C. W., Kollen, B. J., & Kwakkel, G. (2013). Time course of visuospatial neglect early after stroke: A longitudinal cohort study. *Cortex*, *49*(8), 2021–2027.

Nijboer, T. C. W., Kollen, B. J., & Kwakkel, G. (2014). The impact of recovery of visuospatial neglect on motor recovery of the upper paretic limb after stroke. *PLoS One*, *9*(6), e100584.

Nijboer, T. C. W., McIntosh, R. D., Nys, G. M. S., Dijkerman, H. C., & Milner, A. D. (2008). Prism adaptation improves voluntary but not automatic orienting in neglect. *Neuroreport*, *19*(3), 293–298.

Nijboer, T. C. W., Nys, G. M. S., Van der Smagt, M., Van der Stigchel, S., & Dijkerman, H. C. (2011). Repetitive long-term prism adaptation permanently improves the detection of contralesional visual stimuli in a patient with chronic neglect. *Cortex*, *47*(6), 734–740.

Nijboer, T. C. W., Olthoff, L., Van der Stigchel, S., & Visser-Meily, A. (2014). Prism adaptation improves postural imbalance in neglect patients. *Neuroreport*, *25*(5), 307–311.

Nijboer, T. C. W., Van de Port, I., Schepers, V. P., Post, M. W., & Visser-Meily, A. (2013). Predicting functional outcome after stroke: The influence of neglect on basic activities in daily life. *Frontiers in Human Neuroscience*, *7*, 182.

Nijboer, T. C. W., Vree, A., Dijkerman, H. C., & Van der Stigchel, S. (2010). Prism adaptation influences perception but not attention: Evidence from antisaccades. *Neuroreport*, *21*(5), 386–389.

Nobre, A. C., Gitelman, D. R., Dias, E. C., & Mesulam, M. M. (2000). Covert visual spatial orienting and saccades: Overlapping neural systems. *Neuroimage*, *11*(3), 210–216.

Nothdurft, H.-C. (2000). Salience from feature contrast: Temporal properties of saliency mechanisms. *Vision Research*, *40*(18), 2421–2435.

Nummenmaa, L., & Hietanen, J. K. (2006). Gaze distractors influence saccadic curvature: Evidence for the role of the oculomotor system in gaze-cued orienting. *Vision Research*, *46*(11), 3674–3680.

Nys, G. M., Seurinck, R., & Dijkerman, H. C. (2008). Prism adaptation moves neglect-related perseveration to contralesional space. *Cognitive and Behavioral Neurology*, *21*(4), 249–253.

Nys, G. M., Stuart, M., & Dijkerman, H. C. (2010). Repetitive exploration towards locations that no longer carry a target in patients with neglect. *Journal of Neuropsychology*, *4*(1), 33–45.

Olivers, C. N. L., Meijer, F., & Theeuwes, J. (2006). Feature-based memory-driven attentional capture: Visual working memory content affects visual attention. *Journal of Experimental Psychology: Human Perception and Performance*, *32*, 1243–1265.

Olk, B., Hildebrandt, H., & Kingstone, A. (2010). Involuntary but not voluntary orienting contributes to a disengage deficit in visual neglect. *Cortex*, *46*(9), 1149–1164.

Ottes, F. B., Van Gisbergen, J. A. M., & Eggermont, J. J. (1985). Latency dependence of colour-based target vs nontarget discrimination by the saccadic system. *Vision Research*, *25*, 849–862.

Peterson, M. S., Kramer, A. F., & Irwin, D. E. (2004). Covert shifts of attention precede involuntary eye movements. *Perception & Psychophysics*, *66*(3), 398–405.

Pisella, L., Berberovic, N., & Mattingley, J. B. (2004). Impaired working memory for location but not for colour or shape in visual neglect: A comparison of parietal and non-parietal lesions. *Cortex*, *40*(2), 379–390.

Pisella, L., & Mattingley, J. B. (2004). The contribution of spatial remapping impairments to unilateral visual neglect. *Neuroscience and Biobehavioural Reviews*, *28*(2), 181–200.

Pisella, L., Rode, G., Farne, A., Boisson, D., & Rossetti, Y. (2002). Dissociated long lasting improvements of straight ahead pointing and line bisection tasks in two hemineglect patients. *Neuropsychologia*, *40*(3), 327–334.

Posner, M. I. (1980). Orienting of attention, the VIIth Sir Frederic Bartlett Lecture. *Quarterly Journal of Experimental Psychology*, *32*, 3–25.

Posner, M. I., & Cohen, Y. (1984). Components of visual orienting. In H. Bouma, & D. G. Bouwhuis (Eds.), *Attention and performance X: Control of language processes* (pp. 531–556). Hillsdale, NJ: Lawrence Erlbaum.

Posner, M. I., & Petersen, S. E. (1990). The attention system of the human brain. *Annual Review of Neuroscience*, *13*, 25–42.

Postle, B. R., Awh, E., Jonides, J., Smith, E. E., & D'Esposito, M. (1999). The where and how of attention-based rehearsal in spatial working memory. *Cognitive Brain Research*, *20*, 194–205.

Rizzolatti, G., Riggio, L., Dascola, I., & Umilta, C. (1987). Reorienting attention across the horizontal and vertical meridians: Evidence in favor of a premotor theory of attention. *Neuropsychologia*, *25*, 31–40.

Rizzolatti, G., Riggio, L., & Sheliga, B. M. (1994). Space and selective attention. In C. Umilta, & M. Moscovitch (Eds.), *Attention and performance XIV* (pp. 231–265). Cambridge: MIT Press.

Robertson, I. H., Mattingley, J. B., Rorden, C., & Driver, J. (1998). Phasic alerting of neglect patients overcomes their spatial deficit in visual awareness. *Nature*, *395*, 169–172.

Rode, G., Rossetti, Y., & Boisson, D. (1998). Improvement of mental imagery after prism exposure in neglect: A case study. *Behavioural Neurology*, *11*(4), 251–258.

Rossetti, Y., Rode, G., Pisella, L., Farne, A., Li, L., Biosson, D., et al. (1998). Prism adaptation to a rightward optical deviation rehabilitates left hemispatial neglect. *Nature*, *395*(6698), 166–169.

Rubin, E. (1965/1925). *Die Nichtexistenz der Aufmerksamkeit (Psykologiske Tekster, 1).* Copenhagen: Akademisk Forlag.

Rusconi, M. L., Maravita, A., Bottini, G., & Vallar, G. (2002). Is the intact side really intact? Perseverative responses in patients with unilateral neglect: A productive manifestation. *Neuropsychologia*, *40*(6), 594–604.

Saevarsson, S., Kristjánsson, A., Hildebrandt, H., & Halsband, U. (2009). Prism adaptation improves visual search in hemispatial neglect. *Neuropsychologia*, *47*(3), 717–725.

Schindler, I., McIntosh, R. D., Cassidy, T. P., Birchall, D., Benson, V., Ietswaart, M., et al. (2009). The disengage deficit in hemispatial neglect is restricted to between-object shifts and is abolished by prism adaptation. *Experimental Brain Research*, *192*(3), 499–510.

Serino, A., Barbiani, M., Rinaldesi, M. L., & Làdavas, E. (2009). Effectiveness of prism adaptation in neglect rehabilitation: A controlled trial study. *Stroke*, *40*(4), 1392–1398.

Serino, A., Bonifazi, S., Pierfederici, L., & Làdavas, E. (2007). Neglect treatment by prism adaptation: What recovers and for how long. *Neuropsychological Rehabilitation*, 7(6), 657–687.

Sheliga, B. M., Riggio, L., & Rizzolatti, G. (1994). Orienting of attention and eye movements. *Experimental Brain Research*, *98*, 507–522.

Sheliga, B. M., Riggio, L., & Rizzolatti, G. (1995). Spatial attention and eye movements. *Experimental Brain Research*, *105*, 261–275.

Shiraishi, H., Yamakawa, Y., Itou, A., Muraki, T., & Asada, T. (2008). Long-term effects of prism adaptation on chronic neglect after stroke. *Neurorehabilitation*, *23*(2), 137–151.

Silvis, J. D., & Van der Stigchel, S. (2014). How memory mechanisms are a key component in the guidance of our eye movements: Evidence from the global effect. *Psychonomic Bulletin & Review*, *21*(2), 357–362.

Smith, D. T., Rorden, C., & Jackson, S. R. (2004). Exogenous orienting of attention depends upon the ability to execute eye movements. *Current Biology*, *14*(9), 792–795.

Smith, D. T., Rorden, C., & Schenk, T. (2012). Saccade preparation is required for exogenous attention but not endogenous attention or IOR. *Journal of Experimental Psychology: Human Perception and Performance*, *38*(6), 1438–1447.

Smith, D. T., & Schenk, T. (2012). The premotor theory of attention: Time to move on? *Neuropsychologia*, *50*, 1104–1114.

Sommer, M. A., & Wurtz, R. H. (2006). Influence of the thalamus on spatial visual processing in frontal cortex. *Nature*, *444*(7117), 374–377.

Stone, S. P., Patel, P., & Greenwood, R. J. (1993). Selection of acute stroke patients for treatment of visual neglect. *Journal of Neurology, Neurosurgery & Psychiatry*, *56*, 463–466.

Striemer, C. L., & Danckert, J. (2010). Through a prism darkly: Re-evaluating prisms and neglect. *Trends in Cognitive Sciences*, *14*, 308–3016.

Styles, E. A. (1997). *The psychology of attention*. Hove: Psychology Press/Erlbaum.

Theeuwes, J. (1991). Exogenous and endogenous control of attention: The effect of visual onsets and offsets. *Perception & Psychophysics*, *49*(1), 83–90.

Theeuwes, J. (1992). Perceptual selectivity for color and form. *Perception & Psychophysics*, *51*, 599–606.

Theeuwes, J. (1994). Stimulus-driven capture and attentional set: Selective search for color and visual abrupt onsets. *Journal of Experimental Psychology: Human Perception and Performance*, *20*, 799–806.

Theeuwes, J. (2010). Top-down and bottom-up control of visual selection. *Acta Psychologica*, *123*, 77–99.

Theeuwes, J., Kramer, A. F., & Belopolsky, A. V. (2004). Attentional set interacts with perceptual load in visual search. *Psychonomic Bulletin & Review*, *11*, 697–702.

Theeuwes, J., Kramer, A. F., Hahn, S., & Irwin, D. E. (1998). Our eyes do not always go where we want them to go: Capture of eyes by new objects. *Psychological Science, 9*, 379–385.

Tipper, S. P., Howard, L. A., & Houghton, G. (2000). Behavioral consequences of selection from population codes. In S. Monsell, & J. Driver (Eds.), *Attention and performance* (Vol. 18, pp. 223–245). Cambridge: MIT Press.

Tipper, S. P., Howard, L. A., & Jackson, S. R. (1997). Selective reaching to grasp: Evidence for distractor interference effects. *Visual Cognition, 4*, 1–38.

Treisman, A. M., & Gelade, G. (1980). A feature-integration theory of attention. *Cognitive Psychology, 12*, 97–136.

Umeno, M. M., & Goldberg, M. E. (1997). Spatial processing in the monkey frontal eye field. I. Predictive visual responses. *Journal of Neurophysiology, 78*(3), 1373–1383.

Vallar, G., & Perani, D. (1986). The anatomy of unilateral neglect after right-hemisphere stroke lesions. A clinical/CT-scan correlation study in man. *Neuropsychologia, 24*(5), 609–622.

Van der Stigchel, S. (2010). Recent advances in the study of saccade trajectory deviations. *Vision Research, 50*, 1619–1627.

Van der Stigchel, S., Belopolsky, A. V., Peters, J. C., Wijnen, J. G., Meeter, M., & Theeuwes, J. (2009). The limits of top-down control of visual attention. *Acta Psychologica, 132*(2), 201–212.

Van der Stigchel, S., Meeter, M., & Theeuwes, J. (2006). Eye movement trajectories and what they tell us. *Neuroscience & Biobehavioral Reviews, 30*(5), 666–679.

Van der Stigchel, S., Meeter, M., & Theeuwes, J. (2007). Top down influences make saccades deviate away: The case of endogenous cues. *Acta Psychologica, 125*(3), 279–290.

Van der Stigchel, S., Merten, H., Meeter, M., & Theeuwes, J. (2007). The effects of a task-irrelevant visual event on spatial working memory. *Psychonomic Bulletin & Review, 14*(6), 1066–1071.

Van der Stigchel, S., Mills, M., & Dodd, M. D. (2010). Shift and deviate: Saccades reveal that shifts of covert attention evoked by trained spatial stimuli are obligatory. *Attention, Perception & Psychophysics, 72*, 1244–1250.

Van der Stigchel, S., & Nijboer, T. C. W. (2010). The imbalance of oculomotor capture in unilateral visual neglect. *Consciousness and Cognition, 19*(1), 186–197.

Van der Stigchel, S., & Nijboer, T. C. W. (2011). The global effect: What determines where the eyes land? *Journal of Eye Movement Research, 4*(2), 1–13.

Van der Stigchel, S., Rommelse, N. N. J., Deijen, J. B., Geldof, C. J. A., Witlox, J., Oosterlaan, J., et al. (2007). Oculomotor capture in ADHD. *Cognitive Neuropsychology, 24*(5), 535–549.

Van der Stigchel, S., & Theeuwes, J. (2005). The influence of attending to multiple locations on eye movements. *Vision Research, 45*(15), 1921–1927.

Van der Stigchel, S., & Theeuwes, J. (2006). Our eyes deviate away from a location where a distractor is expected to appear. *Experimental Brain Research, 169*, 338–349.

Van der Stigchel, S., & Theeuwes, J. (2007). The relationship between covert and overt attention in endogenous cueing. *Perception & Psychophysics, 69*(5), 719–731.

van Zoest, W., & Donk, M. (2005). The effects of salience on saccadic target selection. *Visual Cognition, 12*(2), 353–375.

van Zoest, W., Donk, M., & Theeuwes, J. (2004). The role of stimulus-driven and goal-driven control in saccadic visual selection. *Journal of Experimental Psychology: Human Perception and Performance, 30*(4), 746–759.

van Zoest, W., Donk, M., & Van der Stigchel, S. (2012). Stimulus-salience and the time-course of saccade trajectory deviations. *Journal of Vision, 12*(8), 16.

Vuilleumier, P., Sergent, C., Schwarz, S., Valenza, N., Girardi, M., Husain, M., et al. (2007). Impaired perceptual memory of locations across gaze-shifts in patients with unilateral spatial neglect. *Journal of Cognitive Neuroscience, 19*(8), 1388–1406.

Walker, M. F., Fitzgibbon, E. J., & Goldberg, M. E. (1995). Neurons in the monkey superior colliculus predict the visual result of impending saccadic eye movements. *Journal of Neurophysiology, 73*(5), 1988–2003.

Walker, R., & Findlay, J. M. (1996). Saccadic eye movement programming in unilateral neglect. *Neuropsychologia, 34*(6), 493–508.

Walker, R., McSorley, E., & Haggard, P. (2006). The control of saccade trajectories: Direction of curvature depends upon prior knowledge of target location and saccade latency. *Perception & Psychophysics, 68*, 129–138.

Wojciulik, E., Husain, M., Clarke, K., & Driver, J. (2001). Spatial working memory deficit in unilateral neglect. *Neuropsychologia, 39*, 390–396.

Wolfe, J. M. (1994). Guided Search 2.0. A revised model of visual search. *Psychonomic Bulletin & Review, 1*, 202–238.

Wolfe, J. M. (1998). Visual search. In H. Pashler (Ed.), *Attention* (pp. 13–74). East Sussex: Psychology Press Ltd..

Yantis, S., & Hillstrom, A. P. (1994). Stimulus-driven attentional capture: Evidence from equiluminant visual objects. *Journal of Experimental Psychology: Human Perception and Performance, 20*, 95–107.

Yarbus, A. (1967). *Eye movements and vision*. New York, NY: Plenum Press.

CHAPTER 6

Tell Me Where to Go: On the Language of Space

Marijn E. Struiksma[1] and Albert Postma[2,3,4]
[1]Utrecht Institute of Linguistics OTS, Utrecht University, Utrecht, The Netherlands
[2]Experimental Psychology, Helmholtz Institute, Utrecht University, Utrecht, The Netherlands
[3]Department of Neurology, University Medical Center, Utrecht, The Netherlands
[4]Korsakov Center Slingedael, Rotterdam, The Netherlands

In everyday life we spend a substantial amount of time exploring our environments looking for vital items, such as food and water (cf. chapter: Multisensory Perception and the Coding of Space). Moreover, once we have found them, we need to remember where they were (see chapter 7: Keeping Track of Where Things Are in Space: The Neuropsychology of Object Location Memory) and how to navigate back to reach them (see chapter 8: Navigation Ability). To achieve these goals different sources of information about the spatial world have to be sampled, stemming from different sensory modalities, such as sight, hearing, and touch. In addition, we can use a range of complex vocabularies to efficiently communicate place and direction information to our peers. By sharing our spatial knowledge we can combine our efforts to explore, understand, and remember the outside world. Effective spatial communication makes it much easier to find and refind the water and food when we are hungry and thirsty. In this chapter we will elaborate on the language of space.

6.1 FROM CATEGORICAL SPACE TO SPATIAL LANGUAGE

Spatial knowledge of the world comprises, among others, object recognition and defining the spatial relations between different objects. Stephen Kosslyn (1987) proposed a distinction between two classes of spatial relations: fine-grained, metric, coordinate spatial relations versus global, abstract, categorical spatial relations (see chapter: A Sense of Space and chapter: On Feeling and Reaching: Touch, Action and Body Space). Categorical spatial relations are thought to capture relative spatial invariants; the abstract, spatial structure of the environment (Jager & Postma, 2003).

Neuropsychology of Space.
DOI: http://dx.doi.org/10.1016/B978-0-12-801638-1.00006-9

For example, a category such as *in front of the library* does not correspond to a single, specific position, but refers to an area of spatial positions that make up a suitable *in front* category. Moreover, the two classes of spatial relations are thought to be mediated by different hemispheric biases; coordinate spatial relations in general depend more on right hemispheric circuitries, while categorical spatial relations rely more on resources in the left side of the brain (Jager & Postma, 2003). The notion of distinct hemispheric lateralization of categorical and coordinate spatial relations has among others been supported by Laeng (1994) who tested 60 unilateral stroke patients, and by various other studies with brain damaged patients (Suegami & Laeng, 2013; Palermo, Bureca, Matano, & Guariglia, 2008; van der Ham, van Wezel, Oleksiak, van Zandvoort, Frijns, Kapelle, & Postma, 2012; van der Ham, van Zandvoort, Frijns, Kappelle, & Postma, 2011).

In light of the foregoing, it is not surprising that a close link between categorical spatial relations and spatial language has been suggested. Kosslyn (1987) already hypothesized that the general tuning during evolution of the left hemisphere for language processing and categorization extended to spatial categories as well. A more extreme option is that perceptual and verbal spatial categories refer to essentially the same thing. In contrast it has been claimed that perceptual and verbal spatial categories are connected but still distinct. Kemmerer and Tranel (Kemmerer, 2006; Kemmerer & Tranel, 2000) defend the latter position, among others on the basis of dissociations observed in two brain damaged patients. A patient with left hemisphere lesions was impaired on verbal spatial categorization tests (processing linguistic prepositions), whereas a right hemisphere patient scored lower only on perceptual spatial category processing (see, however, van der Ham & Postma, 2010; van der Ham, Raemaekers, van Wezel, Oleksiak, & Postma, 2009, for a different view). Below we will further address the nature of the verbal spatial categories.

A main function of spatial language is to communicate the spatial relation between objects, e.g. by using simple sentences that describe the relation between two objects in a scene. This scene might be directly perceivable, or in the case of navigation instructions that in particular also contain directional information, refer to a future situation. Take, for example, the sentence *the statue is in front of the library*, the relation between the *statue* and the *library* is described by using the spatial preposition *in front of*. Spatial prepositions - arguably the verbal spatial categories meant by - such as *in front of*, *on*, *above*, and *to the left of* are part of a

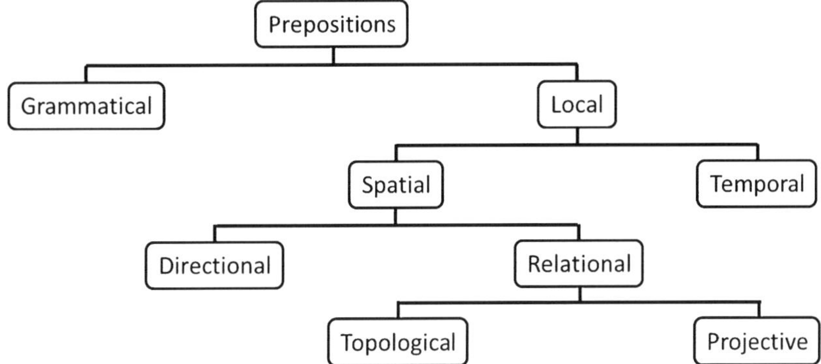

Figure 6.1 Subclasses of prepositions.

closed class of ±80 prepositions in most languages (Landau & Jackendoff, 1993).[1] The class of prepositions is remarkably small if you compare it, for example, to the class of nouns which consists of tens of thousands of instances. Within the class of prepositions several subclasses can be distinguished based on the functions of the prepositions, see Fig. 6.1 (Coventry & Garrod, 2004). The main distinction is between *grammatical* use, e.g. *of* or *for* which are used as a syntactic marker rather than carry meaning, and *local* use, which contains *temporal* and *spatial* uses. Temporal use refers to expressions about time (eg, *see you in ten minutes*). Spatial prepositions can be further divided into *directional* and *relational* prepositions. Directional prepositions describe, as the name suggests, a change in direction or position (e.g., *Jenny went to the theatre* or *the girl pointed to the bike*). Relational prepositions describe the relation between locations of different objects. These relational prepositions can again be further divided into *topological* and *projective* prepositions. Examples of topological prepositions are *in, on,* and *near,* which describe static relations between objects. Projective prepositions on the other hand describe how one object is precisely oriented with respect to the other object (e.g., *to the right, in front of, below*).

Interestingly several notable neurocognitive differences appear to apply to topological and projective prepositions. One of them concerns the mathematical conception of different geometries, contrasting regions and boundary maps to represent the semantics of topological prepositions

[1] Statements such as "in front of" or "to the right" are so-called compound prepositions that consist of two or more words, containing, for example, an adverb and a preposition or a prepositional phrase.

and vectors for projective prepositions (cf. Coventry & Garrod, 2004; O'Keefe, 1996; Regier & Carlson, 2001; Zwarts & Winter, 2000). Topological prepositions are typically short function words, historically more stable, more frequently used, and seem acquired relatively early on by children. Projective prepositions are often morphologically complex, more sensitive to language change, less frequently used, and acquired later in life (see Muysken, 2008, for some of these aspects). Most relevant evidence regarding the nature of the distinction would be to observe neurological dissociations. However, to our knowledge, it has not yet been observed whether different patterns of brain involvement underlie the two types of prepositions (see further in Box 6.1).

BOX 6.1 Confusing "Above" and "Below": Selective Disorders of Processing Spatial Prepositions

Neuropsychological research has reported several interesting patients who show selective disorders in processing locative spatial prepositions. A double dissociation between linguistic and visual–spatial categorical spatial representations was reported by Kemmerer and Tranel (2000). Their first patient had a left frontoparietal lesion including, among others, the left supramarginal gyrus, and was severely impaired on four linguistic tests that assessed the comprehension and production of locative prepositions. These tests included: first a Naming task where the spatial relationship between a figure and a ground had to be named, second a Matching task where the participant had to choose the appropriate preposition to describe the relationship in the picture, third another Matching task where the participant had to choose from three pictures the one that best matched the given preposition, and fourth an Odd-One-Out task where the participant had to pick the picture that did not match the spatial relationship of the other two pictures. The second patient had a right frontoparietal and temporal lesion. The second patient performed normally on the linguistic tests, but was impaired on the set of nonlinguistic visuospatial neuropsychological tests. This set of visuospatial tests consisted of: the Benton Judgment of Line Orientation task where oblique lines had to be matched, the Hooper Visual Organization test where scrambled line objects have to be named, the Taylor Complex Figure test which requires copying a complex abstract line drawing built up from subfigures aligned according to spatial relationships, and finally the Three-Dimensional Block Construction task which is similar to the previous task but incorporates the 3D representation. These two patients constitute a double dissociation indicating that linguistic and visuospatial categorical spatial representations are independent and are

(*Continued*)

BOX 6.1 Confusing "Above" and "Below": Selective Disorders of Processing Spatial Prepositions—cont'd

processed by distinct neural correlates. This double dissociation supports the tripartition suggested by Jager and Postma (2003) and also by van der Ham and Postma (2010).

Another study focusing on the processing of locative spatial prepositions was conducted by Wu and colleagues who tested 14 left hemisphere damaged patients (Wu, Waller, & Chatterjee, 2007). They tested patients on locative relations and thematic role knowledge. Thematic roles signify the relation between who does what to whom during actions. For example, they tested simple sentences such as *the square kicked the circle* to study thematic role knowledge, and *the square is above the circle* to test spatial relations. Since both types of sentences require the extraction of a relation, the authors wondered whether there would be a correlation between performance on these two tasks and the site of the lesion. Although there was a correlation between performance on both tasks and damage to the anterior superior temporal gyrus and the inferior prefrontal cortex, there were also patients who showed a double dissociation. In other words, there were also patients who performed below average on the locative task and not on the thematic role task, and vice versa. Performance on the thematic role task correlated with lesions in the middle temporal and middle superior temporal gyrus. These regions are also involved in motion processing, a function which could also be accessed when processing thematic roles. On the other hand, performance on the locative task correlated with lesions in the inferior frontoparietal cortex, supramarginal gyrus, and posterior temporoparietal junction. These regions are also involved in reaching and grasping, which might be important in understanding spatial relations.

A final interesting group of patients are those with lesions in the left angular gyrus who sometimes show Gerstmann syndrome. Gerstmann syndrome is characterized by finger agnosia, agraphia, acalculia and interesting to the present discussion left/right confusion (Gerstmann, 1957). Their left/right confusion provides an interesting point of departure and infers a link between the angular gyrus and processing a subset of locative prepositions. These patients show difficulty in pointing to the left and right body parts of the experimenter. However, pointing to the left and right of their own body is sometimes preserved (Carota, Di Pietro, Ptak, Poglia, & Schnider, 2004; Mayer, Martory, Pegna, Landis, Delavelle, & Annoni, 1999). This suggests that their comprehension of the locative prepositions and concepts LEFT and RIGHT is intact, but applying them in a task that requires mental manipulation provides difficulties. This conclusion is corroborated by the impaired performance of the patient reported by Carota et al. on a mental rotation task. The angular gyrus is a structure that seems to be involved in mental representation of spatial information, and in particular the spatial manipulation of this representation.

Interestingly, a number of prepositions can be used to describe both temporal and spatial situations. For example, the preposition *in* can be used to describe a point in time, e.g. *see you in ten minutes,* or a spatial configuration, e.g. *the milk is in the glass*. This remarkable feature is not only present in the English language, but also common in many other languages (Haspelmath, 1997). One of the possible explanations of this feature is proposed by the Metaphoric Mapping Theory (Boroditsky, 2000; Heine, Claudi, & Hünnemeyer, 1991; Kemmerer, 2005), which features the Time Is Space metaphor. This metaphor states that a moment in time can be represented by a point in space and can be used to explain the parallel between temporal and spatial usage of prepositions. In other words spatial concepts are used to provide a structure for temporal concepts. Evidence for this theory can be found when studying language development in children. It turns out that young children first learn spatial concepts and later apply these concepts to understand and describe temporal situations (Bowerman, 1983). Table 6.1 illustrates the overlap in the spatial and temporal use of prepositions.

Kemmerer (2005) conducted an intriguing study in four CVA patients on the processing of spatial and temporal meanings of prepositions. Two of the patients were observed to have lower scores on comprehending temporal meanings compared to spatial meanings whereas the other two

Table 6.1 The overlap in how prepositions can be applied to indicate space and time

Space	**Time**
She's *at* the corner	She arrived *at* 1:30
Her book is *on* the table	Her birthday is *on* Monday/October 6th
Her coat is *in* the closet	She left *in* the morning/July/the summer/2003
She left her keys somewhere *around* her desk	She had dinner *around* 6:30
She planted flowers *between* the tree and the bush	She likes to run *between* 4:00 and 5:00
She ran *through* the forest	She worked *through* the evening
She hung the chandelier *over* the table	She worked *over* 8 hours
She swept the crumbs *under* the rug	She worked *under* 8 hours
She painted the picture *in* her studio	She painted the picture *in* an hour

Source: From Kemmerer, D. (2005). The spatial and temporal meanings of English prepositions can be independently impaired. *Neuropsychologia* 43(5), 797–806.

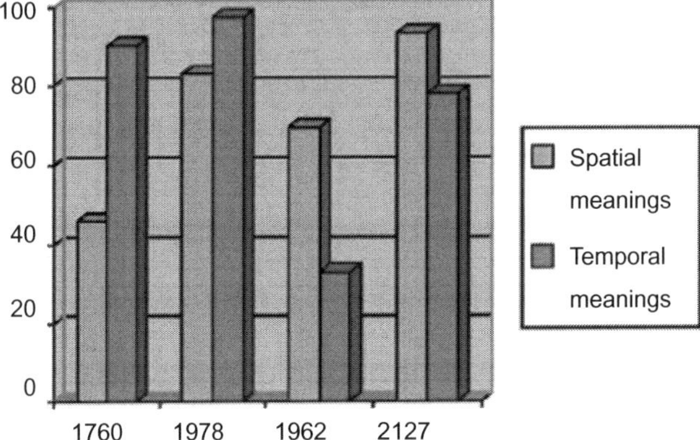

Figure 6.2 Performance scores of the four brain damaged subjects on the Spatial Matching Test, which evaluates knowledge of the spatial meanings of prepositions, and the Temporal Matching Test, which evaluates knowledge of the temporal meanings of the same prepositions. *From Kemmerer, D. (2005). The spatial and temporal meanings of English prepositions can be independently impaired.* Neuropsychologia *43(5), 797–806.*

patients showed the reverse pattern. As we can see in Fig. 6.2 there is a notable double dissociation between patient 1760 and 1962.

On the basis of the results in Fig. 6.2, Kemmerer (2005) points out that such a double dissociation suggests that spatial and temporal meanings of prepositions are processed independently and hence can independently be impaired. Apparently, there is some qualitative distinction between spatial and temporal processing of prepositions. This counters a very strict interpretation of the Time Is Space metaphor, which assumes a dependency. One possibility is that early in life we use the spatial framework to understand time, whereas later on we might obtain a more independent conceptualization of time. Further work is needed to see whether this means full independence or related, but distinct representations. Whatever the case, the flexible use of prepositions to indicate both spatial and temporal relations further suggests that perceptual spatial categories cannot simply be the same as verbal spatial categories but rather form distinct representational subclasses.

6.2 REPRESENTATION OF SPATIAL LANGUAGE

A central question is what the nature of the representation evoked by a spatial statement precisely is. Classic experiments on the representation of spatial language that were conducted in the seventies of the last century used simple spatial sentences, such as *the plus is above the star*, and compared them to a picture containing a plus and a star (Carpenter & Just, 1975; Clark & Chase, 1972). In this sentence–picture verification paradigm participants had to judge whether or not the sentence matched the display in the picture. At that time there were two theorized representational formats: a visual–spatial mental imagery view (Paivio, 1971; Paivio, 1975; Paivio, Yuille, & Madigan, 1968; Kosslyn, 1988; Kosslyn, Ganis, & Thompson, 2003) or a set of abstract propositions (Fodor, 1975; Pylyshyn, 1981). A proposition is the smallest truth-value unit. In the given example the proposition would be [above (plus, star)], which can be either true or false. The discussion in the 70s contrasted models that targeted just one of these two representational formats. These early experiments tested simple spatial sentences such as the one mentioned above, which either matched or mismatched with the given picture, and a slightly more complex sentence: *the plus is not above the star*, which again matched or mismatched the picture. According to the visual–spatial mental imagery model the sentence is automatically converted into a visual–spatial mental image and hence the model predicts similar response times for the matching *above* and matching *not above* sentences and slightly higher response times when the sentences do not match the picture. The propositional model on the other hand predicts an increase in response times for increasing number of processing steps, such as additional propositions or mismatching representations. Thus the matching *above* sentence is the easiest, followed by the *above* sentence that mismatches with the picture. The proposition for the *not above* sentences is [not [above (plus, star)]], which contains an additional proposition for *not* compared to the *above* proposition. This additional proposition requires extra processing time and hence the propositional model predicts slower response times for the *not above* sentences than the *above* sentences and the slowest response time for the mismatching *not above* sentence. The results from the early experiments demonstrated the pattern of increasing response times predicted by the propositional model (Carpenter & Just, 1975; Clark & Chase, 1972).

However, at the same time there were also models that combined multiple representational formats, such as the dual coding theory where both representations are available in parallel (Paivio, 1971). MacLeod and colleagues (1978) showed that the pattern that fit the propositional model reported by Clark and Chase (1972) did not apply to all participants.

A closer inspection of their data revealed two distinct groups of participants. For one group the data fit the propositional model, however, for the other group the data was poorly fit by that model. In contrast, the data of the latter group better fit the visual–spatial mental imagery model. These findings show that there are different strategies possible at least between different groups of participants.

Paivio took it even further and suggested that these different representation strategies are simultaneously available within most individuals. In line with this conjecture, Noordzij and colleagues performed a series of studies based on the sentence–picture verification paradigm (Noordzij, van der Lubbe, Neggers, & Postma, 2004; Noordzij, Van der Lubbe, & Postma, 2005; Noordzij, Van der Lubbe, & Postma, 2006) showing strategic variation. Noordzij and colleagues adapted the sentence–picture verification paradigm to test whether participants could adopt different strategies. They manipulated the expectancy of the modality of the second stimulus. In the classical experiments a simple spatial sentence was always compared to a picture. To be able to test different strategies Noordzij and colleagues presented 80% of the trials as a sentence–picture verification and 20% as a sentence–sentence verification, and vice versa. The responses of interest were those to the unexpected modality of the second stimulus. These responses revealed that the spatial sentence is always represented in an abstract propositional format, however, in a visual–spatial context participants strategically form an additional visual–spatial representation. The authors argued that these findings could not be explained by the models that were available at that time and proposed the strategic model where an abstract propositional code is generated by default and strategically a visual–spatial mental image can be created.

As mentioned above, the debate on spatial information representation has contrasted an abstract propositional view, with a visual–spatial mental imagery view, or with a combination of the two views. One of the leading figures in the field of representing information is Lawrence Barsalou who claimed that representations of concepts are grounded in a modality-specific perceptual symbols system (Barsalou, 1999). The main idea behind his perceptual symbols system is that perceptual traces of the perception of concepts are stored in perceptual symbols. For example, the representation of the concept CHAIR consists of traces of visual perception of chairs, but also what chairs are used for and how it feels to touch or sit on a chair. In order to understand the concept CHAIR, these perceptual symbols are re-enacted through perceptual simulations, which are analogue to their modal referents. Thus, in the example of the concept CHAIR, in order to understand this concept participants reenact the visual information that is linked to chairs as well as other modality-specific experiences, for example, a chair made of wood that feels hard to sit on. Directly related to the perceptual symbols model there is the embodied cognition approach emphasizing that there is a close link between perception, e.g. modality-specific information, and linguistic or conceptual representation (Pulvermüller, 2005; Zwaan, 2004), or in other words that cognition is grounded in perceptual representations. The meaning of words is not just based on lexical information but also entails information on the sensorimotor pathways it refers to. Translating this grounded view to spatial representations results in a spatial representation that is built up from multiple modalities conveying spatial information. Such a multimodal representation would involve at least visual–spatial information and propositional information, as was demonstrated by the experiments described above.

One of the possibilities of how spatial information is processed by the brain is that each modality has its own spatial processing system extracting the relevant information and hence resulting in a spatial representation involving various brain regions related to the processing of modality-specific information, as shown by the multimodal representation in Fig. 6.3A. This option suggests that the spatial information from different modalities is processed independently. This assumption does not seem the most parsimonious solution, however. The fact that the same spatial information can be obtained from multiple different modalities suggests a level of convergence. Moreover, a certain level of convergence is essential for consistency in spatial locations and enables, for example, flexible comparison of objects from different viewpoints. A possible representation that allows for this type of convergence is a supramodal representation as shown in Fig. 6.3B.

In a supramodal mental representation a bidirectional link to modality-specific information is maintained, but essential spatial information is extracted (Barsalou, 1999; Cattaneo & Vecchi, 2008). Such a supramodal representation activates brain regions that are not uniquely processing a single sensory modality but are rather modality-general. A key element of a supramodal representation is the bidirectional connection with modality-specific information. This bidirectional connection provides access to different sensory characteristics of descriptions of a fictitious spatial scene. For example, the following description allows you to draw the scene, and also

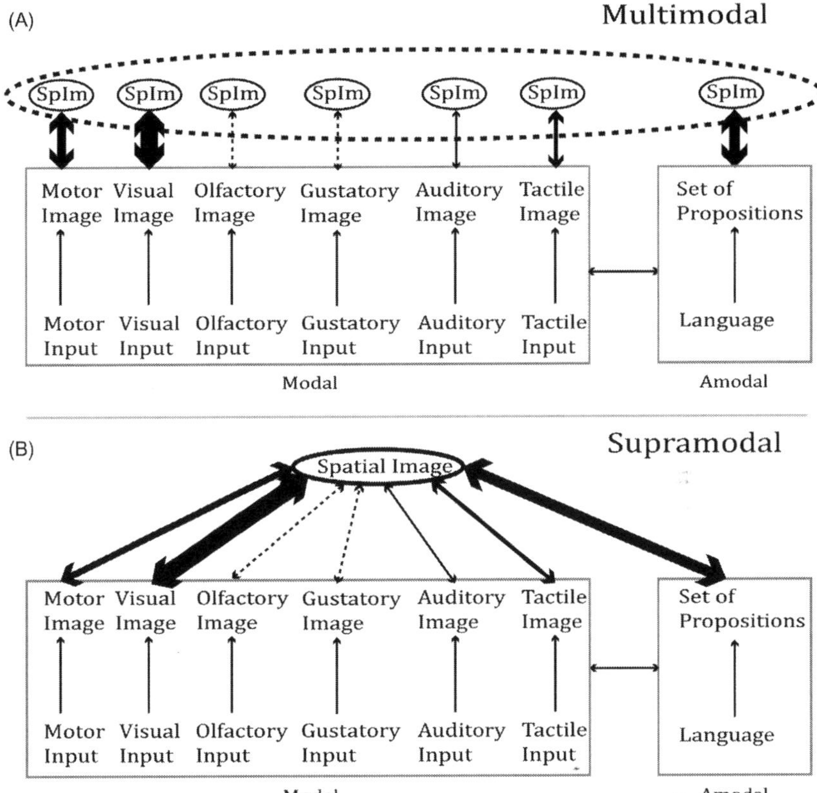

Figure 6.3 Two different models of how different sources of information can contribute to the generation of a spatial representation (*adapted from* Struiksma, M. E., Noordzij, M. L. & Postma, A. (2009). What is the link between language and spatial images? behavioral and neural findings in the blind and sighted. *Acta Psychologica, 132*(2), 145–156.). The line width represents a schematic weighting of the contribution of the different sources as indicated by the thickness of the arrows. *SpIm*, Spatial Image. Panel A shows a multimodal representation established in modality-specific brain areas. Together these form the multimodal representation. Panel B shows a supramodal representation, which exceeds modality-specific input to generate a spatial image, but maintains a bidirectional link with modality-specific input.

to pick up the kiwi based on its location and texture: *the girl picked up the kiwi, which was to the left of the orange in the glass bowl.*

Currently, there is no univocal answer to what extent spatial information is represented modality-specific and independently for different modalities as assumed by the multimodal representation, or modality-general as assumed by the supramodal representation. However, a growing body of behavioral and neuroimaging research, and in particular research on blind participants, appears to suggest a certain degree of convergence and to offer more support for the latter. For example, the results from Noordzij et al. (2005) explained above show that the abstract propositional information is available even when the majority of the second stimuli is a picture and thus would favor a visual—spatial mental image. This finding suggests that these two representations are not independent which could also be explained by a supramodal representation that can be read out in different modalities. Another interesting behavioral finding follows from a study by Cattaneo and Vecchi (2008). They used a task in which participants had to study a 5 × 5 matrix with several locations marked. After the encoding phase they had to reproduce the marked locations on an empty matrix. These matrices could be studied and recalled both visually or haptically. Cattaneo and Vecchi conducted unimodal, visual or haptic, and cross-modal, visual-to-haptic and vice versa, versions of the task. Interestingly, the pattern of results was highly similar for the unimodal and cross-modal versions. This suggests that the relevant spatial information was available to both output modalities, irrespective of the input modality. Again such convergence can be explained by a supramodal representation. Furthermore, in a haptic parallel setting task participants had to set a test bar parallel to a reference bar (Zuidhoek, Kappers, Van der Lubbe, & Postma, 2003). When a delay was introduced performance increased. The authors claimed that with a delay participants could employ a more visual based strategy to reproduce the orientation of the bar, which in this case benefitted performance. This finding again indicates that transfer of spatial information between modalities occurs which requires a level of convergence. Interestingly, when the same task was performed by blind participants, early blind participants did not benefit from a delay whereas late blind participants benefited only slightly. Thus, visual experience helps in identifying the orientation of the bar by touch, and when available, these visual mechanisms are recruited automatically.

6.3 REFERENCE FRAMES

Although, the research we have discussed so far deals with simple spatial sentences, understanding such a spatial sentence is not simple at all. When communicating about spatial relations it is important to use the same point of view as the addressee, also known as employing the same reference frame. For example, when you want to convey the message *the bird is above the tree* this could point to different locations depending on the orientation of the tree, standing up, or lying down.

When a spatial utterance, such as the one about the bird and the tree, refers to a directly visible scene verbal and perceptual information have to be compared with each other. Seminal work on the coupling between linguistic and visual information has been done by Carlson and colleagues (Carlson-Radvansky & Irwin, 1994; Carlson-Radvansky & Logan, 1997; Logan, 1994). Carlson-Radvansky and Logan (1997) suggested a model encompassing the various processing steps required in spatial language comprehension (based on theories from Carlson-Radvansky & Irwin, 1994; Levelt, 1984; Logan & Sadler, 1996; Tversky, 1991). According to this model, when a spatial sentence and a scene co-occur several processes are triggered by one's aim to understand the situation. For example, based on the verbal message spatial indexing links an object from the perceptual representation to a symbol in the conceptual representation, and identifies the reference object (*tree* in the example above). In addition, multiple reference frames, or points of view, can be imposed coordinating the mapping between language and perception.

Imposing a reference frame is an important element in spatial cognition in general. It is critical for spatial language comprehension. In order for communication to be successful it is essential that the reference frames of the interlocutor and the listener align. Only then can the spatial situation correctly be understood. Reference frames consist of three axes, which parse up space into different directions specifying location, and have several parameters that can be adjusted: e.g. origin, orientation, direction, and distance (Carlson-Radvansky & Logan, 1997; Carlson & Van Deman, 2004). The relevant axis used to match a spatial sentence to a scene differs according to which of the three reference frames is adopted: *absolute*, *relative*, or *intrinsic* (Carlson, 1999; Levinson, 1996). The *absolute* (A) reference frame uses environmental characteristics, such as gravity and cardinal directions, to determine the orientation of the axes. In the *relative* (R) reference frame the orientation of the axes is based on the viewer, while in the *intrinsic* (I) reference frame the reference object defines the relevant axis (Fig. 6.4). In the canonical situation these three reference frames are aligned (ARI), for instance, when the tree, in the example above, is upright and the viewer is upright. However, when the tree is lying down, the *intrinsic* (I) reference frame is misaligned with the *absolute* and *relative* (AR) reference frame and when the viewer is lying down the *relative* (R) frame is misaligned with the *absolute* and *intrinsic* (AI). These specific situations can

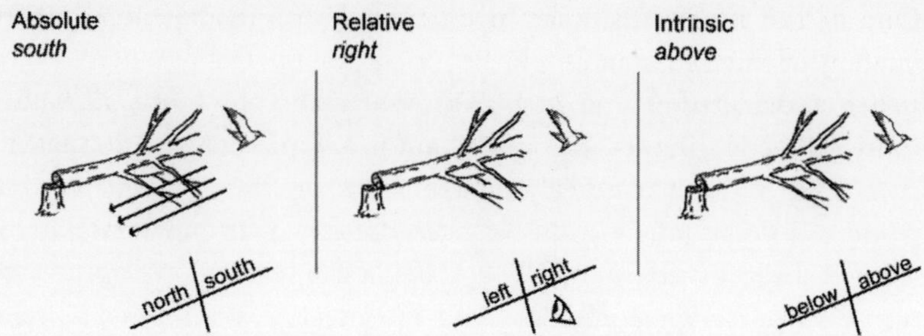

Figure 6.4 Examples of how the intrinsic, relative, and absolute reference frame apply in verifying statements regarding the bird and the tree. *Illustration inspired by Levinson, S. (1996). Frames of reference and Molyneux's question: Crosslinguistic evidence. In P. Bloom (Ed.),* Language and space *(pp. 109–169). Cambridge, MA: MIT Press.*

provide insight in the availability and use of the different reference frames. Notice that the choice of reference frame applies to spatial perception and memory situations as well, but it poses particular challenges in communication because now at least two individuals are involved.

Cross-linguistic evidence has demonstrated that reference frame preferences can differ across cultures. Dutch and European languages prefer a *relative* frame of reference, while certain Mayan languages and the Australian Aboriginal community prefer, or might even only have access to, the *absolute* frame of reference (Levinson, 1996; Pederson et al., 1998). Haun, Rapold, Janzen, and Levinson (2011) studied Dutch and Namibian children who differed in their dominant linguistic reference frames and also in performance on nonlinguistic spatial memory tasks, suggesting these competencies are related, possibly with one driving the other. Notice that even within western societies differences exist in reference frame preferences and accompanying linguistic descriptions. Hund, Schmettow, and Noordzij (2012) reported American students to use more cardinal spatial terms (e.g. north, east), associated with an *abstract* reference frame, when giving directions, whereas Dutch students preferred landmark terms in combination with a *relative* reference frame.

These reference frame preferences are not limited to language use, but are also found across cognitive domains and modalities in a wide variety of nonverbal tasks (see chapter: A Sense of Space). This observation implies that reference frames are an essential part of spatial representations and are not modality-specific. The choice of reference frame poses particular challenges in communication because now at least always two individuals are involved.

One of the modalities, apart from vision, that is also often used to convey spatial information is the haptic modality. From touch we can deduce the orientation and spatial configuration of objects as well as relations between objects. A situation not often investigated thus far, involves how we communicate about what we feel with our hands. The supramodal representation discussed above suggests that reference frames should also be accessible when comparing a sentence to a haptic situation. In a sentence verification task we directly compared a haptic scene to a verbal description (Struiksma, Noordzij, & Postma, 2011) in both blindfolded sighted and blind individuals. This study showed that for the preposition *above* blind and sighted participants have a similar, marked preference for the *relative* reference frame. Still the *intrinsic* reference frame is also available. For verifying whether the preposition *in front of* applies to a situation where they felt a configuration of a shoe with a ball, there were striking differences between blind and sighted participants. While the sighted participants still showed a considerable acceptability of the *relative* reference frame, the blind participants favored more strongly the *intrinsic* reference frame. The blind participants showed greater sensitivity to the orientation of the shoe, thereby adopting the *intrinsic* reference frame of the shoe for their judgments. Taken together, the results from this study showed that reference frames can flexibly be used also in the haptic domain. This resembles results from visual language matching studies. Greater reliance on haptic experience might induce certain preferences for the use of particular reference frames in communication in the blind. In line with this, when describing the spatial layout of an array of objects on a board, previously inspected by touch, blind participants used more object related language which implies an *intrinsic* reference frame compared to sighted participants who used more board related references suggesting a preference for an external reference frame (Postma, Zuidhoek, Noordzij, & Kappers, 2007). In contrast, it should be mentioned here that previous research with blind participants has shown that in other situations where communication is not critical, the blind tend to use a body-centered coordinate system which is associated with the *relative* reference frame for encoding proprioceptive, vestibular, touch and movement information (Millar, 1994; Röder, Kusmierek, Spence, & Schicke, 2007) (see Box 6.2).

BOX 6.2 "Put the Blue Rectangle on the Red Circle": Using the Token Test to Diagnose Problems in Understanding of Spatial Instructions in Aphasic Patients

Language disorders have well been documented after left hemisphere damage. Much less work has been conducted on the question of whether specific spatial language deficits may occur as well. As an exception there are several studies with aphasic patients on the processing of prepositions. Typically, impairments are reported, the degree to which depending on task demands and type and severity of aphasia. Comprehension seems less vulnerable than production, possibly because of additional phonological and syntactic demands. Friederici and colleagues (Friederici, 1981, 1982; Friederici, Schonle, & Garrett, 1982) found Broca's aphasic patients to be more impaired than Wernicke's aphasic patients in both comprehension and production, but elsewhere this pattern seems absent or even reversed (Goodglass, Gleason, & Hyde, 1970; Mack, 1981). More recent work by Kemmerer and Tranel (Kemmerer & Tranel, 2000, 2003; Tranel & Kemmerer, 2004) suggests that limitations in handling prepositions are typical but not a necessary characteristic of aphasia. In addition to the foregoing it seems likely that certain types of prepositions are more often affected than others, candidate factors are frequency and complexity. Matzig, Druks, Neeleman, and Graig (2010) systematically compared different instances of prepositions in patients suffering Broca's aphasia and anomic aphasia but did not find a clear pattern. Surprisingly, when prepositions have syntactic functions (e.g. *of*, *to*, *by*) they tended to be preserved, possibly suggesting some spared potential for syntactic processing in the patients. We recommend that future neuropsychological studies look further into the extent to which projective and topological prepositions get disordered (see also Box 6.1).

In order to further determine the neural basis of preposition comprehension and production we may profit from extended patient lesion studies. To run these studies it would be useful to have a test that quickly screens possible problems in dealing with spatial language terms, followed by more dedicated special purpose tests that focus on particular classes of items, e.g. types of prepositions. De Renzi and Vignolo (1962) published the Token test, now a classical neuropsychological instrument (Figure 6.5). It is a frequently used test to assess language comprehension deficits in case of suspected aphasia. It particularly could serve as this screening instrument to capture potential deficits in spatial language understanding and usage, though it has not often been employed in that role. The test requires 20 tokens, varying in shape (circle and square), size (small large), and color (red, yellow, green, blue, and white), so that every possible combination is represented. The test has 62 commands, each of which requires the manipulation of,

(*Continued*)

BOX 6.2 "Put the Blue Rectangle on the Red Circle": Using the Token Test to Diagnose Problems in Understanding of Spatial Instructions in Aphasic Patients—cont'd

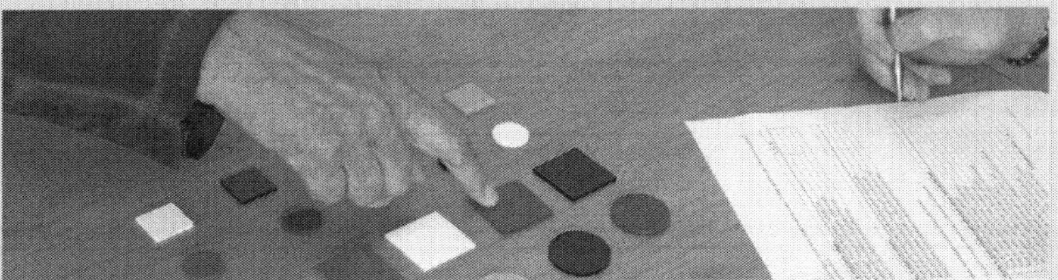

Figure 6.5 Example of an assignment in the Token test. *Courtesy of IHGR www.tokentest.eu*

or attention to, one or more of the shapes. For example, one may ask *Touch the green rectangle.* In more complex items, the patient might be instructed to *Put the red square under the red circle.* There now exist several shortened and adapted versions of the test (McNeil & Prescott, 1978). The appealing side of the test is that, though simple and easy to conduct, it measures multiple linguistic dimensions together: among others lexical meaning (which object does a word designate), grammatical structure, conjunction and the understanding of prepositions (such as in the red square and red circle example). The latter is quite interesting, since it informs us about potential problems in spatial language understanding. Laeng (1994) compared coordinate and categorical spatial relation processing in left and right hemisphere patients and among other related this to scores on the Token test. Notably he did not find any correlation, again suggesting perceptual categorical spatial relations might be something else than verbal categorical spatial relations. Kemmerer and Tranel (2003) observed a double dissociation in two patients on preposition processing and verb processing tests. Both patients failed on the Token test as well. It would have been interesting to see whether particularly the items that measure spatial relation comprehension were affected in the patient with preposition processing deficits.

6.4 THE NEURAL REPRESENTATION OF SPATIAL LANGUAGE

How does the brain process spatial language instructions? One of the first neuroimaging studies on processing locative spatial prepositions was a PET study that compared naming spatial relations between tools and utensils with simple naming of the tools and utensils (Damasio, Grabowski, Tranel, Ponto, Hichwa, & Damasio, 2001). This comparison revealed significantly stronger activation in the left supramarginal gyrus for naming spatial relations. Bilateral supramarginal gyrus activity was also found in a study testing deaf participants who used American Sign Language (Emmorey, Damasio, McCullough, Grabowski, Ponto, Hichwa, & Bellugi, 2002). The supramarginal gyrus was activated when comparing spatial relations using classifier constructions, signing objects and their relative locations, to simply naming objects. The involvement of the right hemisphere is probably because signing these classifier constructions uses space topographically and also activates a coordinate representation (see Box 6.3). The activation in the left supramarginal gyrus provides additional evidence that this structure is a plausible key candidate in processing locative spatial relations.

In a lesion study Tranel and Kemmerer (2004) tested 78 patients on four tasks measuring semantic processing of spatial prepositions. The tasks were the Naming task, the Matching task and the Odd-One-Out task described in Box 6.1 and an additional Verification task where the patients had to determine whether a picture with abstract figures correctly displayed the given preposition. A lesion overlap analysis revealed that the highest region of overlap for those patients who scored lowest on the tasks

BOX 6.3 Sign Language: A Direct Form of Spatial Communication?

Sign language refers to a systematic communication system in which meaning is conveyed by manual and bodily signs in contrast to conventional spoken, acoustic language (and its written counter parts). One of the unique features of sign language is its "iconicity." Iconicity is typically taken as the intuitively experienced similarity between a symbol (a sign or a word) and its referent (see, however, Emmorey (2014) for a structured mapping theory of iconicity). Iconicity can occur in spoken language as well. For example, the English word *peep* may by the name itself directly refer to the activity of producing a high sound. Arguably, the amount of iconicity in spoken language is limited to only certain instances and special classes of words, e.g. "onomatopoeia" (cf. Perniss, Thompson, & Vigliocco, 2010). In contrast, sign language encompasses a much larger extent of iconicity. Signs may offer straightforward tokens of shape, location or direction linked to an object or an activity. Fig. 6.6 illustrates examples of iconic and noniconic referencing in British Sign Language. Likewise in referent tracking in discourse (e.g. in the utterance *The man went to the café. He drank a cup of coffee*) the referent "man/he" maintains location in egocentric or allocentric space in both signing and gesturing.

Following up on the foregoing, we may consider spatial language to be communicated in a particularly direct manner in sign language.

(Continued)

BOX 6.3 Sign Language: A Direct Form of Spatial Communication?—cont'd

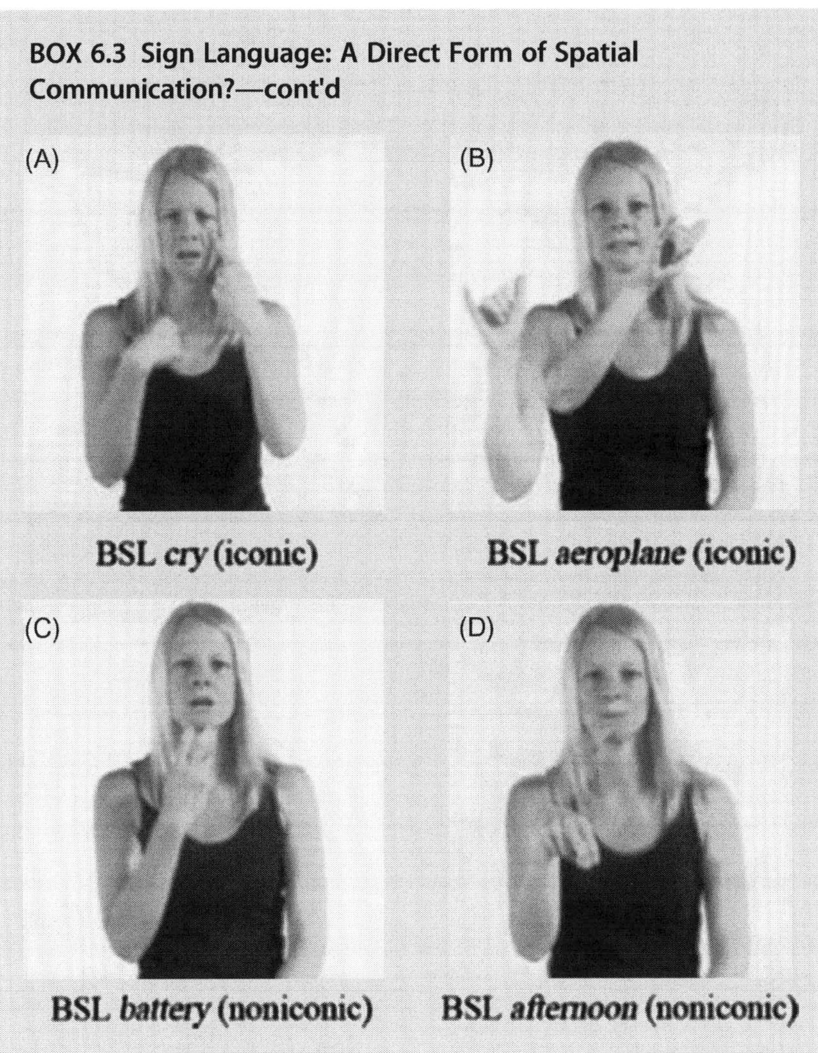

Figure 6.6 Examples in British Sign Language of iconic signs meaning (A) "Cry" and (B) "Aeroplane" and of noniconic signs meaning (C) "Battery" and (D) "Afternoon." *From Perniss, P., Thompson, R. L., & Vigliocco, G. (2010). Iconicity as a general property of language: Evidence from spoken and signed languages.* Front Psychol *1, 227.*

Emmorey et al. (2005) point out that in sign language spatial relations contained in locative expressions are typically conveyed by handshapes that specify the shape of the objects involved with the positions of the hands indicating the schematic spatial relation. Moreover, gradient, though not

(*Continued*)

BOX 6.3 Sign Language: A Direct Form of Spatial Communication?—cont'd

necessarily metric, spatial detail can also easily be expressed by signs. We may speculate here that semantic fields, or vector representations thought to be associated with the meaning of spatial prepositions (see main text; Zwarts & Winter, 2000), may directly be mimicked in sign language. Fig. 6.7 gives an example.

Interestingly in a neuroimaging experiment in which 10 bilingual participants had to describe a particular spatial relation between objects, either in spoken English or by sign language, Emmorey et al. (2005) observed bilateral

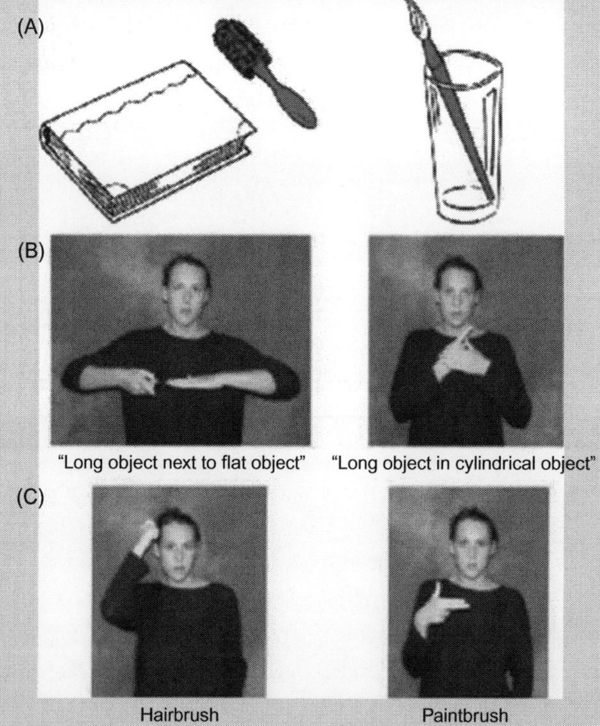

Figure 6.7 Illustrations of (A) sample stimuli, including objects and spatial configurations. (B) American Sign Language locative classifier constructions depicting the spatial relations in sample stimuli from (A). (C) American Sign Language nouns for the two figure objects in (A). *From Emmorey, K., Grabowski, T., McCullough, S., Ponto, L.L., Hichwa, R.D., & Damasio, H. (2005). The neural correlates of spatial language in English and American Sign Language: A PET study with hearing bilinguals.* Neuroimage *24(3), 832–840.*

(*Continued*)

BOX 6.3 Sign Language: A Direct Form of Spatial Communication?—cont'd

parietal activation. Right superior parietal activation was however higher in the signed situation. Related to this MacSweeney, Capek, Campbell, and Woll (2008) in their review on the neurobiology of sign language also discuss a variety of evidence indicating extended right hemisphere involvement when processing spatial language expressions in signed language.

Together it seems that space is emphasized twice in sign language: first because the signs convey spatial information in an analog fashion; second because the communication medium has a visuospatial nature. We thus might view signing as a direct form of spatial communication. It is interesting to further consider one of the consequences of this strengthened emphasis: do other cognitive abilities profit from sign language usage? There is evidence in that direction. Emmorey and colleagues (Emmorey & Kosslyn, 1996; Emmorey, Kosslyn, & Bellugi, 1993) observed improved mental imagery performance in hearing and deaf ASL signers. Van Dijk, Kappers, and Postma (2013) demonstrated better haptic learning of spatial configurations in a shape slot filling task in deaf and hearing signers compared to hearing nonsigners. Apparently substantial experience in signed communication may stimulate certain spatial skills. New support for the old Sapir-Whorf hypothesis?

was in the left frontal operculum and the left supramarginal gyrus. A recent lesion overlap analysis in both left and right hemisphere damaged patients revealed that left hemisphere patients, including lesions in the supramarginal gyrus, suffered particular problems in matching categorical pictorial relations to the correct spatial language terms (i.e. prepositions) (Amorapanth et al., 2012).

The research thus far did not answer the question at what point in time during the process the left supramarginal gyrus becomes active. Does this activation represent the link to a spatial word, a spatial computation, or the parsing of a picture? Noordzij, Neggers, Ramsey, and Postma (2008) further explored these questions. They employed a sentence–picture and sentence–sentence verification task in the MRI scanner. The verification task was presented using an event-related design, which made it possible to tease apart the activation belonging to processing the first and second stimulus. By varying the modality of the second stimulus the researchers could distinguish between activity linked to a spatial word and a spatial picture. The results revealed significant activation in the left supramarginal gyrus for spatial sentences compared to nonspatial sentences when the first stimulus was a sentence. This activation was found for trials in which the second stimulus was another sentence, but also for trials in which the second stimulus was a picture. Thus, irrespective of the modality of the second stimulus the supramarginal gyrus was activated for spatial sentences, implying a role in the processing of the spatial language term in the first stimulus. Interestingly, the supramarginal gyrus was also activated during the processing of the second stimulus for the spatial minus nonspatial contrast. Again this activation occurred irrespective of the modality of the second stimulus. Together these findings suggest that the left supramarginal gyrus is involved in generating a supramodal representation that allows for flexible comparison to either sentence or pictorial spatial information.[2]

A possible, alternative explanation to the results by Noordzij and colleagues is that the input format is responsible for the left supramarginal gyrus activation, since the sentences and pictures were always presented visually. Hence, the left supramarginal gyrus would then be a hub where visual spatial information is processed. Such a modality-specific hub fits with a multimodal representation of spatial information. However, if the left supramarginal gyrus also processes nonvisual spatial information, then a supramodal representation seems more plausible. In order to discriminate between the supramodal and multimodal account a follow-up study was conducted testing congenitally blind participants (Struiksma, Noordzij, Neggers, & Postma, 2011). Congenitally blind individuals have no (memory of) visual experience, therefore, they provide an interesting group of participants. According to a multimodal representation we would expect to find different patterns of activation for blind and sighted participants in a sentence–sentence verification task, since blind participants cannot deal with visuospatial/pictorial inputs. Since the task had to be adapted to an auditory version to be able to test the blind participants we might also find a different pattern of activation for the sighted participants, compared to the results from Noordzij et al. (2008) where sighted participants were tested in the visual modality (i.e. pictures and printed text). According to

[2] We should mention here that in an EEG study Noordzij et al. (2006) did find strategic effects. Immediately after reading a first spatial sentence stimulus, larger slow waves occurred when participants expected a pictorial second stimulus where the spatial relation had to be matched to the first stimulus, accompanied by a posterior occipital source. This effect did not occur when the first spatial sentence had to be matched to another spatial sentence. This slow wave effect might be related to generating a visual mental image and as such be independent from the supramarginal activation reported in the fMRI studies.

the multimodal account an auditory task would then activate an auditory spatial image representation that is different from what has been found before with the visual materials. However, if the sighted participants convert an auditory spatial sentence to a supramodal spatial representation, the activation patterns would remain the same, that is, they might still activate the left supramarginal gyrus.

To summarize, according to a multimodal representation view we might expect to find different activations between blind and sighted participants when they adopt different modality-specific representations, or we might expect similar findings for the blind and sighted, but still different from the results reported in the Noordzij study where the input modality was different. The supramodal representation account on the other hand predicts similar activation in the left supramarginal gyrus for blind and sighted participants, as this representation is modality independent and this occurs irrespective of the input or output modality. The results from the fMRI study with blind participants (Struiksma et al., 2011) clearly support the latter representation. They found significant left supramarginal gyrus activation in both blind and sighted participants for the spatial minus nonspatial contrast in the auditory sentence–sentence verification task (Fig. 6.8). Notice the specific supramarginal gyrus activation was not limited to spatial prepositions but extended to relational, quasispatial statements in general (e.g. the phrase *taller than*).

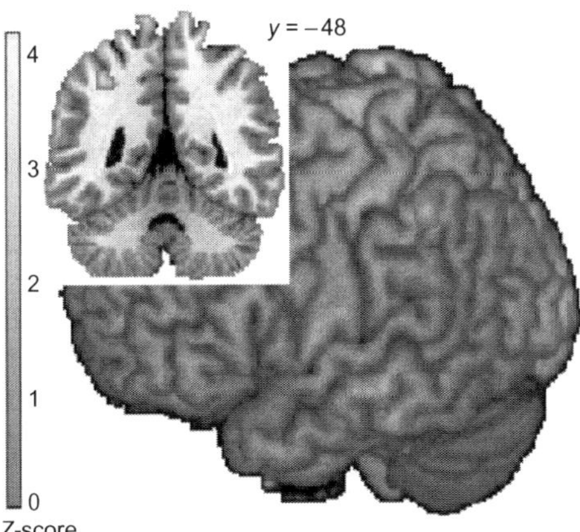

Figure 6.8 Activation of the left supramarginal gyrus in the contrast between a sentence with a spatial preposition (*left of*) and a sentence with a conjunction (*together with*) in blind and sighted participants. *From Struiksma, M. E., Noordzij, M. L., Neggers, S. F. W., & Postma, A. (2011). Spatial language processing in the blind: Evidence for a supramodal representation and cortical reorganization.* PLoS ONE [E], 6*(9), e24253.*

Taken together, the results from neuropsychological patient studies and neuroimaging studies with sighted and blind participants provide converging evidence that the left supramarginal gyrus plays a key role in processing spatial language and generating a supramodal representation. However, it seems implausible that processing spatial language relies only on the left supramarginal gyrus. Indeed, several studies discussed in this chapter have shown that a left posterior parietal network comprising of the left supramarginal gyrus, the anterior superior temporal gyrus, angular gyrus and extending into the parietal lobule has been associated with processing spatial information and spatial language in particular (Amorapanth, Widick, & Chatterjee, 2010; Amorapanth, Kranjec, Bromberger, Lehet, Widick, Woods, Kimberg, & Chatterjee, 2012; Damasio, Grabowski, Tranel, Ponto, Hichwa, & Damasio, 2001; Emmorey, Damasio, McCullough, Grabowski, Ponto, Hichwa, & Bellugi, 2002; Emmorey, McCullough, Mehta, Ponto, & Grabowski, 2013; Noordzij, Neggers, Ramsey, & Postma, 2008; Struiksma, Noordzij, Neggers, & Postma, 2011; Wu, Waller, & Chatterjee, 2007).

6.5 FROM SIMPLE STATEMENTS TO EXTENDED, MORE COMPLEX SPATIAL DESCRIPTIONS

Thus far we have restricted the discussion to simple spatial sentences focusing mainly on locative spatial prepositions. Typically a single spatial relation is communicated here. But of course everyday communication is not limited to locative spatial prepositions and simple sentences. One example where more complex spatial language is used is in wayfinding situations. You might have experienced looking for a nice restaurant and asking for directions. The ultimate goal of this action is for your interlocutor to describe to you how to get to the restaurant and for you to build up or address a spatial mental representation of the town and the route to get from your current position to the restaurant.

When giving directions you can adopt different strategies. For example, when someone is on foot, without a map, the apparent strategy is to provide directions from a first-person, or egocentric perspective, giving a mental tour through the town. This can be done using a route perspective in describing the relation between prominent landmarks and the observer in a linear fashion using indications such as left, right, straight on, and continue. Alternatively, when someone has a map available a birds-eye view, or allocentric perspective, is more apparent in which the environment is described in a hierarchical fashion using cardinal directions, such as north, east, south, and west to relate landmarks to each other instead of to the observer

(Hund, Haney, & Seanor, 2008; Taylor & Tversky, 1992). The first-person type description is also referred to as having a route perspective, while the birds-eye view is also called a survey perspective.

In order to navigate successfully to the restaurant, wayfinding information needs to be converted into a spatial mental representation (Taylor & Tversky, 1992; Tversky, 1991; Zwaan & Radvansky, 1998). The fact that different perspectives can be used to describe the way to the restaurant suggests that those might result in different mental representations. However, as argued before, spatial information can be encoded from different modalities resulting in a supramodal spatial representation. A substantial body of research has focused on different aspects of complex spatial descriptions and how they are encoded into memory and the reported results are mixed. For the case of perspective there are several studies that report convergence into a single representation, but there are also studies that report a preservation of different perspectives.

For example, Taylor and Tversky (1992) have shown that different study perspectives can give identical results. In a series of experiments they studied what type of information is incorporated into a spatial mental representation. They contrasted the idea of a visuospatial image with the idea that these representations are like structural descriptions that represent the gist or verbatim record of the text. In order to test this contrast they constructed descriptions with route or survey perspectives and tested a group of participants on each perspective. Participants had to answer verbatim and inference questions about the environments described. The questions used both the learned and alternative perspective. Their hypothesis was that the construction of a spatial mental representation relied on a structural description and therefore perspective information would be incorporated in the representations and yield different results for the two perspectives. Taylor and Tversky found the contrary: there was no difference between the two groups, suggesting that spatial information was extracted regardless of the perspective used. In the same study Taylor and Tversky also showed that participants who had read descriptions performed similarly compared to participants who had viewed an actual map, indicating that they had built up a functionally equivalent spatial mental representation. Along the same line Denis and Zimmer (1992) have shown that there is substantial overlap between spatial mental representations built up from visual experience and those derived from spatial descriptions. These results suggest that participants can build up a functional equivalent spatial mental representation from route or survey descriptions as well as viewing a map or actual visual experience.

Although there seems to be evidence that a functional equivalent mental representation can be built up, there are also studies that show that perspective differences remain visible. An example of such a study is a behavioral study by Hund et al. (2008) that examined what type of descriptions participants provided when giving directions to an imaginary recipient. Hund et al. found that when describing a large-scale environment, participants adequately incorporated the need of the recipient. When the recipient was thought to be traveling through the city by car, the participants were more likely to provide directions from a route perspective. However, when the recipient was thought to be viewing a map, they would provide directions from a survey perspective. In another study, Noordzij and Postma (2005) showed that the spatial mental representation that participants had built up from spatial descriptions also entailed metric spatial information. Even though participants who had learned the route description had constructed a spatial mental representation with analog metric detail, those who had learned the survey description had built up a representation with more fine-grained spatial detail.

According to Brunyé and Taylor (2008) participants who received a single study cycle with a route description had more difficulty in verifying inference statements when a perspective switch had taken place. This effect was robust over three study cycles. On the other hand, participants who had a single study cycle with a survey description performed significantly better on the inference statements and map drawing task. In summary, the encoding of a route description has shown to take longer and produce a higher load on visuospatial and central executive memory compared to the encoding of a survey description (Brunyé & Taylor, 2008; Deyzac, Logie, & Denis, 2006; Hubona, Everett, Marsh, & Wauchope, 1998). The resultant spatial representation from a route description has shown to be less flexible and has yielded more problems with switching perspective.

Whether or not perspective differences remain, these studies make clear that spatial information can be conveyed using spatial language and that, with sufficient exposure, this information can be used to build up a spatial mental representation with isomorphic properties to the real world. However, the encoding process differs in a number of ways between a route and a survey description. Possibly, the abovementioned behavioral differences found during the construction of a mental representation from a route and survey description are the result of the manner in which spatial information is conveyed in these descriptions. A route description consists of a series of imagined movements, provided by a set of instructions using an egocentric perspective. In line with this Brunyé, Mahoney, and Taylor (2010) showed that reading speed became higher with increases in accompanying movement sounds (running vs walking) but only for route perspective texts and not for texts from a survey perspective. Moreover, with ample exposure to route representations, also knowledge about the larger allocentric configuration can be inferred, although this only holds for simple environments. On the other hand, a survey description presents the relations between landmarks that only allow construction of an allocentric representation. The allocentric information from a survey description is more abstract and therefore requires less working memory resources and takes less time to encode (Brunyé & Taylor, 2008). Consequently, already with a few study cycles participants show flexibility to compute novel routes. Despite initial differences during encoding, it seems that after sufficient learning, spatial mental models built from route and survey descriptions can result in functional equivalent mental representations that give rise to similar performance levels on a number of spatial cognition tasks.

What about possible brain correlates of route and survey descriptions? We will first briefly turn to work from the nonverbal, spatial memory and navigation domain. At present, a wide range of neuroimaging studies has revealed that that different aspects of a spatial scene and spatial memory are processed in parallel systems in a large, overlapping frontal-parietal network, but also including markedly distinct neural correlates (Aguirre & D'Esposito, 1997; Burgess, 2008; Doeller, King, & Burgess, 2008; Hartley, Maguire, Spiers, & Burgess, 2003; Janzen & Weststeijn, 2007; Zaehle, Jordan, Wüstenberg, Baudewig, Dechent, & Mast, 2007). The distinction between egocentric and allocentric components has also been studied using neuroimaging paradigms and has demonstrated that these components are processed in different areas in the brain (Burgess, 2006; Maguire, Burgess, Donnett, Frackowiak, Frith, & O'Keefe, 1998; see also chapter: Navigation Ability). One of the main structures involved in egocentric navigation memory is the caudate nucleus. It is involved in following a well-known route (Hartley, Maguire, Spiers, & Burgess, 2003; Janzen & Weststeijn, 2007), egocentric response strategies (Maguire, Burgess, Donnett, Frackowiak, & O'Keefe, 1998), remembering turns (Iaria, Petrides, Dagher, Pike, & Bohbot, 2003) and landmarks (Doeller, King, & Burgess, 2008). The hippocampus is one of the main structures dealing with allocentric spatial navigation (for a review see Burgess, Maguire, & O'Keefe, 2002). The hippocampus is associated with: survey knowledge (Latini-Corazzini, Nesa, Ceccaldi, Guedj, Thinus-Blanc, Cauda, Dagata, & Péruch,, 2010; Mellet, Bricogne, Crivello, Mazoyer, Denis, & Tzourio-Mazoyer, 2002; Neggers,

Van der Lubbe, Ramsey, & Postma, 2006; Wolbers & Buchel, 2005), information about boundary locations (Doeller, King, & Burgess, 2008; Iaria, Petrides, Dagher, Pike, & Bohbot, 2003), navigational accuracy (Maguire, Burgess, Donnett, Frackowiak, Frith, & O'Keefe, 1998), and flexible wayfinding (Hartley, Maguire, Spiers, & Burgess, 2003).

The majority of spatial memory studies and almost all neuroimaging studies into navigation have used visual stimuli, for example, by means of virtual reality environments. Zaehle and colleagues (2007) are one of the few who distinguished between verbal descriptions of egocentric and allocentric spatial relations for a set of objects. They found a common frontoparietal network and distinct hippocampal activation associated with the allocentric coding of space, a pattern similar to visual paradigms. This finding suggests that the supramodal representation presented earlier might also apply to more complex spatial language processing. According to this model verbal descriptions of spatial scenes should provide a functionally equivalent representation. The results by Zaehle et al. seem to support this model, but further research is needed to substantiate this claim. An important next step would be to see in how far verbal spatial descriptions activate similar brain networks as found for real world/virtual reality navigation.

6.6 CONCLUSION

In this chapter we have discussed spatial prepositions and how they are used in simple sentences and more complex descriptions. In order to correctly understand a spatial sentence the reference frames of the interlocutors have to be aligned. Using the correct reference frame a spatial sentence may serve as an instruction to search for an object with respect to a reference object. A growing body of research, particularly testing neurological patients and blind participants, demonstrates that different input modalities can feed into a spatial mental representation. As such, whereas the saying "a picture is worth a thousand words" may be true, the opposite statement "a spatial sentence is worth at least one (spatial) picture" most certainly applies as well (Noordzij, 2005).

REFERENCES

Aguirre, G. K., & D'Esposito, M. (1997). Environmental knowledge is subserved by separable dorsal/ventral neural areas. *Journal of Neuroscience*, *17*(7), 2512–2518.

Amorapanth, P. X., Widick, P., & Chatterjee, A. (2010). The neural basis for spatial relations. *Journal of Cognitive Neuroscience*, *22*(8), 1739–1753.

Amorapanth, P. X., Kranjec, A., Bromberger, B., Lehet, M., Widick, P., Woods, A. J., . . . Chatterjee, A. (2012). Language, perception, and the schematic representation of spatial relations. *Brain and Language, 120*(3), 226–236.

Amorapanth, P., Kranjec, A., Bromberger, B., Lehet, M., Widick, P., Woods, A. J., & Chatterjee, A. (2012). Language, perception, and the schematic representation of spatial relations. *Brain and Language, 120*(3), 226–236.

Barsalou, L. W. (1999). Perceptions of perceptual symbols. *Behavioral and Brain Sciences, 22* (4), 637–660.

Boroditsky, L. (2000). Metaphoric structuring: Understanding time through spatial metaphors. *Cognition, 75*(1), 1–28.

Bowerman, M. (1983). In D. Rogers, & J. A. Sloboda (Eds.), *Hidden meanings: The role of covert conceptual structures in children's development of language* (pp. 445–470). US: Springer.

Brunyé, T. T., & Taylor, H. A. (2008). Extended experience benefits spatial mental model development with route but not survey descriptions. *Acta Psychologica, 127*(2), 340–354.

Brunye, T. T., Mahoney, C. R., & Taylor, H. A. (2010). Moving through imagined space: Mentally simulating locomotion during spatial description reading. *Acta Psychologica, 134*(1), 110–124.

Burgess, N. (2006). Spatial memory: How egocentric and allocentric combine. *Trends in Cognitive Sciences, 10*(12), 551–557.

Burgess, N. (2008). Spatial cognition and the brain. *Annals of the New York Academy of Sciences, 1124*(1), 77–97.

Burgess, N., Maguire, E. A., & O'Keefe, J. (2002). The human hippocampus and spatial and episodic memory. *Neuron, 35*(4), 625–641.

Carlson, L. A. (1999). Selecting a reference frame. *Spatial Cognition and Computation, 1*(4), 365–379.

Carlson, L. A., & Van Deman, S. R. (2004). The space in spatial language. *Journal of Memory and Language, 51*(3), 418–436.

Carlson-Radvansky, L. A., & Irwin, D. E. (1994). Reference frame activation during spatial term assignment. *Journal of Memory and Language, 33*(5), 646–671.

Carlson-Radvansky, L. A., & Logan, G. D. (1997). The influence of reference frame selection on spatial template construction. *Journal of Memory and Language, 37*(3), 411–437.

Carota, A., Di Pietro, M., Ptak, R., Poglia, D., & Schnider, A. (2004). Defective spatial imagery with pure gerstmann's syndrome. *European Neurology, 52*(1), 1–6.

Carpenter, P. A., & Just, M. A. (1975). Sentence comprehension: a psycholinguistic processing model of verification. *Psychological Review, 82*(1), 45–73.

Cattaneo, Z., & Vecchi, T. (2008). Supramodality effects in visual and haptic spatial processes. *Journal of Experimental Psychology: Learning, Memory and Cognition, 34*(3), 631–642.

Clark, H. H., & Chase, W. G. (1972). On the process of comparing sentences against pictures. *Cognitive Psychology, 3*(3), 472–517.

Coventry, K. R., & Garrod, S. C. (2004). *Saying, seeing and acting. The psychological semantics of spatial prepositions*. Hove and New York: Psychology Press Taylor & Francis Group.

Damasio, H., Grabowski, T. J., Tranel, D., Ponto, L. L., Hichwa, R. D., & Damasio, A. R. (2001). Neural correlates of naming actions and of naming spatial relations. *NeuroImage, 13*(6), 1053–1064.

Denis, M., & Zimmer, H. D. (1992). Analog properties of cognitive maps constructed from verbal descriptions. *Psychological Research, 54*(4), 286–298.

De Renzi, E., & Vignolo, L. A. (1962). The Token test: A sensitive test to detect receptive disturbances in aphasics. *Brain*, *85*, 665–678.

Deyzac, E., Logie, R. H., & Denis, M. (2006). Visuospatial working memory and the processing of spatial descriptions. *British Journal of Psychology*, *97*(2), 217–243.

Doeller, C. F., King, J. A., & Burgess, N. (2008). Parallel striatal and hippocampal systems for landmarks and boundaries in spatial memory. *Proceedings of the National Academy of Sciences*, *105*(15), 5915–5920.

Emmorey, K., Damasio, H., McCullough, S., Grabowski, T. J., Ponto, L. L. B., Hichwa, R. D., & Bellugi, U. (2002). Neural systems underlying spatial language in american sign language. *NeuroImage*, *17*(2), 812–824.

Emmorey, K., McCullough, S., Mehta, S., Ponto, L. L. B., & Grabowski, T. J. (2013). The biology of linguistic expression impacts neural correlates for spatial language. *Journal of Cognitive Neuroscience*, *25*(4), 517–533.

Emmorey, K. (2014). Iconicity as structure mapping. *Philosophical Transactions of the Royal Society of London. Series B, Biological Sciences*, *369*(1651).

Emmorey, K., Grabowski, T., McCullough, S., Ponto, L. L., Hichwa, R. D., & Damasio, H. (2005). The neural correlates of spatial language in English and American Sign Language: A PET study with hearing bilinguals. *Neuroimage*, *24*(3), 832–840.

Emmorey, K., & Kosslyn, S. M. (1996). Enhanced image generation abilities in deaf signers: A right hemisphere effect. *Brain and Cognition*, *32*(1), 28–44.

Emmorey, K., Kosslyn, S. M., & Bellugi, U. (1993). Visual imagery and visual–spatial language: Enhanced imagery abilities in deaf and hearing ASL signers. *Cognition*, *46*(2), 139–181.

Fodor, J. A. (1975). *The language of thought*. Cambridge, MA: Harvard University Press.

Friederici, A. D. (1981). Production and comprehension of prepositions in aphasia. *Neuropsychologia*, *19*(2), 191–199.

Friederici, A. D. (1982). Syntactic and semantic processes in aphasic deficits: The availability of prepositions. *Brain and Language*, *15*(2), 249–258.

Friederici, A. D., Schonle, P. W., & Garrett, M. F. (1982). Syntactically and semantically based computations: Processing of prepositions in agrammatism. *Cortex*, *18*(4), 525–534.

Gerstmann, J. (1957). Some notes on the gerstmann syndrome. *Neurology*, 7(12), 866.

Goodglass, H., Gleason, J. B., & Hyde, M. R. (1970). Some dimensions of auditory language comprehension in aphasia. *Journal of Speech and Hearing Research*, *13*(3), 595–606.

Hartley, T., Maguire, E. A., Spiers, H. J., & Burgess, N. (2003). The well-worn route and the path less traveled: Distinct neural bases of route following and wayfinding in humans. *Neuron*, *37*(5), 877–888.

Haspelmath, M. (1997). *From space to time: Temporal adverbials in the world's languages*. Newcastle, UK: Lincom Europa.

Haun, D. B., Rapold, C. J., Janzen, G., & Levinson, S. C. (2011). Plasticity of human spatial cognition: Spatial language and cognition covary across cultures. *Cognition*, *119*(1), 70–80.

Heine, B., Claudi, U., & Hünnemeyer, F. (1991). *Grammaticalization*. Chicago, IL: University of Chicago Press.

Hubona, G. S., Everett, S., Marsh, E., & Wauchope, K. (1998). Mental representations of spatial language. *International Journal of Human-Computer Studies*, *48*(6), 705–728.

Hund, A. M., Haney, K. H., & Seanor, B. D. (2008). The role of recipient perspective in giving and following wayfinding directions. *Applied Cognitive Psychology*, *22*(7), 896–916.

Hund, A. M., Schmettow, M., & Noordzij, M. L. (2012). The impact of culture and recipient perspective on direction giving in the service of wayfinding. *Journal of Environmental Psychology*, *32*, 327–336.

Iaria, G., Petrides, M., Dagher, A., Pike, B., & Bohbot, V. D. (2003). Cognitive strategies dependent on the hippocampus and caudate nucleus in human navigation: Variability and change with practice. *Journal of Neuroscience, 23*(13), 5945–5952.

Jager, G., & Postma, A. (2003). On the hemispheric specialization for categorical and coordinate spatial relations: A review of the current evidence. *Neuropsychologia, 41*, 504–515.

Janzen, G., & Weststeijn, C. G. (2007). Neural representation of object location and route direction: An event-related fMRI study. *Brain Research, 1165*, 116–125.

Kemmerer, D. (2005). The spatial and temporal meanings of English prepositions can be independently impaired. *Neuropsychologia, 43*(5), 797–806.

Kemmerer, D. (2006). The semantics of space: Integrating linguistic typology and cognitive neuroscience. *Neuropsychologia, 44*(9), 1607–1621.

Kemmerer, D., & Tranel, D. (2000). A double dissociation between linguistic and perceptual representations of spatial relationships. *Cognitive Neuropsychology, 17*(5), 393–414.

Kemmerer, D., & Tranel, D. (2003). A double dissociation between the meanings of action verbs and locative prepositions. *Neurocase: Case Studies in Neuropsychology, Neuropsychiatry, and Behavioural Neurology, 9*(5), 421–435.

Kosslyn, S. M. (1987). Seeing and imagining in the cerebral hemispheres: A computational approach. *Psychological Review, 94*(2), 148–175.

Kosslyn, S. M. (1988). Aspects of a cognitive neuroscience of mental imagery. *Science, 240* (4859), 1621–1626.

Kosslyn, S. M., Ganis, G., & Thompson, W. L. (2003). Mental imagery: Against the nihilistic hypothesis. *Trends in Cognitive Sciences*, 7(3), 109–111.

Laeng, B. (1994). Lateralization of categorical and coordinate spatial functions: A study of unilateral stroke patients. *Journal of Cognitive Neuroscience, 6*(3), 189–203.

Landau, B., & Jackendoff, R. (1993). "What" and "where" in spatial language and spatial cognition. *Behavioral and Brain Sciences, 16*, 217–265.

Latini-Corazzini, L., Nesa, M. P., Ceccaldi, M., Guedj, E., Thinus-Blanc, C., Cauda, F., ... Péruch, P. (2010). Route and survey processing of topographical memory during navigation. *Psychological Research, 74*(6), 545–559.

Levelt, W. J. M. (1984). Some perceptual limitations on talking about space. In A. J. van Doorn, W. A. van der Grind, & J. J. Koenderink (Eds.), *Limits in perception* (pp. 323–358). Utrech: VNU Science Press.

Levinson, S. (1996). Frames of reference and Molyneux's question: Crosslinguistic evidence. In P. Bloom (Ed.), *Language and space* (pp. 109–169). Cambridge, MA: MIT Press.

Logan, G. D. (1994). Spatial attention and the apprehension of spatial relations. *Journal of Experimental Psychology: Human Perception and Performance, 20*(5), 1015–1036.

Logan, G. D., & Sadler, D. D. (1996). A computational analysis of the apprehension of spatial relations. In P. Bloom, M. A. Peterson, L. Nadel, & M. Garrett (Eds.), *Language and space* (pp. 493–529). Cambridge, MA: MIT Press.

MacLeod, C. M., Hunt, E. B., & Mathews, N. N. (1978). Individual differences in the verification of sentence-picture relationships. *Journal of Verbal Learning & Verbal Behavior, 17*(5), 493–507.

Mack, J. L. (1981). The comprehension of locative prepositions in nonfluent and fluent aphasia. *Brain and Language, 14*(1), 81–92.

MacSweeney, M., Capek, C. M., Campbell, R., & Woll, B. (2008). The signing brain: The neurobiology of sign language. *Trends in Cognitive Sciences, 12*(11), 432–440.

Maguire, E. A., Burgess, N., Donnett, J. G., Frackowiak, R. S., Frith, C. D., & O'Keefe, J. (1998). Knowing where and getting there: A human navigation network. *Science, 280*(5365), 921–924.

Matzig, S., Druks, J., Neeleman, A., & Graig, G. (2010). Spared syntax and impaired spell-out: The case of prepositions. *Journal of Neurolinguistics*, *23*(4), 354–382.

Mayer, E., Martory, M., Pegna, A. J., Landis, T., Delavelle, J., & Annoni, J. (1999). A pure case of gerstmann syndrome with a subangular lesion. *Brain*, *122*(6), 1107–1120.

McNeil, M. R., & Prescott, T. E. (1978). *The revised Token test*. Austin, TX: Pro Ed Inc.

Mellet, E., Bricogne, S., Crivello, F., Mazoyer, B., Denis, M., & Tzourio-Mazoyer, N. (2002). Neural basis of mental scanning of a topographic representation built from a text. *Cerebral Cortex*, *12*(12), 1322–1330.

Muysken, P. (2008). *Functional categories*. Cambridge: Cambridge University Press.

Millar, S. (1994). *Understanding and representing space. Theory and evidence from studies with blind and sighted children*. Oxford: Clarendon Press.

Neggers, S. F. W., Van der Lubbe, R. H. J., Ramsey, N. F., & Postma, A. (2006). Interactions between ego- and allocentric neuronal representations of space. *NeuroImage*, *31*(1), 320–331.

Noordzij, M. L. (2005). *Communicating spatial information from verbal descriptions.* (PhD thesis). Utrecht: Utrecht University.

Noordzij, M. L., van der Lubbe, R. H. J., Neggers, S. F. W., & Postma, A. (2004). Spatial tapping interferes with the processing of linguistic spatial relations. *Canadian Journal of Experimental Psychology*, *58*(4), 259–271.

Noordzij, M. L., Van der Lubbe, R. H. J., & Postma, A. (2005). Strategic and automatic components in the processing of linguistic spatial relations. *Acta Psychologica*, *119*(1), 1–20.

Noordzij, M. L., Van Der Lubbe, R. H., & Postma, A. (2006). Electrophysiological support for strategic processing of spatial sentences. *Psychophysiology*, *43*(3), 277–286.

Noordzij, M. L., Neggers, S. F. W., Ramsey, N. F., & Postma, A. (2008). Neural correlates of locative prepositions. *Neuropsychologia*, *46*(5), 1576–1580.

Noordzij, M. L., & Postma, A. (2005). Categorical and metric distance information in mental representations derived from route and survey descriptions. *Psychological Research*, *69*(3), 221–232.

O'Keefe, J. (1996). The spatial prepositions in English, vector grammar and the cognitive map theory. In P. Bloom, M. A. Peterson, L. Nadel, & M. F. Garrett (Eds.), *Language and space* (pp. 277–316). Cambridge, MA: MIT Press.

Paivio, A. (1971). *Imagery and verbal processes*. New York: Holt, Rinehart and Winston.

Paivio, A. (1975). Perceptual comparisons through the mind's eye. *Memory & Cognition*, *3*(6), 635–647.

Paivio, A., Yuille, J. C., & Madigan, S. A. (1968). Concreteness, imagery, and meaningfulness values for 925 nouns. *Journal of Experimental Psychology*, *76*(1), Suppl: 1-25.

Palermo, L., Bureca, I., Matano, A., & Guariglia, C. (2008). Hemispheric contribution to categorical and coordinate representational processes: A study on brain-damaged patients. *Neuropsychologia*, *46*(11), 2802–2807.

Pederson, E., Levinson, S., Danziger, E., Kita, S., Wilkins, D., & Senft, G. (1998). Semantic typology and spatial conceptualization. *Language*, *74*(3), 557–589.

Perniss, P., Thompson, R. L., & Vigliocco, G. (2010). Iconicity as a general property of language: Evidence from spoken and signed languages. *Frontiers in Psychology*, *1*, 227.

Postma, A., Zuidhoek, S., Noordzij, M. L., & Kappers, A. M. L. (2007). Differences between early-blind, late-blind, and blindfolded-sighted people in haptic spatial-configuration learning and resulting memory traces. *Perception*, *36*, 1253–1265.

Pulvermüller, F. (2005). Brain mechanisms linking language and action. *Nature Reviews. Neuroscience*, *6*(7), 576–582.

Pylyshyn, Z. W. (1981). The imagery debate: Analogue media versus tacit knowledge. *Psychological Review*, *88*(1), 16–45.

Regier, T., & Carlson, L. A. (2001). Grounding spatial language in perception: An empirical and computational investigation. *Journal of Experimental Psychology. General, 130*(2), 273–298.

Röder, B., Kusmierek, A., Spence, C., & Schicke, T. (2007). Developmental vision determines the reference frame for the multisensory control of action. *Proceedings of the National Academy of Sciences, 104*(11), 4753–4758.

Struiksma, M. E., Noordzij, M. L., & Postma, A. (2009). What is the link between language and spatial images? behavioral and neural findings in the blind and sighted. *Acta Psychologica, 132*(2), 145–156.

Struiksma, M. E., Noordzij, M. L., Neggers, S. F. W., & Postma, A. (2011). Spatial language processing in the blind: Evidence for a supramodal representation and cortical reorganization. *PLoS ONE, 6*(9), e24253.

Struiksma, M. E., Noordzij, M. L., & Postma, A. (2011). Reference frame preferences in haptics differ for the blind and sighted in the horizontal but not in the vertical plane. *Perception, 40*(6), 725–738.

Suegami, T., & Laeng, B. (2013). A left cerebral hemisphere's superiority in processing spatial-categorical information in a non-verbal semantic format. *Brain and Cognition, 81*(2), 294–302.

Taylor, H. A., & Tversky, B. (1992). Descriptions and depictions of environments. *Memory & Cognition, 20*(5), 483–496.

Tranel, D., & Kemmerer, D. (2004). Neuroanatomical correlates of locative prepositions. *Cognitive Neuropsychology, 21*(7), 719–749.

Tversky, B. (1991). Spatial mental models. In G. H. Bower (Ed.), *The psychology of learning and motivation: Advances in research and theory* (Vol. 27, pp. 109–145). San Diego: Academic Press.

van der Ham, I. J., & Postma, A. (2010). Lateralization of spatial categories: A comparison of verbal and visuospatial categorical relations. *Memory & Cognition, 38*(5), 582–590.

van der Ham, I. J., Raemaekers, M., van Wezel, R. J., Oleksiak, A., & Postma, A. (2009). Categorical and coordinate spatial relations in working memory: An fMRI study. *Brain Research, 1297*, 70–79.

van der Ham, I. J., van Wezel, R. J., Oleksiak, A., van Zandvoort, M. J., Frijns, C. J., Kappelle, L. J., & Postma, A. (2012). The effect of stimulus features on working memory of categorical and coordinate spatial relations in patients with unilateral brain damage. *Cortex, 48*(6), 737–745.

van der Ham, I. J., van Zandvoort, M. J., Frijns, C. J., Kappelle, L. J., & Postma, A. (2011). Hemispheric differences in spatial relation processing in a scene perception task: A neuropsychological study. *Neuropsychologia, 49*(5), 999–1005.

van Dijk, R., Kappers, A. M., & Postma, A. (2013). Haptic spatial configuration learning in deaf and hearing individuals. *PLoS One, 8*(4), e61336.

Wolbers, T., & Buchel, C. (2005). Dissociable retrosplenial and hippocampal contributions to successful formation of survey representations. *Journal of Neuroscience, 25*(13), 3333–3340.

Wu, D. H., Waller, S., & Chatterjee, A. (2007). The functional neuroanatomy of thematic role and locative relational knowledge. *Journal of Cognitive Neuroscience, 19*(9), 1542–1555.

Zaehle, T., Jordan, K., Wüstenberg, T., Baudewig, J., Dechent, P., & Mast, F. W. (2007). The neural basis of the egocentric and allocentric spatial frame of reference. *Brain Research, 1137*, 92–103.

Zuidhoek, S., Kappers, A. M. L., Van der Lubbe, R. H. J., & Postma, A. (2003). Delay improves performance on a haptic spatial matching task. *Experimental Brain Research, 149*(3), 320–330.

Zwaan, R. A. (2004). The immersed experiencer: Toward an embodied theory of language comprehension. In B. H. Ross (Ed.), *The psychology of learning and motivation* (pp. 35–62). New York: Academic Press.

Zwaan, R. A., & Radvansky, G. A. (1998). Situation models in language comprehension and memory. *Psychological Bulletin, 123*(2), 162–185.

Zwarts, J., & Winter, Y. (2000). Vector space semantics: A modeltheoretic analysis of locative prepositions. *Journal of Logic, Language and Information, 9*, 171–213.

CHAPTER 7

Keeping Track of Where Things Are in Space: The Neuropsychology of Object Location Memory

Albert Postma[1,2,3] and Ineke J.M. van der Ham[1,4]
[1]Experimental Psychology, Helmholtz Institute, Utrecht University, Utrecht, The Netherlands
[2]Department of Neurology, University Medical Center, Utrecht, The Netherlands
[3]Korsakov Center Slingedael, Rotterdam, The Netherlands
[4]Department of Health, Medical and Neuropsychology Leiden University, Leiden, The Netherlands

We are regularly confronted with the challenge to find back personal belongings. In the example in Chapter 1, A Sense of Space, you had to relocate the car keys first before you could start your trip to your friend's new house. A special form of spatial memory is very relevant in this situation: object location memory. Object location memory critically requires associating objects to locations in space. In contrast to other forms of spatial memory such as navigation (see chapter 6: Tell Me Where to Go: On the Language of Space), there is not a specific trajectory or route toward target locations that has to be followed. The order in which object locations need to be retrieved may be critical, though, depending on the task at hand. Often object location layouts are remembered from a single observer perspective. This opens the possibility that object locations are stored by means of simple visual snapshot mechanism. If you code your keys locations always from the perspective of the same door by which you enter the room where they are hidden, a mental snapshot of the layout might suffice (cf. Burgess, Spiers, & Paleologou, 2004). Fortunately our memories are more flexible: learning perspective and retrieval perspective do not have to coincide. Hence updated egocentric spatial memory and allocentric memory mechanisms are used as well (cf. Burgess et al., 2004; Wang & Simons, 1999).

7.1 SPATIAL WORKING MEMORY AND THE VISUOSPATIAL SKETCHPAD

How long does an object location memory last? Many of the paradigms typically used employ a rather brief period of encoding and retention time

Neuropsychology of Space.
DOI: http://dx.doi.org/10.1016/B978-0-12-801638-1.00007-0

(Bohbot et al., 1998; Burgess et al., 2004; Kessels, de Haan, Kappelle, & Postma, 2002; Kessels, Postma, Wester, & de Haan, 2000), spanning a few seconds up to a couple of minutes. One reason to limit time periods is simply out of convenience. It shortens total test duration and allows the option to present multiple test trials, potentially accompanied by different test conditions. Moreover, one might argue that object location memory in daily life also often involves only brief periods. Examples such as finding where you left your glasses or keys apply to just a few moments after you have put them down. For this limited time range, especially spatial working memory (SWM) functioning seems to be relevant.

Ever since William James' classical notion that our mind possesses both a primary (short-term, conscious awareness) and a secondary (long-term, not-activated knowledge) memory system (James, 1890), researchers have been concerned with the possible division between a temporary memory mechanism and a more durable storage capacity (see also chapter 4: Multisensory Perception and the Coding of Space). Various theoretical accounts of working memory and the division with long-term memory have been put forward in the years following, ranging from viewing working memory as the currently activated part of long-term memory, to attentional resource limited accounts, to more structural system based descriptions. Arguably the most dominant model of working memory in the last decades has been the multi-component model by Baddeley and colleagues postulating separate subsystems for different types of information and for distinct control operations. In the subsequent sections we will follow the outline of the Baddeley model (Baddeley, 2000, 2012; Baddeley & Hitch, 1974).

A central claim in the Baddeley model most relevant for this chapter in particular and the book as a whole is that the memory systems of the brain can be divided on the basis of information modality. A major division is that between verbal contents on the one hand and visuospatial contents on the other. As can be seen in Fig. 7.1 a dedicated working memory component has been postulated for processing verbal information: the phonological loop, depicted here by the phonological store and the inner speech link. Similarly a specialized visuospatial component of working memory is supposed to exist as well: the so-called visuospatial sketchpad (the visual cache and the inner scribe). This component is responsible for maintaining visual patterns, such as the visual matrix array depicted in Fig. 7.1, or for spatial sequences. Moreover we might think of it as the projection buffer for mental images, though there is some discussion on that (Zimmer, 2012). Among others it has been suggested that

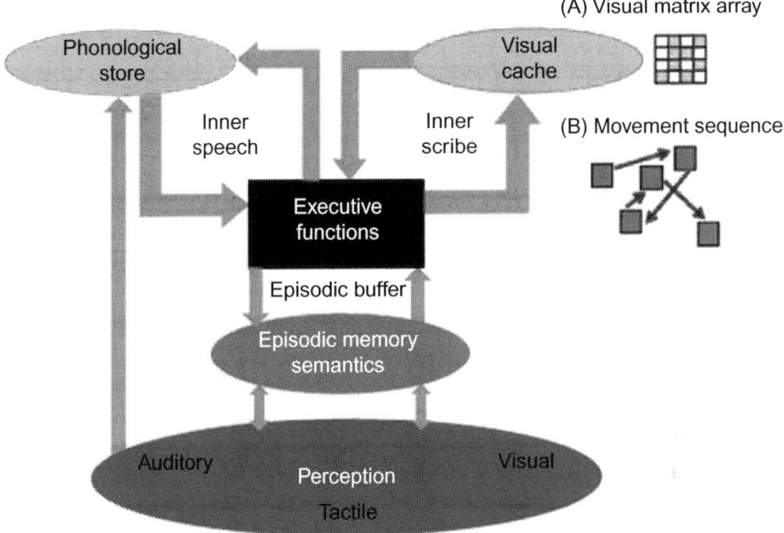

Figure 7.1 Notice that according to Logie, perceptual auditory inputs can enter the phonological store both in a direct fashion and after preprocessing/categorization by the semantic system, whereas only visual inputs are processed in the visual cache after first being analyzed in the visual semantic system. Both, by means of the inner speech loop and the inner scribe verbal and visuospatial working memory contents, can be rehearsed. Eventually the central executive and the episodic buffer allow further processing of these materials in order to be coded in more permanent format in (recent) episodic memory. *From Logie, R. H. (2011). The functional organization and capacity limits of working memory.* Current Directions in Psychological Science *20, 240.*

image generation and transformation depend in particular on the central executive (cf. Cattaneo, Fastame, Vecchi, & Cornoldi, 2006), the attentional controller of the working memory complex, taking care of coordination, selection, inhibition and updating.

Evidence for distinct working memory mechanisms dedicated to either verbal or visuospatial information processing has been offered by several behavioral, neuroimaging, and neuropsychological studies (Baddeley, 2007; Jonides et al., 1996; Logie, 1995; Logie, 2011). Interestingly, although not really surprising, a clear pattern of brain lateralization seems to be present with left hemispheric areas typically involved in verbal working memory tasks, and right fronto-parietal areas linked to visuospatial working memory processing. Notably a variety of tasks have been employed in these studies ranging from span tasks to N back tasks to pattern recognition paradigms. Hence apparent controversies might partly stem from differences in test procedures and task details.

To assess SWM in clinical neuropsychology the Corsi Block tapping task has long been used (Corsi, 1972; Kessels, van Zandvoort, Postma, Kappelle, & de Haan, 2000), in which an experimenter taps a sequence of a particular length over (a subset of) the 9 blocks organized in a quasi random layout on a rectangular board of 22 × 20 cm. The participant subsequently has to reproduce the presented sequence. Each sequence length is tested in two separate trials. At least one of these trials has to be performed correctly in order to proceed to the next sequence length. If a participant fails on both trials for a given length the experiment will be ended. The working memory span is the longest sequence length for which at least one trial was repeated correctly. Kessels, van Zandvoort et al. (2000) reported that a group right hemispheric stroke patients performed more poorly than a comparable patient group with left sided lesions. In a recent lesion overlap study Chechlacz, Rotshtein, and Humphreys (2014) further pinned down the neural correlates of Corsi block span performance in the posterior parietal areas of the brain, as well as in the middle temporal and middle occipital gyrus, all clearly right lateralized. The authors point out that they did not observe dorsolateral prefrontal involvement, as could have been expected. The fact that they only looked at simple forward span performance could have been responsible for this. Another measure frequently derived from the Corsi block tapping test is the backward span in which participants have to reproduce the just presented sequence in the reverse order. It has been argued that this procedure loads more heavily on visuospatial working memory and even on central executive functioning.

A more recent development is the use of a digital version of the Corsi block tapping task presented on a tablet computer (Brunetti et al., 2014; Claessen et al., 2015). Such an approach allows for a more precise examination of performance, as response times can be accurately measured. Moreover, it has also shown that there may be crucial differences between the forward and backward tapping condition, as performance on these tasks is differentially affected in the digital version (Claessen et al., 2015). In the digital version of the task, performance on the forward condition dropped to the level of the backward condition, whereas for the traditional version, forward performance is typically higher than performance on the backward condition. Furthermore, this digital approach also revealed additional information about the processes assessed in the Corsi task. Probably, the predictive value of the pointing movements performed by the experimenter affects working memory quality. In the digital equivalents used so far, the blocks light up sequentially, without any predictive, pointing-like movement involved. Intuitively, it may seem that simply turning blocks on and off by changing their color would seem like the digital equivalent, yet additional experiments are necessary to isolate the potential impact of dynamic pointing in the traditional Corsi setting.

Given the architecture in Fig. 7.1 one may wonder whether the contents of visuospatial working memory are visual or spatial. Fig. 7.1 separates a visual cache from the inner scribe. It has been suggested that the former acts as a temporary buffer for maintaining colors, shapes and forms, and objects. In turn the inner scribe subserves a more dynamic, sequential spatial mechanism and would particularly be involved in refreshing information. There is considerable evidence for some sort of separation between processing the two types of information in visuospatial spatial working memory (Cattaneo et al., 2006; McAfoose & Baune, 2009). This further fractionation of working memory within the visuospatial component raises one particular question: How is the visual content of the visual cache refreshed by sequential, spatial recycling of the inner scribe? If at a certain moment I have a particular color shade in mind how can this be kept active by the alleged rehearsal function of the inner scribe. One speculation here is that we can only reactivate shape or color content within a particular place. Hence rehearsal of places by the inner scribe has as a natural collateral the reactivation of item information.

Related to the foregoing it has been discussed whether a pattern needs to be sequential in order to be considered spatial or whether a simultaneously presented pattern of multiple separate locations should also be regarded as spatial. With regard to this question, Zimmer, Speiser, and Seidler (2003) demonstrated that spatial interference by repeatedly manually tapping a spatial pattern did not interfere with an object location memory test (with simultaneously presented objects) whereas it did hamper performance on the Corsi block tapping test. It should be noted here that interference was offered during a retention period. It might have yielded different effects when combined with the encoding phase. Recently, Wansard et al. (2015) reported double dissociations between sequential and simultaneous spatial working memory (concerning the mode of presentation of spatial patterns in a matrix) in neglect patients. In our opinion the question here involves not as much the presentation mode (sequential or simultaneous) but rather how the input needs to be attended in order to be encoded in memory. If a simultaneously presented array can be integrated into a single coherent gestalt, it yields a different type of processing in working memory than in case one needs to inspect separate parts of the input sequentially during encoding, even though all parts are presented at the same time (see also Zimmer, 2008) (Box 7.1).

BOX 7.1 Visuo spatial Working Memory in Extrapersonal Space: Evidence for a Separate Cognitive System?

Many of the tasks discussed in this chapter, and in particular the SWM tests, run in peripersonal space, that is, within reach of your hands. However, as already reviewed in Chapter 1, A Sense of Space, there is abundant evidence that space is not a unitary whole but instead may be carved up in a number of radial divisions surrounding the body, that are potentially controlled by separate neurocognitive mechanisms. Extending this idea to spatial memory, this raises the question of whether spatial memory works the same in near space compared to extrapersonal or far space. Or in other words, do we search for an object close to our body in the same way as when we search for it in the bookshelf at the far end of the room, 4 m away. Interestingly Piccardi and colleagues designed a visuospatial working memory test mimicking the Corsi block tapping test to be used in extrapersonal space with nine locations (squares) in an area of 2.5×3 m^2, the so-called Walking Corsi Test (Piccardi et al., 2013; Piccardi et al., 2008). The experimenter walks a path of a certain length. The participant begins at the same starting point with the same initial viewpoint and has to reproduce the sequence (see Fig. 7.2).

In a group of patients that had undergone unilateral, temporal lobe surgery Piccardi et al. (2010) reported the peripersonal and extrapersonal working memory tests to be related in the sense that in most patients the two test scores were either both impaired or both spared (see also Piccardi, Bianchini et al., 2014). However, a few selective cases were observed as well hinting at the possibility of separate memory mechanisms underlying the two tests. In line with this Bianchini et al. (2014) demonstrated selective deficits on the extrapersonal space test in early Alzheimer patients. One explanation for the latter could be that the large scale variant is more difficult. Among others it might be that the task requires bodily reorienting with full body turns in the sequence. Hence some form of egocentric updating would take place. Partly this is confirmed by the fact that women had larger peripersonal spans than extrapersonal spans, as well as young children (see also chapter 9: How Children Learn to Discover Their Environment: An Embodied Dynamic Systems Perspective on the Development of Spatial Cognition). Piccardi, Palermo et al. (2014) argued that children growing up have to learn to master environmental, navigation space, whereas body space control is mature earlier in life already. We may doubt however whether the Walking Corsi Test is really assessing topographical or navigational skills. It clearly does not involve processing of landmarks and environmental geometry (see Chapter 8: Navigation ability). More definitive support for the existence of two separate sequential spatial (working) memory systems, for peripersonal and extrapersonal space, respectively, should follow from a task setup in which sequence presentation is achieved by lighting up the squares or blocks in the display and in which sequence reproduction is

(*Continued*)

BOX 7.1 Visuo spatial Working Memory in Extrapersonal Space: Evidence for a Separate Cognitive System?—cont'd

(A)

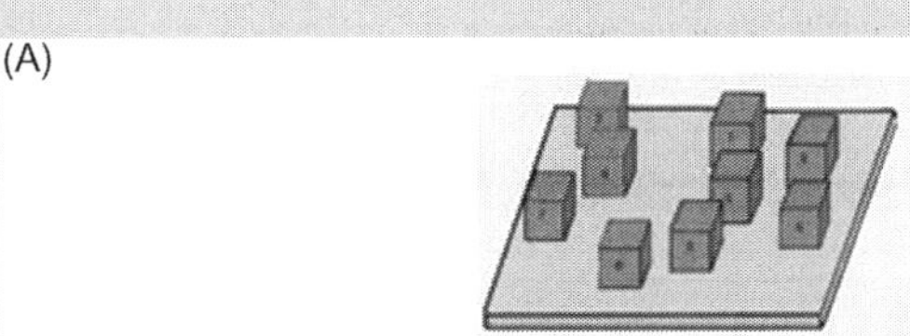

(B)

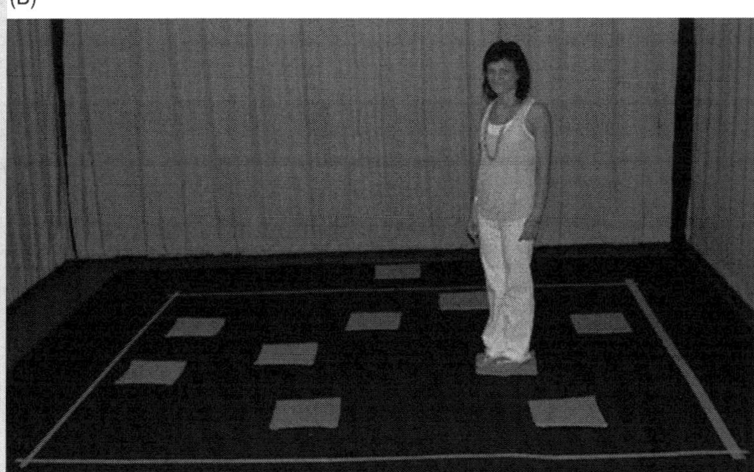

Figure 7.2 Examples from the Corsi block tapping test (A) and the Walking Corsi Test (B). In the former the experimenter taps a pattern of a certain length across the blocks and the participants have to reproduce this by the tapping the same pattern. In the latter the experimenter starts at the square in the middle of the far side of the room, and then walks a pattern of a certain length across the squares. The participant has to reproduce this by walking the same, starting from the same position. Size of frame spanning the gray squares is 3 × 2.50 m; squares are 30 × 30 cm. *From Piccardi, L., Berthoz, A., Baulac, M., Denos, M., Dupont, S., Samson, S., & Guariglia, C. (2010). Different spatial memory systems are involved in small- and large-scale environments: Evidence from patients with temporal lobe epilepsy.* Experimental Brain Research 206(2), *171–177, Figure 1.*

done by having participants use a pointer to indicate the target locations in the correct order. Finding double dissociations this way will offer more convincing evidence. The next step would be to consider which daily life activities in particular recruit the two systems. We may speculate that the extrapersonal SWM system supports sequential route learning during navigation (see Chapter 8: Navigation ability).

A central question regarding working memory in general has been how the transfer of information into long-term memory runs. The notion that simple rehearsal in either the phonological loop or the visuospatial sketchpad suffices has long been discarded. Building on from the levels of processing approach in the 1970s (Craik & Lockhart, 1972), it now typically is held that special classes of processing operations in working memory are responsible for long-term memory transfer (ie, for transfer into a more permanent format). The central executive seems a logical candidate to control these processing operations. The problem then however could be assigning too many "magical powers" to the central executive without really explaining what exactly is going on (ie, without really describing the transfer processes). In more recent years therefore a new component has been added to the working memory system: the episodic buffer. It is described to form a limited capacity component responsible for combining information from the other working memory components in multimodal codes, allowing conscious awareness, and for connecting to long-term memory and integrating information into new, temporally stable episodic memory representations (Baddeley, 2000). We wish to point out here that the original problem has shifted from the central executive to the episodic buffer. That is, the episodic buffer has now been assigned certain critical functional properties. However we hardly have begun to understand how these properties are realized in concrete processing terms. In Box 7.2, we further illustrate how the episodic buffer might work in the spatial domain in particular.

7.2 REPRESENTATIONAL MECHANISMS AND LEARNING PERSPECTIVES IN OBJECT LOCATION MEMORY

Storing spatial information in the episodic buffer allows for longer time periods to retain and use the information. As such the question of which representational formats are involved becomes more important. In an ingenious series of studies Burgess et al. (2004) and Wang and Simons (1999) set out to disentangle three possible types of representational formats or memory mechanisms to remember object locations in the world. A most basic one concerns a visual snapshot mechanism, somewhat close to taking a mental picture of the object array when you first study them. Notice that in this case the perspective during learning is critical. A second mechanism would be to code locations with respect to

BOX 7.2 Measures of Spatial Working Memory and the Episodic Buffer

The CANTAB, Cambridge Neuropsychological Test Automated Battery, is a computerized, widespread neuropsychological test battery. It offers a variety of short tests for diversity of cognitive domains. It has successfully been applied to various clinical groups, including Alzheimer's disease, autism, Down's syndrome, epilepsy, Huntington's, multiple sclerosis, stroke, Parkinson's disease, and traumatic brain injury (cf. Dowson et al., 2004; Morris, Evenden, Sahakian, & Robbins, 1987; Morris et al., 1988; Owen, Downes, Sahakian, Polkey, & Robbins, 1990; Owen, Sahakian, Semple, Polkey, & Robbins, 1995; Sahakian et al., 1988). Interestingly it also includes a variety of short-term visuospatial memory tests. The Spatial Span Test (SST) is comparable to the Corsi block tapping test. As it is computerized, it has the advantage of easy scoring of errors and latencies. Moreover it has removed experimenter-related variability, for example, in the speed with which they tap the blocks. The Spatial Recognition Test (SRT) presents five squares serially at different locations. In the reverse order of presentation pairs of boxes are given and the participant has to pick the correct one from the originally presented sequence. Both the SST and SRT assess maintaining information in SWM (visual cache and inner scribe). The temporal component is lower for the SRT. The SWM module requires participants to find a blue token in an array of boxes and use these to fill up an empty column placed to the right of the array, while not returning to boxes where a blue token has already been found (after having been found in a box, in the next search this box is empty again. Hence opening it will cause an error). This continues until all of the boxes have been filled once and this has been detected by the participant. Notice this test requires more complex working memory operations, among others strategy of search, updating (switching between filled, possibly filled, and empty boxes), besides remembering spatial location information.

Van Asselen and colleagues (van Asselen, Kessels, Wester, & Postma, 2005) designed a variant of the SWM (Morris et al., 1987) and the Executive Golf task employed by Feigenbaum, Polkey, and Morris (1996): the so-called Box task. Here an array of boxes has to be searched for a distinct target object. After this has been found a new object is hidden in one of the unfilled boxes. This can even be one of the boxes that on the previous searches has already been opened without success. Interestingly, van Asselen et al. (2005) distinguished two types of errors: within search errors, that is, reopening a box that had already been inspected in the same search; and between search errors, indicating reopening a box that had been found to contain an object during one of the previous searches for that array of boxes (see Fig. 7.3). Within search errors occur on a relatively short time span. Between search errors fall within a longer period of time (ie, one can reopen a box during the search for the seventh

(*Continued*)

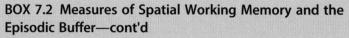

BOX 7.2 Measures of Spatial Working Memory and the Episodic Buffer—cont'd

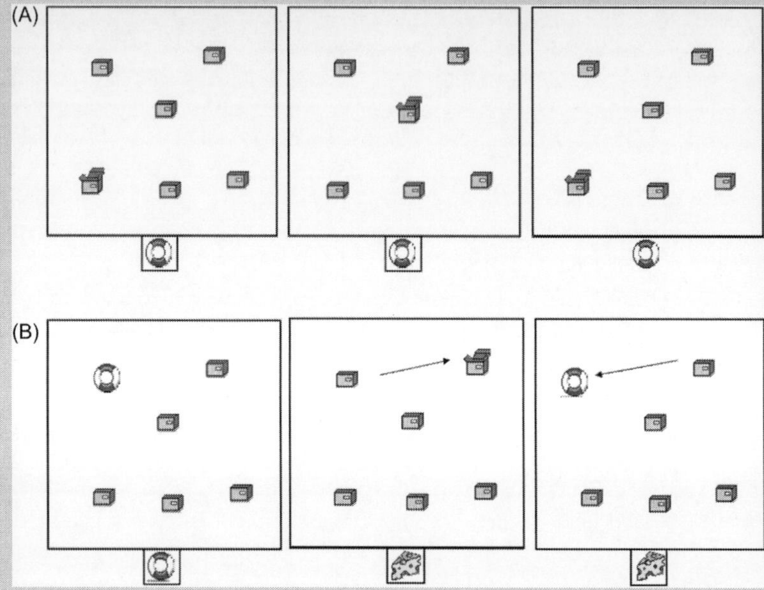

Figure 7.3 Errors in the Box task where a hidden object has to be found by opening the boxes. Once it is found, a new object is hidden in one of the remaining boxes, even in the ones previously already opened. (A) Within search errors occur within the same search, reflecting keeping information "on line" by the visuospatial sketchpad. (B) Between search take place across searches by reopening a box where in one of the preceding searches already an object has been hidden. This reflects maintaining information over longer intervals and integrating different kinds of information by the visuospatial sketchpad and the episodic buffer.

object that contains the first object in the search series). Moreover, between search errors depend on integrating information across searches. For these reasons, the authors suggested that between search errors might specifically load on the episodic buffer.

van Asselen et al. (2005) showed that Korsakoff patients made both more within search errors and between errors than healthy controls, with larger differences for the latter (see also Oudman et al., 2011). Interestingly, adding a cue by showing boxes that have different colors instead of uniform boxes, benefited control participants by lower between search errors rates, but did not help the patients (see Fig. 7.4). We may speculate that on the short time range it suffices to keep track of the locations where you have been before. On longer time ranges other types of information become also important, such as the shape or color of the location markers. The integration of different forms of information

(*Continued*)

BOX 7.2 Measures of Spatial Working Memory and the Episodic Buffer—cont'd

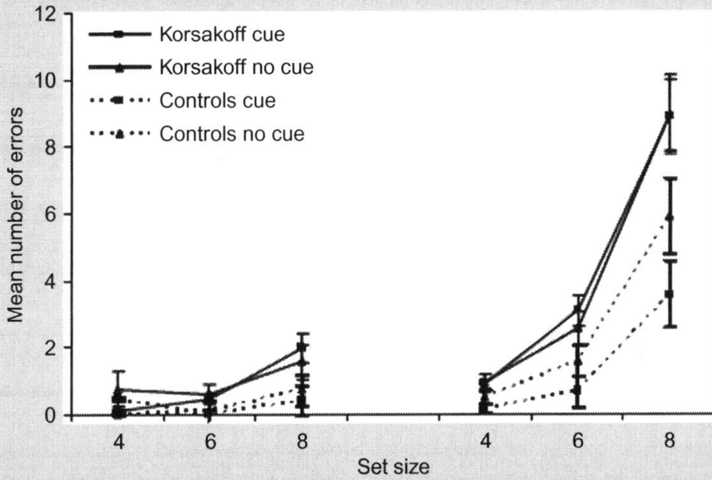

Figure 7.4 Within search errors and between search errors for different numbers of boxes (set sizes) in Korsakoff patients and healthy controls. When an additional cue is given by differentiating the boxes by colors between search errors in the controls are lower. *From van Asselen, M., Kessels, R. P., Wester, A. J., & Postma, A. (2005). Spatial working memory and contextual cueing in patients with Korsakoff amnesia.* Journal of Clinical and Experimental Neuropsychology *27(6), 645–655.*

cues and of information across searches in particular could involve the episodic buffer. In a lesion overlap study in stroke patients van Asselen et al. (2006) reported right posterior parietal and right dorsolateral prefrontal cortex lesions to increase within search error rates. In addition to these areas, bilateral hippocampal damage caused more between search errors.

Whether between search errors indeed reflect the working of the episodic buffer in a spatial domain setting remains open to discussion. The critical test would be to see whether participants after having found all the targets for a given array of boxes in the Box task are also able to relocate these objects either in empty space or in a space in which the locations are marked. If the SWM engaged by the Box task functions primarily as a "blackboard" all the information should be erased once the current task is completed (ie, once all the items for a given array have been found). If however the episodic buffer is recruited as well some spatial information should be transferred to more stable long term, declarative memory, meaning that afterward participants still are able to recall part of the display they have previously searched. Moreover, it can be conjectured that better object relocation performance should correlate with episodic buffer efficiency, or, in other words, object relocation error rates should correlate positively with the between search error rates.

your own body, that is, egocentrically. Here also your personal perspective is important but it also allows keeping track of self-movements in space during the retention period as well. Hence as long as you mentally can accommodate personal position changes—that is, egocentric updating—egocentric object location memory might function even when switching perspective. The final option is that of an allocentric memory in which you code locations to external references outside the object array itself, such as the room frame. In the studies by Wang & Simons and by Burgess and colleagues, participants studied an array of objects on a circular table. During a brief delay the table was hidden and one object was displaced. Moreover, during the delay both the subject (participant) and the table could remain in the same place (N, no move), either the table was turned (T), the subject moved (S), or both subject and table moved in the same direction (ST). Notice in both the first (N) and the last situation (ST) the visual snapshot remains the same. As can be seen in Fig. 7.5, memory benefits from maintaining the visual snapshot. However, when the perspective during test is aligned with the self-motion (S) performance is better than in the case when the visual snapshot alignment is achieved by both participant motion and table motion (ST). This strongly suggests that we rely more on an updated eogocentric object location representation that follows our bodily movements in space.

What about the allocentric representational possibility? As mentioned we may also store object locations in memory with respect to an external reference. This would give an allocentric, arguably more stable representation. Burgess and colleagues therefore introduced an external visual cue that was either stable throughout the series of trials or movable. Fig. 7.6 illustrates the setup and findings of this study. We can see that alignment with the external cue-card also yields a memory advantage, somewhat in between egocentric and snapshot alignment. Apparently we possess different representational frameworks on which we can base our object location memories and that have a different weighing on the ultimate performance. In a recent fMRI study Sulpizio, Committeri, Lambrey, Berthoz, and Galati (2013) compared view point changes in object location memory with respect to an environmental-absolute (room), an object-relative (array of objects), and an egocentric (viewer) frame. They observed fronto-parietal areas to be relevant for spatial transformations of the egocentric frame. Coding with respect to object and environments frames activated frontal eye fields, left precuneus,

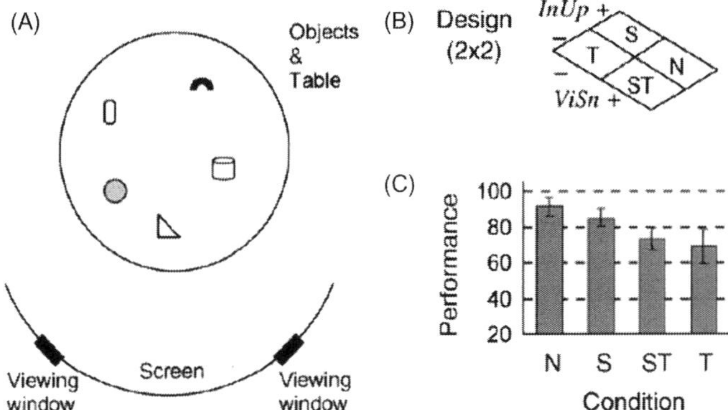

Figure 7.5 Spatial updating paradigm from Wang and Simons (1999) as taken from **Burgess et al (2004)**, figure 1. (A) Participants were presented with an array of five objects on a circular table top for 3 seconds. The table was obscured during a 7 seconds delay and one of the objects was moved to a new position. Participants had to indicate which of the objects had moved. Importantly between presentation and test, the table or the participant's viewpoint could change by a 47 degrees rotation by the center of the table making four possible conditions: no change (N), subject/participant rotation (S), table rotation (T), subject/participant rotation & table rotation in the same direction (ST). In the N and T conditions, participants moved halfway to the other viewpoint and back again to control for any disruptive effects of movement. Participants were warned that the table would be rotated in the conditions T and ST. (B) 2 × 2 factorial design: the test can be consistent (+) or inconsistent (−) with visual snapshot representations (ViSn) or egocentric representations internally updated by self-motion (InUp). (C) Results from 16 participants each performing 20 trials of each condition. Error bars are 95% confidence intervals. Consistency with both egocentric representations that are internally updatable by self-motion (InUp) and visual snapshot (ViSn) representations improves performance, with the effects of the former being greater than the effects of the latter. *Text and figure adapted from Wang, R. F., & Simons, D. J. (1999). Active and passive scene recognition across views.* Cognition *70(2), 191–210.*

lingual/parahippocampal gyrus and the retrosplenial complex, with the last two areas specifically involved in environmental frame processing.

There is a growing body of studies involving neurological patients and object location memory tasks (see also Box 7.3 and Zimmermann & Eschen, in press, for a recent review). In our opinion, the differential assessment of the various representation frames in patients needs further attention in future investigations. Abrahams, Pickering, Polkey, and Morris (1997) had patients always change positions before starting to search for hidden objects in a circular array, arguing that this would in particular require allocentric coding. On the other hand, as we have seen

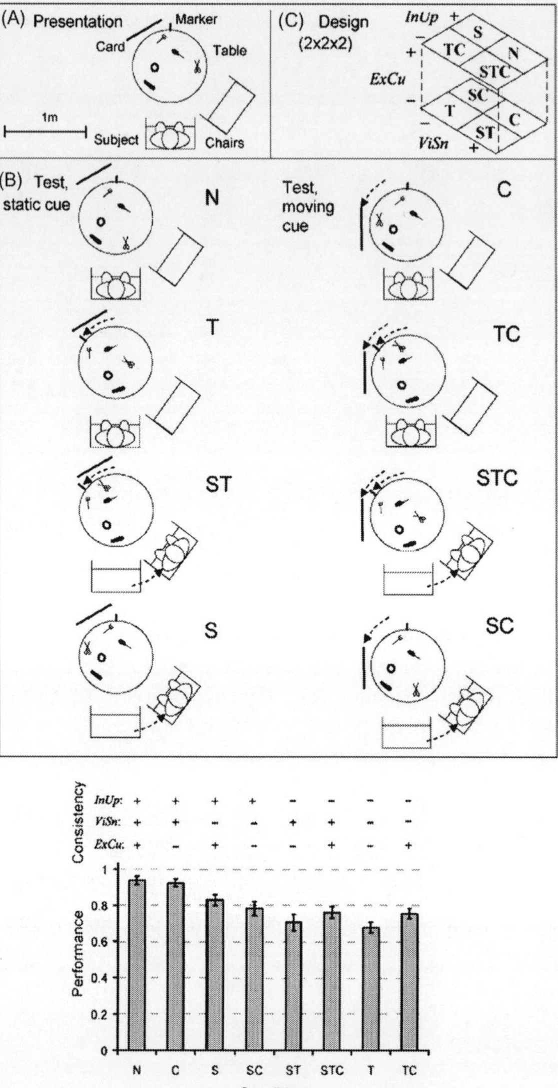

Figure 7.6 Spatial updating paradigm and results, *figure and text from* Burgess, N., Spiers, H. J., & Paleologou, E. (2004). Orientational manoeuvres in the dark: Dissociating allocentric and egocentric influences on spatial memory. Cognition, 94(2), 149–166. Available from http://dx.doi.org/10.1016/j.cognition.2004.01.001, Figures 2 and 3). (A) Experimental apparatus and conditions. (a) Presentation: Plan view of the experimental setup for an example trial in the presentation phase, surrounding black curtains not shown. The objects occupy five of the nine possible locations on the table, the marker is not seen by the participant. (b) Test: Examples of the setup for the each of the corresponding conditions following the given example presentation trial in (a). The scissors have been moved, occupying one of the four possible remaining locations in the various trials. The letters refer to the experimental conditions indicating what has been rotated relative to the presentation phase (a) (see *dashed arrow*): no change (N), cue-card (C), table (T), subject/participant (S), subject/participant & table (ST), table & cue-card (TC),

(*Continued*)

BOX 7.3 The Classical Smith & Milner Studies on Object Location Memory

Mandler, Seegmiller, and Day (1977) designed a spatial memory test that has turned out to become a highly influential experimental paradigm in subsequent years, in particular by its application in various patient studies by Mary Lou Smith and Brenda Milner from McGill University and the Montreal Neurological Hospital. In the paradigm participants viewed an array of 16 toy objects on a board (60 cm) for some time, and either immediately or after a delay participants had first to recall the objects and next they had to relocate the objects on the empty board. Fig. 7.7 shows the version of the task used by Nunn et al. (1999).

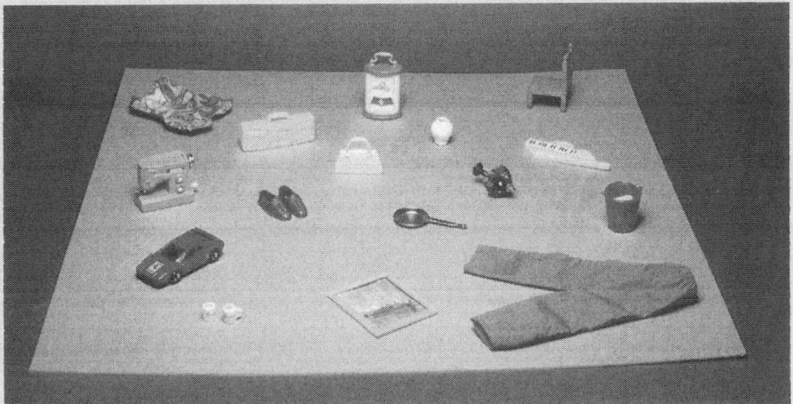

Figure 7.7 Object layout in the object location memory tasks employed in the studies by Smith and Milner, and Nunn. *From Nunn, J. A., Graydon, F. J., Polkey, C. E., & Morris, R. G. (1999). Differential spatial memory impairment after right temporal lobectomy demonstrated using temporal titration.* Brain 122 *(Pt 1), 47–59.*

Smith and Milner (1981) tested 17 right and 17 left hemispherectomy patients both immediately after exposure and after a 24-hour delay. Major results of this study are given in Fig. 7.8. We can see that the left hemisphere group performed more poorly on object recall than the right hemisphere and

(*Continued*)

◀ subject/participant & cue-card (SC), subject/participant & table & cue-card (STC). (B) Performance in the extended spatial updating paradigm. Above which conditions are consistent with which representations. Below: Columns show the mean performance of the 16 participants, error bars are standard errors of the mean. The letters refer to the experimental conditions indicating what has been moved in the test relative to the presentation phase (a) (see *dashed arrow*): no change (N), cue-card (C), table (T), subject/participant (S), subject/participant & table (ST), table & cue-card (TC), subject/participant & cue-card (SC), subject/participant & table & cue-card (STC).

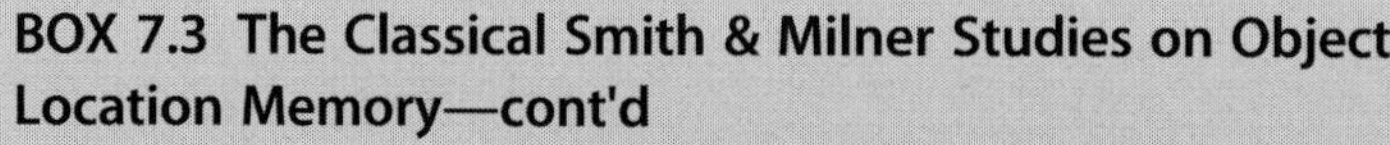

BOX 7.3 The Classical Smith & Milner Studies on Object Location Memory—cont'd

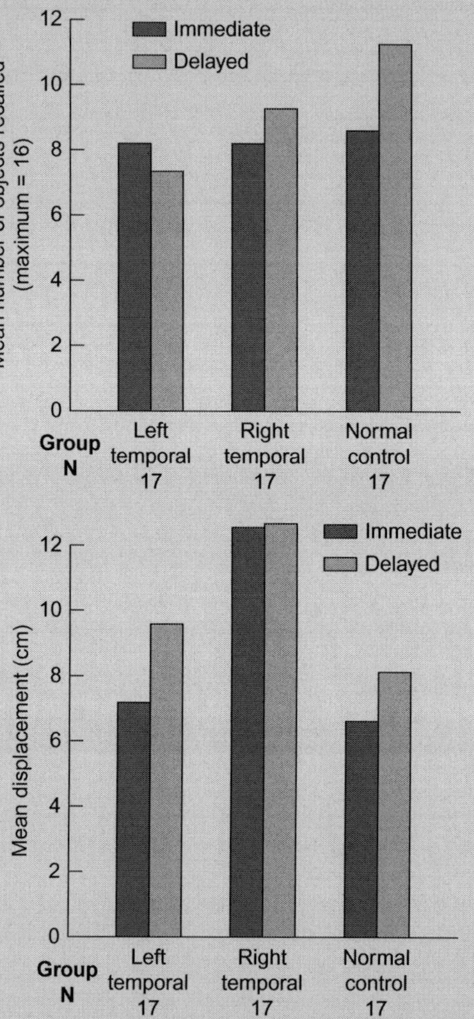

Figure 7.8 Object recall and relocation scores by temporal lobe patients and healthy controls. *From Smith, M. L., & Milner, B. (1981). The role of the right hippocampus in the recall of spatial location.* Neuropsychologia *19(6), 781–793.*

the control group. In contrast the right hemisphere group performed worse on the object relocation measure.

To better understand the foregoing results it is important to notice that Smith and Milner asked their participants in the object recall test to write

(*Continued*)

BOX 7.3 The Classical Smith & Milner Studies on Object Location Memory—cont'd

down or name the object names. This means that recall depends very much on verbal labeling and verbal memory ability. Hence it is not surprising that in particular left hemisphere patients scored weakly on object recall. In contrast, Nunn et al. (1999) found right temporal lobe patients to have deficits in the object name recall as well. So this task is not just verbal but also visual. We may also observe in Fig. 7.8 that both right hemisphere patients and controls do better on delayed object recall. The most likely explanation is that the immediate relocation test offered again an exposure to the objects, which might have profited the subsequent delayed object recall

The Smith and Milner study was unique in its type. It was one of the first allowing testing of spatial memory in a simple, single trial learning manner within a clinical setting. Previously, mostly small scale, stylus mazes had been used that capitalize on verbalization of route turns. Part of the strength of the Smith and Milner studies was also that they demonstrated an intriguing pattern of brain lateralization emphasizing the role of the right hemisphere in processing spatial information. All of the patients had undergone temporal lobe surgery to relieve epileptic seizures. A further precision of the relevant neural circuitry was attempted by dividing patients in subgroups with limited hippocampal removal and those with larger hippocampectomy. In particular the right hemisphere patients with larger removal of the hippocampus suffered on the object location memory scores (Smith & Milner, 1981; see also Smith & Milner, 1989).

It should be mentioned that at present more refined and quantified methods exist for taking into account the role of well-described brain areas and lesion patterns in specific cognitive domains. Voxels containing some form of neural damage are marked on the brains scans of relatively large patient groups and registered on to standardized brain maps. In the lesion overlap and subtraction methodology, patients are divided in groups that are impaired on the target cognitive task against those that are not. Next the lesion overlap in both groups is computed and the nonimpaired group overlap is subtracted from the overlap in the impaired group revealing the brain areas that are typically damaged in patients that perform poorly on the target task whereas they are also typically spared in patients with normal performance levels (Rorden & Karnath, 2004; van Asselen, Kessels et al., 2009). In another recent approach instead of taking cognition as the grouping factor and lesion site as the outcome, now the voxel damage is taken as the grouping factor and cognition as outcome. In so-called voxel-based lesion-symptom mapping, voxels that are lesioned in at least a minimum of patients (typically three or more) are considered and the group of patients in which this voxel is lesioned is contrasted on the cognitive test under scrutiny with the group of patients in which the voxel

(*Continued*)

BOX 7.3 The Classical Smith & Milner Studies on Object Location Memory—cont'd

is spared. Since typically tens of thousands of voxels are tested specialized corrections for multiple comparisons need to be applied. For each voxel it can be determined in how far it loads on the particular cognitive function (Bates et al., 2003; Biesbroek et al., 2015).

Special Aspects of the Smith and Milner Studies

The paradigm used by Smith and Milner is cumbersome in a way. Setting up and especially measuring the distance error is difficult and time-consuming. Consequently, only a few test trials can be given. Whereas the fact that multiple objects are given allows computation of a continuous, graded memory measure, it seems preferable to have multiple trials to control for lapses of attention, to have the possibility to give different test conditions, and to compute a wider variety of task aspects. For these reasons computerized versions of the task have been developed, most notably the Object Relocation Program (Kessels, Postma, & de Haan, 1999; Postma & De Haan, 1996). This program offers the possibility to present multiple trials with different objects sets, spatial layouts, presentations times, presentation modes (serial vs parallel) and with different delays and test conditions (grids vs free space, marked locations, positions only; temporal order vs spatial order; object recognition). Outcome scores can easily be computed. Of course the perceived stimulus very much depends upon the computer screen used and the distance to the screen. One interesting question concerns whether the physical task used in the Smith and Milner studies differs from the computerized version by being three-dimensional whereas the latter is two-dimensional. It is indeed the case that the three-dimensional physicality of the toy objects might make a difference. Still the relocation space is also two-dimensional and therefore should be comparable to the computerized version.

Smith and Milner (1981) computed two spatial test scores. The absolute relocation score is the distance between the original object location and its reconstructed place. This gives a metric or coordinate place estimation. They also used a relative score, taking into account the relations with the neighboring objects (Fig. 7.9).

Another, more simple method is to define a circular area around the object (cf. Crane & Milner, 2005). Placement within the circular area will be taken as a correct score even though the exact position does not have to match. Sometimes an area of twice the object size is taken. This is however rather arbitrary. Both of the relative measures discussed offer the possibility to calculate proportions of correct scores, which might be useful for making comparisons across test scores. It can be discussed whether they reflect some categorical position measure, that conceptually has been distinguished from more absolute distance measures.

(Continued)

BOX 7.3 The Classical Smith & Milner Studies on Object Location Memory—cont'd

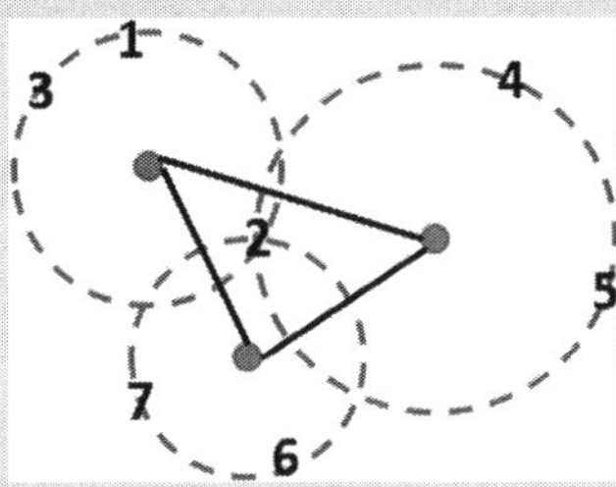

Figure 7.9 The numbers indicate object positions. For each object a number of circles can be drawn containing the target object and two other adjacent objects on the perimeter, with the restriction that no other objects are located within this circle. The centers of these circles in turn can be connected to make a polygon shape with the target object in the center. Here this is done for object 2, with the so-called "neighborhood" for object 2 marked by the triangle. One way to compute relative position score could have been to see whether object 2 was relocated within the triangle area or not, However, Smith and Milner (1981) applied a different relative position measure. They determined which were the "neighbors" for each object—that is, those objects whose neighborhoods were adjacent to the neighborhood of the target object—and contrasted this with the thus observed neighbors in the reconstructed object location array. In this way they could establish a relative position score depending on the spatial relations between objects.

Interestingly, Smith and Milner (1981) employed an incidental learning instruction. During the initial exposure to the object array participants had to give a judgment of the price of the toy objects. As such the subsequent memory tests were unexpected. The prize judgment did ensure proper inspection and attention being given to the objects without a deliberate intention to store them in memory for later usage. Smith and Milner (1984) observed frontal lobe patients do worse on price estimation without however deficits in object relocation. So it seems rather that it is the effort invested in the estimation process and not its eventual outcome that is important. From a general neuropsychological viewpoint the usage of the incidental coding condition was highly valuable. It resembles more closely memory circumstances in the real world. That is, much of our daily life events are acquired and retained automatically and unsupervised. This type of learning might specifically apply to the pick up of spatial location information (Chalfonte, Verfaellie, Johnson, & Reiss, 1996; Hasher & Zacks, 1979; Postma & Kessels, 2006; Shoqeirat & Mayes, 1991).

In a later study Smith and Milner included another condition that might in particular be relevant for spatial memory in the real world. They used an

(*Continued*)

BOX 7.3 The Classical Smith & Milner Studies on Object Location Memory—cont'd

interference condition by presenting the same (pictures of) objects three times in different positional arrays (Smith, Leonard, Crane, & Milner, 1995). Relocation performance in the later trials suffered from the already learned object locations associations in the first trial indicating a clear sign of proactive interference or negative transfer. In particular patients with frontal lobe damage were susceptible to this form of interference. In the real, spatial world we are continuously confronted by situations in which interference occurs. Remembering where you parked your car in the vicinity of your office in the morning might suffer from having parked it the previous day in another location. When taking a route to an irregular destination you need to avoid taking the wrong more habitual turn to your favorite pub. Future work should focus further on interference mechanisms in spatial memory and how certain clinical groups deal with interference in memory (cf. Elmes, 1988; Dewar, Della Sala, Beschin, & Cowan, 2010; Oberauer & Vockenberg, 2009).

in the foregoing, flexible egocentric updating is also possible in this situation. An example of a direct comparison of perspective effects is given in the study by King, Trinkler, Hartley, Vargha-Khadem, and Burgess (2004), in which a spatial memory test had to be done for scenes studied in a VR environment, using either a same perspective at test as during learning against a shifted perspective. Fig. 7.10 illustrates that patient John, suffering developmental amnesia because of focal hippocampal damage in particular, has problems in relocating objects when viewpoints are shifted. This might suggest impaired allocentric memory against spared egocentric/visual snapshot memory.

7.3 FRACTIONATION OF OBJECT LOCATION MEMORY: ITEM PROCESSING, LOCATION PROCESSING, AND BINDING

Irrespective of which representational format is recruited by an object location memory task (snapshot, egocentric, allocentric) and irrespective of the time course in the task (short term vs long term), it is clear that multiple processing components are involved. Typically one needs to identify and remember which items/objects were shown, the locations that were occupied in the task space, and finally one has to bind these two streams of information. Postma, Kessels, and van Asselen (2008) have

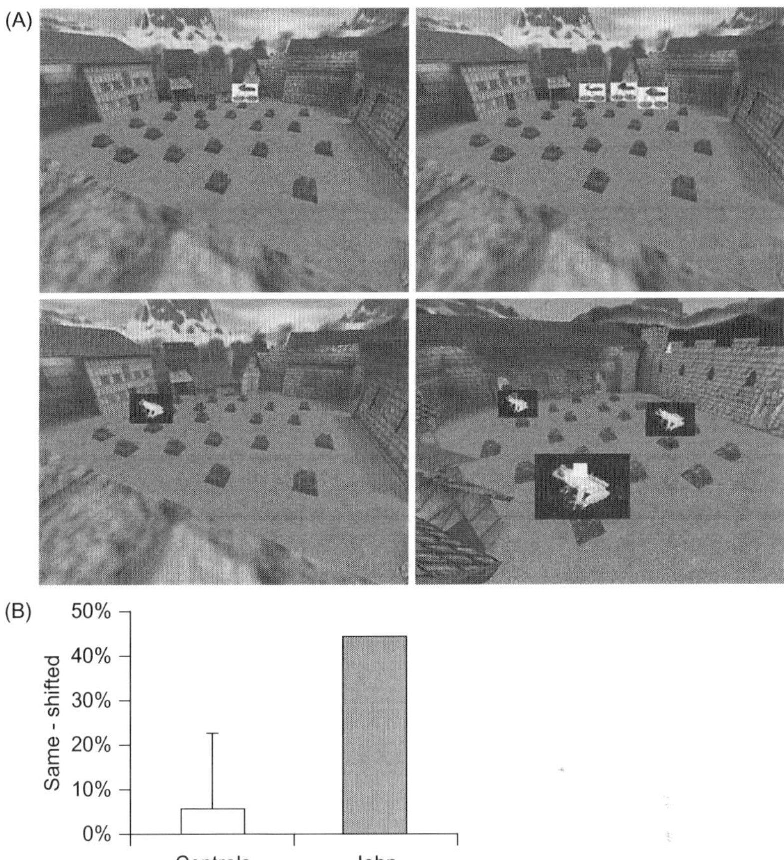

Figure 7.10 Learning and test perspectives in spatial memory task by hippocampal patient John and controls. *From* King, J. A., Trinkler, I., Hartley, T., Vargha-Khadem, F., & Burgess, N. (2004). The hippocampal role in spatial memory and the familiarity–Recollection distinction: A case study. Neuropsychology, 18(3), 405–417. Available from http://dx.doi.org/10.1037/0894-4105.18.3.405. (A) Examples are given of the stimuli used in the paper by King et al. (2004) (Figure 2). In the upper panel, study phase and test phase of a same view trial are shown. Distractors are chosen quite close to the target location in order to increase task difficulty and match it to the difficulty in the shifted view trials (see lower panel), for which distracters are further away from the target location. (B) The increase in error rate for the shifted view trials relative to the same view trials. It is clear that patient John suffers in the shifted view trials.

presented a tentative model of the architecture of object location memory, mainly based upon patient studies (Fig. 7.11).

The model presented in Fig. 7.11 sketches three main processing components—object processing, spatial location processing, binding object to

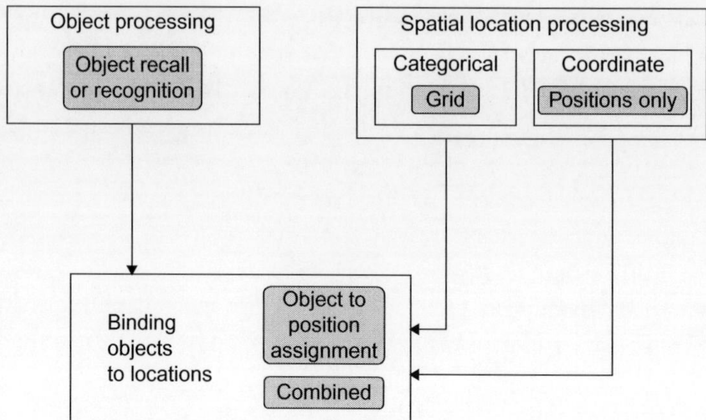

Figure 7.11 Hypothesized functional components of object location memory. *Adapted from Postma, A., Kessels, R. P., & van Asselen, M. (2008). How the brain remembers and forgets where things are: The neurocognition of object-location memory.* Neuroscience and Biobehavioral Reviews 32*(8), 1339–1345.*

locations. The second component is also further differentiated according to the grain of the spatial code involved (cf. Kosslyn, 1987; van der Ham, Postma, & Laeng, 2014, see Chapter 2: On inter and intra hemispheric differences in visuospatial perception). A coordinate code is thought to give an exact, metric placeholder. A categorical code is a global or relative position indication: for example, the target location can be found in the right upper corner of the display. Notice that a multitude of positions correspond to this categorical code. They share the more or less abstract, invariant property of all being in the right top corner.

Starting with the first component—object processing—Postma, Kessels et al. (2008) suggest that ventral cortical areas and prefrontal dorsolateral areas are mostly involved in pure object memory per se, often with bilateral contributions. It may be mentioned here that in order to test object memory one can either use a visual recognition test or use a verbal, free recall test. Hence the test method employed can already cause substantial differences in the brain areas implicated. Part of the relevant ventral brain areas is formed by the lateral occipital complex, LOC, that is generally thought to have a role in object identification (Grill-Spector, Kourtzi, & Kanwisher, 2001). In turn free recall measures of object memory involve object naming. Hence verbal labeling and verbal rehearsal processes become engaged, possibly leading to object memory deficits after left hemispheric, frontal lesions (see also Box 7.3).

What about spatial location processing in object location memory? Postma, Kessels et al. (2008) and van Asselen, Kessels et al. (2009) point out that the right posterior parietal and hippocampal areas support coordinate position memory. Categorical position memory can be assessed by testing positions in a grid, in which the cells of the grids are designed to form distinct spatial categories. The visual matrix shown in Fig. 7.1 as such can be considered a categorical test as well. van Asselen, Kessels, Kappelle, and Postma (2008) observed performance on a categorical position task to be specifically affected in left hemisphere patients. However, more precise lesion location information was lacking in this study. It has been speculated that the left posterior parietal cortex is central to categorical location processing.[1] As yet further studies are needed on this processing component.

Categorical space is more often sampled by measurements of the third object location memory component, the binding process. One exemplary test is the Location Learning Test (LLT) developed by Bucks and colleagues (Bucks & Willison, 1997). Participants study a 5 × 5 grid with 10 objects presented on small cards. They later have to relocate the objects by placing the object cards in the correct cell. Multiple test trials are given in order to obtain learning curves. Delayed recall is also tested. Kessels, Nys, Brands, van den Berg, and Van Zandvoort (2006) compared large groups of stroke and diabetic patients to healthy controls. Patients' groups performed more poorly on several of the LLT measures. Notably, right hemisphere stroke patients had lower scores than left hemisphere patients. This is somewhat remarkable since the authors themselves acknowledge that the LLT is not a proper spatial memory test since verbal coding strategies can be employed as well. The literature appears mixed with respect to lateralization. Some studies report left hippocampal and parietal involvement on aggregate object location memory scores (Kessels, Hendriks, Schouten, Van Asselen, & Postma, 2004; Kessels, Kappelle, de Haan, & Postma, 2002); others demonstrate in particular right hippocampal lesions to degrade performance (Crane & Milner, 2005; Nunn, Graydon, Polkey, & Morris, 1999). There are several reasons for this mixed pattern. It might depend on the precise type of binding measured: grids, versus binding to

[1] We should mention here that the Corsi block tapping test can also be considered a categorical location test. The exact places of the blocks are not important, only their relative locations and relative order. For this test instead right hemisphere involvements has been found—see above (Chechlacz et al., 2014).

premarked positions, to binding by free relocation. Another reason is that aggregate object location memory scores encompass not only the binding component but also the other two components. In turn this could reveal a larger neural circuitry playing a role (Postma, Kessels et al., 2008). Pure binding effects—controlling either experimentally or statistically for object identity processing and spatial location processing contributions (Dent & Smyth, 2005)—should be collected in future studies in order to get a clear idea of how the binding processes are anchored in the brain. As of yet, most of the work seems to hint toward bilateral medial temporal lobe and parietal involvement.

7.4 UNCONSCIOUSLY MANAGING TO RETRACE WHERE THINGS ARE: IMPLICIT OBJECT LOCATION MEASURES

The aforementioned discussion of short-term and long-term object location mainly concerned the formation of explicit, highly aware memories. That is, we are fully conscious of where things are placed in our surroundings (though not necessarily accurate). An interesting question is whether we also can rely on more unconscious, implicit and automatically operating spatial memory influences. The distinction between implicit and explicit memory systems has long been acknowledged in the neuropsychological literature. A notorious starting point without doubt is Clarapede's famous anecdote of an amnesic patient who withdrew her hand from Clarapede when previously being pricked by a hidden pin without however being able to recognize the persons involved or recalling the foregoing event at all (Clarapede 1907; see Nicolas, 1996). Studies on implicit memory include multiple procedures (priming, conditioning) and materials. We will discuss some examples from the spatial information processing domain in more length here.

Chun and colleagues (Chun, 2000; Chun & Jiang, 1998) devised a particularly attractive implicit spatial memory task: the contextual cueing task. In this task multiple trials are given of a search task, in which a target item has to be found among an array of distractors (see also chapter: Multisensory Perception and the Coding of Space). Unknowingly to the participants, some of the search arrays/trials are repeated throughout the experiment. Participants get faster for these repeated arrays than for completely new ones. A final critical test is done at the end of the experiment. New and repeated arrays are given and participants now have to indicate whether they recognize an array as having seen and searched previously. They perform at chance, strongly suggesting that there is no conscious memory. The fact that they are faster on the repeated items does indicate that in contrast implicit learning of the spatial context actually is taking place. Further studies indicate that in particular the learning of spatial relations is important (Olson & Chun, 2002), though repetition of item information might also make a contribution (van Asselen, Sampaio, Pina, & Castelo-Branco, 2011). Brockmole and Henderson (2006) employed the contextual cueing procedure in a more natural, daily life setting.

Oudman and colleagues (Oudman, Van der Stigchel, Wester, Kessels, & Postma, 2011) employed the implicit cueing paradigm in a group of Korsakov patients. They observed longer general search times in patients but the implicit cueing effects were comparable to those obtained in healthy controls. Notably patients did clearly suffer performance impairments on a conscious SWM task that also included search aspects (see Box 7.2). Other studies in contrast reported implicit spatial memory deficits in different groups of patients. Chun and Phelps (1999) found medial temporal lobe/hippocampal patients to be lacking with respect to the implicit cueing effect. We may presume that they would also have performed poorly on an explicit spatial memory task if it had been given. van Asselen, Almeida et al. (2009) tested Parkinson patients. As we can see in Fig. 7.12 these patients lacked the ability for implicit context learning. On the other hand some residual learning capacities seem intact. Over all the trials both patients and controls get faster. This arguably reflects some form of visuomotor procedural learning, that is not directly spatial however. Similar findings were obtained in a group of Huntington patients (van Asselen et al., 2012). Together these patient studies paint a bit confusing picture of the brain areas possibly underlying implicit (spatial) context cueing. The studies by van Asselen and colleagues suggest a special role for the basal ganglia. In contrast Chun and Phelps (1999) point toward the medial temporal lobes. If both circuitries are involved it raises the question of why selective damage to one circuitry cannot be compensated by the other intact circuitry. This calls for a closer investigation of which particular tasks, aspects are controlled by the basal ganglia and the hippocampus, respectively. To further complicate things the paper by Oudman et al. (2011) shows that patients with widespread cortical and subcortical damage including diencephalic, fronto-parietal, and medial temporal areas do not have any problems in implicit spatial context learning at all.

We may dwell a bit further on the exact nature of the contextual cueing task here. Partly it seems a sort of procedural visuomotor

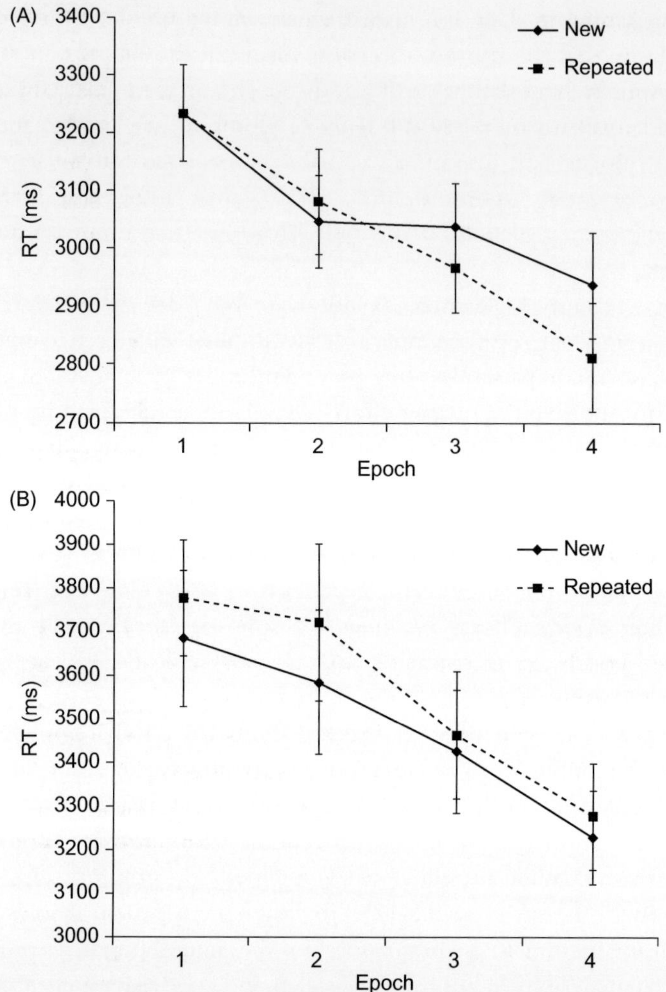

Figure 7.12 Learning curves for new search displays and repeated search displays across blocks of trials (epochs). It can be seen that in the healthy controls search times for repeated and new items start to diverge from epoch 3. This was not the case in Parkinson patients (van Asselen, Almeida et al., 2009).

learning task specifically depending on the ability to pick up spatial regularities in the environment. On the other hand Tseng and Lleras (2013) emphasize that it is a relatively fast process. Differences in search performance on old and new arrays arise already within less than five exposures. As such it resembles more a spatial-based repetition priming mechanism. In line with the latter option, a situation with which we are often confronted in daily life occurs when we directly but unconsciously start searching in the correct direction for a target object even after the first encounter. A technique that is especially suited to assess these automatic and unaware memory influences consists of eye movement tracking. Richardson and Spivey (2000) had participants listen to simple semantic statements offered at different spatial locations (quadrants at a screen). When later asked to answer questions with respect to these statements, participants typically looked in the direction of the quadrant where the statement was originally offered. Richardson and Spivey (2000) argue that our cognitive system employs spatial indexes to retrieve information even in a task where spatial location is not relevant and the to-be-retrieved information is not linked to a location by the information content. This behavior thus seems to run automatically. Spivey and Geng (2001) further demonstrated the automaticity of this spatial indexing process by showing participants to make spontaneous, directional eye movements when recalling or imaging objects that were not there. Admittedly the critical test of this being really an implicit measure should consist of observing eye movement toward previously inspected locations in the absence of consciously remembering the target location. This would more convincingly demonstrate that residual spatial information traces, that are not consciously accessible, still guide our eye movement system in a compelling, automatic fashion. One line of evidence in that direction is given by Laeng et al. (2007) who demonstrated that three amnesic patients who could not explicitly remember the contents of an event still directed their gaze to the location on the screen where information related to the event had previously been given. Together the foregoing indicates that our eyes might remember important spatial places that our minds already long have forgotten. In particular this could be vital to searching and finding objects in space.

An elegant third type of test for implicit object location processing is offered by Caldwell and Masson (2001). They started with the notion formulated by Jacoby (1991) that our behavior at the same time can be guided by both conscious memory influences and unconscious memory influences, the former reflecting the working of explicit memory systems and the latter that of implicit memory systems. In order to separate these joint influences in the observed, aggregate behavior Jacoby (1991) designed an elegant procedure that was adapted by Caldwell and Masson (2001) for object location memory tasks. The basic principle is to have participants study multiple object locations that later have to be relocated. At test for half of the trials—the include-trials—the task is to pick the old location that was studied in the learning phase from a multiple possible choice locations. In the other half of the trials—the exclude-trials—the task is to choose a new location in the multiple choice test. Notice that for both types of trials one has to use the conscious memories of where the object has been before in order to perform correctly. This illustrates the flexibility of our conscious memories: we can express them in a variety of ways depending on the current conditions or instructions. If however there is no conscious memory, any existing unconscious memory influences might play a role. The assumption is that these unconscious influences are rather inflexible, habit based: they will always guide you back to the old location, independent from the instructions holding for that situation. Consequently, in the include-trials conscious and unconscious influences will work together in retrieving the old locations. In the exclude-trials they will instead work oppositely, with the conscious influences making you pick a new location and the unconscious causing you to return to the old places contrary to the instructions. The latter effects can only be observed when there is no conscious memory at the time (illustrating that conscious memory dominates the unconscious influence). Effectively the conscious and unconscious estimates can be computed from calculating the proportion old locations both for the include-trials and for the exclude-trials. This proportion is taken to equate to $C + (1\text{-}C)U$ for the include-trials, and to $(1\text{-}C)U$ for the exclude-trials (with C being the conscious memory estimate and U the unconscious memory estimate).

Interestingly, Caldwell and Masson (2001) observed age differences for the conscious object location memory estimate but not for the unconscious form. In contrast, by showing the object multiple times during the study phase either in the same location or in new locations, different habit strengths were created. Unconscious memory was found to relate to habit strength but conscious memory did not. In a subsequent study, Postma, Antonides, Wester, and Kessels (2008) demonstrated spared unconscious object location memory against a severely impaired conscious counterpart in Korsakov patients. Similar patterns were found in Alzheimer patients (Kessels, Feijen, & Postma, 2005). On a critical note it should be mentioned here that the process dissociation procedure as employed in spatial memory also suffers problems. Among others, one further assumption is that the conscious and unconscious memory estimates are independent. This has not always been tested however. Moreover in particular the unconscious estimate reflecting a tendency to go back to the old locations independent from the present instructions should effectively be higher than chance in order to show a real memory effect (chance resembling the fact that because of the multiple choice object location memory test, one can by luck pick the old location). This has not always been observed though (Kessels et al., 2005; Postma, Antonides et al., 2008).

Together, the foregoing discussion of implicit forms of spatial memory strongly suggests that we often have a gut feeling of where things are that escapes conscious reflection and awareness. It seems interesting to further investigate just how far these gut feelings can form the basis for a residual memory capacity that may support amnesic patients in various daily life activities. At the same time we should acknowledge that in more complex spatial memory situations, such as in navigation tasks, it may be doubted in how far implicit memory can really be helpful. It might help us to pick the correct turn at the start of the route. However, any of the subsequent turns in which there is no implicit memory will lead us completely off track in case we go the wrong direction.

REFERENCES

Abrahams, S., Pickering, A., Polkey, C. E., & Morris, R. G. (1997). Spatial memory deficits in patients with unilateral damage to the right hippocampal formation. *Neuropsychologia*, *35*(1), 11–24. Available from http://dx.doi.org/10.1016/S0028-3932(96)00051-6.

Baddeley, A. (2012). Working memory: Theories, models, and controversies. *Annual Review of Psychology*, *63*, 1–29. Available from http://dx.doi.org/10.1146/annurev-psych-120710-100422.

Baddeley, A. D. (2000). The episodic buffer: A new component of working memory? *Trends in Cognitive Sciences*, *4*(11), 417–423. Retrieved from http://www.ncbi.nlm.nih.gov/pubmed/11058819.

Baddeley, A. D. (2007). Working memory, thought and action. Oxford, England: Oxford University Press.

Baddeley, A. D., & Hitch, G. (1974). Working memory. In G. H. Bower (Ed.), *The psychology of learning and motivation: Advances in research and theory* (Vol. 8, pp. 47–89). New York: Academic Press.

Bates, E., Wilson, S. M., Saygin, A. P., Dick, F., Sereno, M. I., Knight, R. T., & Dronkers, N. F. (2003). Voxel-based lesion-symptom mapping. *Nature Neuroscience*, *6* (5), 448–450. Available from http://dx.doi.org/10.1038/nn1050.

Bianchini, F., Di Vita, A., Palermo, L., Piccardi, L., Blundo, C., & Guariglia, C. (2014). A selective egocentric topographical working memory deficit in the early stages of Alzheimer's disease: A preliminary study. *American Journal of Alzheimer's Disease and Other Dementias*, *29*(8), 749–754. Available from http://dx.doi.org/10.1177/1533317514536597.

Biesbroek, J. M., van Zandvoort, M. J., Kappelle, L. J., Schoo, L., Kuijf, H. J., Velthuis, B. K., Biessels, G. J., & Postma, A. (2015). Distinct anatomical correlates of discriminability and criterion setting in verbal recognition memory revealed by lesion-symptom mapping. *Human Brain Mapping*, *36*(4), 1292–1303. Available from http://dx.doi.org/10.1002/hbm.22702.

Bohbot, V. D., Kalina, M., Stepankova, K., Spackova, N., Petrides, M., & Nadel, L. (1998). Spatial memory deficits in patients with lesions to the right hippocampus and to the right parahippocampal cortex. *Neuropsychologia, 36*(11), 1217–1238. Retrieved from http://www.ncbi.nlm.nih.gov/pubmed/9842767.

Brockmole, J. R., & Henderson, J. M. (2006). Using real-world scenes as contextual cues for search. *Visual Cognition, 13*, 99–108.

Brunetti, R., Del Gatto, C., & Delogu, F. (2014). eCorsi: implementation and testing of the Corsi block-tapping task for digital tablets. *Frontiers in Psychology, 5*, 939. Available from http://dx.doi.org/10.3389/fpsyg.2014.00939.

Bucks, R. S., & Willison, J. R. (1997). Development and validation of the Location Learning Test (LLT): A test of visuo-spatial learning designed for use with older adults and in dementia. *Clinical Neuropsychologist, 11*, 273–286.

Burgess, N., Spiers, H. J., & Paleologou, E. (2004). Orientational manoeuvres in the dark: Dissociating allocentric and egocentric influences on spatial memory. *Cognition, 94*(2), 149–166. Available from http://dx.doi.org/10.1016/j.cognition.2004.01.001.

Caldwell, J. I., & Masson, M. E. (2001). Conscious and unconscious influences of memory for object location. *Memory & Cognition, 29*(2), 285–295. Retrieved from http://www.ncbi.nlm.nih.gov/pubmed/11352211.

Cattaneo, Z., Fastame, M. C., Vecchi, T., & Cornoldi, C. (2006). Working memory, imagery and visuo-spatial mechanisms. In T. Vecchi, & G. Bottini (Eds.), *Imagery and spatial cognition: Methods, models and cognitive assessment*. Amsterdam: John Benjamins Publishing Company.

Chalfonte, B. L., Verfaellie, M., Johnson, M. K., & Reiss, L. (1996). Spatial location memory in amnesia: Binding item and location information under incidental and intentional encoding conditions. *Memory (Hove, England), 4*(6), 591–614. Available from http://dx.doi.org/10.1080/741940998.

Chechlacz, M., Rotshtein, P., & Humphreys, G. W. (2014). Neuronal substrates of Corsi Block span: Lesion symptom mapping analyses in relation to attentional competition and spatial bias. *Neuropsychologia, 64C*, 240–251. Available from http://dx.doi.org/10.1016/j.neuropsychologia.2014.09.038.

Chun, M. M. (2000). Contextual cueing of visual attention. *Trends in Cognitive Sciences, 4*(5), 170–178. Retrieved from http://www.ncbi.nlm.nih.gov/pubmed/10782102.

Chun, M. M., & Jiang, Y. (1998). Contextual cueing: Implicit learning and memory of visual context guides spatial attention. *Cognitive Psychology, 36*(1), 28–71. Available from http://dx.doi.org/10.1006/cogp.1998.0681.

Chun, M. M., & Phelps, E. A. (1999). Memory deficits for implicit contextual information in amnesic subjects with hippocampal damage. *Nature Neuroscience, 2*(9), 844–847. Available from http://dx.doi.org/10.1038/12222.

Claessen, M. H., van der Ham, I. J., & van Zandvoort, M. J. (2015). Computerization of the standard corsi block-tapping task affects its underlying cognitive concepts: A pilot study. *Applied Neuropsychology Adult, 22*(3), 180–188. Available from http://dx.doi.org/10.1080/23279095.2014.892488.

Corsi, P. M. (1972). Human memory and the medial temporal region of the brain. *Dissertation Abstracts International: Section B. Sciences and Engineering, 34*(2), 891.

Craik, F. I. M., & Lockhart, R. S. (1972). Levels of processing: A framework for memory research. *Journal of Verbal Learning and Verbal Behavior, 11*, 671–684.

Crane, J., & Milner, B. (2005). What went where? Impaired object-location learning in patients with right hippocampal lesions. *Hippocampus, 15*(2), 216–231. Available from http://dx.doi.org/10.1002/hipo.20043.

Dent, K., & Smyth, M. M. (2005). Verbal coding and the storage of form–position associations in visual–spatial short-term memory. *Acta Psychologica, 120*(2), 113–140. Available from http://dx.doi.org/10.1016/j.actpsy.2005.03.004.

Dewar, M., Della Sala, S., Beschin, N., & Cowan, N. (2010). Profound retroactive interference in anterograde amnesia: What interferes? *Neuropsychology, 24*(3), 357–367. Available from http://dx.doi.org/10.1037/a0018207.

Dowson, J. H., McLean, A., Bazanis, E., Toone, B., Young, S., Robbins, T. W., & Sahakian, B. J. (2004). Impaired spatial working memory in adults with attention-deficit/hyperactivity disorder: Comparisons with performance in adults with borderline personality disorder and in control subjects. *Acta Psychiatrica Scandinavica, 110*(1), 45–54. Available from http://dx.doi.org/10.1111/j.1600-0447.2004.00292.x.

Elmes, D. G. (1988). Interference in spatial memory. *Journal of Experimental Psychology, 14*, 668–675.

Feigenbaum, J. D., Polkey, C. E., & Morris, R. G. (1996). Deficits in spatial working memory after unilateral temporal lobectomy in man. *Neuropsychologia, 34*(3), 163–176. Retrieved from http://www.ncbi.nlm.nih.gov/pubmed/8868274.

Grill-Spector, K., Kourtzi, Z., & Kanwisher, N. (2001). The lateral occipital complex and its role in object recognition. *Vision Research, 41*(10-11), 1409–1422. Retrieved from http://www.ncbi.nlm.nih.gov/pubmed/11322983.

Hasher, L., & Zacks, R. T. (1979). Automatic and effortful processes in memory. *Journal of Experimental Psychology: General, 108*, 356–388.

Jacoby, L. L. (1991). A process dissociation framework: Separating automatic from intentional uses of memory. *Journal of Memory & Language, 30*, 513–541.

James, W. (1890). *The principles of psychology.* London: MacMillan.

Jonides, J., Reuter-Lorenz, P. A., Smith, E. E., Awh, E., Barnes, L. L., Drain, M., & Schumacher, E. (1996). Verbal and spatial working memory in humans. In D. L. Medin (Ed.), *The psychology of learning and motivation* (Vol. 35, pp. 165–192). New York: Academic Press.

Kessels, R. P., de Haan, E. H., Kappelle, L. J., & Postma, A. (2002). Selective impairments in spatial memory after ischaemic stroke. *Journal of Clinical and Experimental Neuropsychology, 24*(1), 115–129. Available from http://dx.doi.org/10.1076/jcen.24.1.115.967.

Kessels, R. P., Feijen, J., & Postma, A. (2005). Implicit and explicit memory for spatial information in Alzheimer's disease. *Dementia and Geriatric Cognitive Disorders, 20*(2–3), 184–191. Available from http://dx.doi.org/10.1159/000087233.

Kessels, R. P., Hendriks, M., Schouten, J., Van Asselen, M., & Postma, A. (2004). Spatial memory deficits in patients after unilateral selective amygdalohippocampectomy. *Journal of the International Neuropsychological Society: JINS, 10*(6), 907–912. Retrieved from http://www.ncbi.nlm.nih.gov/pubmed/15637783.

Kessels, R. P., Jaap Kappelle, L., de Haan, E. H., & Postma, A. (2002). Lateralization of spatial-memory processes: Evidence on spatial span, maze learning, and memory for object locations. *Neuropsychologia, 40*(8), 1465–1473, [pii] S0028393201001993.

Kessels, R. P., Nys, G. M., Brands, A. M., van den Berg, E., & Van Zandvoort, M. J. (2006). The modified Location Learning Test: Norms for the assessment of spatial memory function in neuropsychological patients. *Archives of Clinical Neuropsychology: The Official Journal of the National Academy of Neuropsychologists, 21*(8), 841–846. Available from http://dx.doi.org/10.1016/j.acn.2006.06.015.

Kessels, R. P., Postma, A., & de Haan, E. H. (1999). Object relocation: A program for setting up, running, and analyzing experiments on memory for object locations. *Behavior Research Methods, Instruments, & Computers: A Journal of the Psychonomic Society, Inc., 31*(3), 423–428. Retrieved from http://www.ncbi.nlm.nih.gov/pubmed/10502864.

Kessels, R. P., Postma, A., Wester, A. J., & de Haan, E. H. (2000). Memory for object locations in Korsakoff's amnesia. *Cortex, 36*(1), 47–57. Retrieved from http://www.ncbi.nlm.nih.gov/pubmed/10728896.

Kessels, R. P., van Zandvoort, M. J., Postma, A., Kappelle, L. J., & de Haan, E. H. (2000). The Corsi Block-Tapping Task: Standardization and normative data. *Applied Neuropsychology, 7*(4), 252–258. Available from http://dx.doi.org/10.1207/S15324826AN0704_8.

King, J. A., Trinkler, I., Hartley, T., Vargha-Khadem, F., & Burgess, N. (2004). The hippocampal role in spatial memory and the familiarity—Recollection distinction: A case study. *Neuropsychology, 18*(3), 405–417. Available from http://dx.doi.org/10.1037/0894-4105.18.3.405.

Kosslyn, S. M. (1987). Seeing and imagining in the cerebral hemispheres: A computational approach. *Psychological Review, 94*(2), 148–175. Retrieved from http://www.ncbi.nlm.nih.gov/pubmed/3575583.

Laeng, B., Waterloo, K., Johnsen, S. H., Bakke, S. J., Lag, T., Simonsen, S. S., & Hogsaet, J. (2007). The eyes remember it: Oculography and pupillometry during recollection in three amnesic patients. *Journal of Cognitive Neuroscience, 19*(11), 1888–1904. Available from http://dx.doi.org/10.1162/jocn.2007.19.11.1888.

Logie, R. H. (1995). *Visuo-spatial working memory.* Hove, England: Erlbaum.

Logie, R. H. (2011). The functional organization and capacity limits of working memory. *Current Directions in Psychological Science, 20*(4), 240–245. Available from http://dx.doi.org/10.1177/0963721411415340.

Mandler, J. M., Seegmiller, D., & Day, J. (1977). On the coding of spatial information. *Memory & Cognition, 5*(1), 10–16. Available from http://dx.doi.org/10.3758/BF03209185.

McAfoose, J., & Baune, B. T. (2009). Exploring visual–spatial working memory: A critical review of concepts and models. *Neuropsychology Review, 19*(1), 130–142. Available from http://dx.doi.org/10.1007/s11065-008-9063-0.

Morris, R., Evenden, J., Sahakian, B., & Robbins, T. (1987). Computer-aided assessment of dementia: Comparative studies of neuropsychological deficits in Alzheimer-type dementia and Parkinson's disease. In S. Stahl, S. Iversen, & E. Goodman (Eds.), *Cognitive neurochemistry* (pp. 21–36). Oxford, UK: Oxford University Press.

Morris, R. G., Downes, J. J., Sahakian, B. J., Evenden, J. L., Heald, A., & Robbins, T. W. (1988). Planning and spatial working memory in Parkinson's disease. *Journal of Neurology, Neurosurgery, and Psychiatry, 51*(6), 757–766. Retrieved from http://www.ncbi.nlm.nih.gov/pubmed/3404183.

Nicolas, S. (1996). Experiments on implicit memory in a Korsakoff patient by Claparede (1907). *Cognitive Neuropsychology, 13*(8), 1193–1199.

Nunn, J. A., Graydon, F. J., Polkey, C. E., & Morris, R. G. (1999). Differential spatial memory impairment after right temporal lobectomy demonstrated using temporal titration. *Brain, 122*(Pt 1), 47–59. Retrieved from http://www.ncbi.nlm.nih.gov/pubmed/10050894.

Oberauer, K., & Vockenberg, K. (2009). Updating of working memory: Lingering bindings. *The Quarterly Journal of Experimental Psychology (Hove), 62*(5), 967–987. Available from http://dx.doi.org/10.1080/17470210802372912.

Olson, I. R., & Chun, M. M. (2002). Perceptual constraints on implicit learning of spatial context. *Visual Cognition, 9*, 273–302.

Oudman, E., Van der Stigchel, S., Wester, A. J., Kessels, R. P., & Postma, A. (2011). Intact memory for implicit contextual information in Korsakoff's amnesia. *Neuropsychologia, 49*(10), 2848–2855. Available from http://dx.doi.org/10.1016/j.neuropsychologia.2011.06.010.

Owen, A. M., Downes, J. J., Sahakian, B. J., Polkey, C. E., & Robbins, T. W. (1990). Planning and spatial working memory following frontal lobe lesions in man. *Neuropsychologia, 28*(10), 1021–1034. Retrieved from http://www.ncbi.nlm.nih.gov/pubmed/2267054.

Owen, A. M., Sahakian, B. J., Semple, J., Polkey, C. E., & Robbins, T. W. (1995). Visuospatial short-term recognition memory and learning after temporal lobe excisions, frontal lobe excisions or amygdalo-hippocampectomy in man. *Neuropsychologia, 33*(1), 1–24. Retrieved from http://www.ncbi.nlm.nih.gov/pubmed/7731533.

Piccardi, L., Berthoz, A., Baulac, M., Denos, M., Dupont, S., Samson, S., & Guariglia, C. (2010). Different spatial memory systems are involved in small- and large-scale environments: Evidence from patients with temporal lobe epilepsy. *Experimental Brain Research, 206*(2), 171–177. Available from http://dx.doi.org/10.1007/s00221-010-2234-2.

Piccardi, L., Bianchini, F., Argento, O., De Nigris, A., Maialetti, A., Palermo, L., & Guariglia, C. (2013). The Walking Corsi Test (WalCT): Standardization of the topographical memory test in an Italian population. *Neurological Sciences: Official Journal of the Italian Neurological Society and of the Italian Society of Clinical Neurophysiology, 34*(6), 971–978. Available from http://dx.doi.org/10.1007/s10072-012-1175-x.

Piccardi, L., Bianchini, F., Nori, R., Marano, A., Iachini, F., Lasala, L., & Guariglia, C. (2014). Spatial location and pathway memory compared in the reaching vs. walking domains. *Neuroscience Letters, 566*, 226–230. Available from http://dx.doi.org/10.1016/j.neulet.2014.03.005.

Piccardi, L., Iaria, G., Ricci, M., Bianchini, F., Zompanti, L., & Guariglia, C. (2008). Walking in the Corsi test: Which type of memory do you need? *Neuroscience Letters, 432*(2), 127–131. Available from http://dx.doi.org/10.1016/j.neulet.2007.12.044.

Piccardi, L., Palermo, L., Leonzi, M., Risetti, M., Zompanti, L., D'Amico, S., & Guariglia, C. (2014). The Walking Corsi Test (WalCT): A normative study of topographical working memory in a sample of 4- to 11-year-olds. *The Clinical Neuropsychologist, 28*(1), 84–96. Available from http://dx.doi.org/10.1080/13854046.2013.863976.

Postma, A., Antonides, R., Wester, A. J., & Kessels, R. P. (2008). Spared unconscious influences of spatial memory in diencephalic amnesia. *Experimental Brain Research, 190*(2), 125–133. Available from http://dx.doi.org/10.1007/s00221-008-1456-z.

Postma, A., & De Haan, E. H. (1996). What was where? Memory for object locations. *The Quarterly Journal of Experimental Psychology Section A: Human Experimental Psychology, 49*(1), 178–199. Available from http://dx.doi.org/10.1080/713755605.

Postma, A., Kessels, R. P., & van Asselen, M. (2008). How the brain remembers and forgets where things are: The neurocognition of object-location memory. *Neuroscience and Biobehavioral Reviews, 32*(8), 1339–1345. Available from http://dx.doi.org/10.1016/j.neubiorev.2008.05.001.

Postma, A., & Kessels, R. P. C. (2006). Do we only remember where we left our things when we expect to need them again: Expectancy manipulations and object location memory. In T. Vecchi, & G. Bottini (Eds.), *Imagery and spatial cognition: Methods, models and cognitive assessment*. Amsterdam/Philadelphia: John Benjamins Publishers.

Richardson, D. C., & Spivey, M. J. (2000). Representation, space and Hollywood Squares: Looking at things that aren't there anymore. *Cognition, 76*(3), 269–295. Retrieved from http://www.ncbi.nlm.nih.gov/pubmed/10913578.

Rorden, C., & Karnath, H. O. (2004). Using human brain lesions to infer function: A relic from a past era in the fMRI age? *Nature Reviews Neuroscience, 5*(10), 813–819. Available from http://dx.doi.org/10.1038/nrn1521.

Sahakian, B. J., Morris, R. G., Evenden, J. L., Heald, A., Levy, R., Philpot, M., & Robbins, T. W. (1988). A comparative study of visuospatial memory and learning in Alzheimer-type dementia and Parkinson's disease. *Brain, 111*(Pt 3), 695–718. Retrieved from http://www.ncbi.nlm.nih.gov/pubmed/3382917.

Shoqeirat, M. A., & Mayes, A. R. (1991). Disproportionate incidental spatial-memory and recall deficits in amnesia. *Neuropsychologia*, *29*(8), 749–769. Retrieved from http://www.ncbi.nlm.nih.gov/pubmed/1944876.

Smith, M. L., Leonard, G., Crane, J., & Milner, B. (1995). The effects of frontal- or temporal-lobe lesions on susceptibility to interference in spatial memory. *Neuropsychologia*, *33*(3), 275–285. Retrieved from http://www.ncbi.nlm.nih.gov/pubmed/7791996.

Smith, M. L., & Milner, B. (1981). The role of the right hippocampus in the recall of spatial location. *Neuropsychologia*, *19*(6), 781–793. Retrieved from http://www.ncbi.nlm.nih.gov/pubmed/7329524.

Smith, M. L., & Milner, B. (1984). Differential effects of frontal-lobe lesions on cognitive estimation and spatial memory. *Neuropsychologia*, *22*(6), 697–705. Retrieved from http://www.ncbi.nlm.nih.gov/pubmed/6441896.

Smith, M. L., & Milner, B. (1989). Right hippocampal impairment in the recall of spatial location: Encoding deficit or rapid forgetting? *Neuropsychologia*, *27*(1), 71–81. Retrieved from http://www.ncbi.nlm.nih.gov/pubmed/2496329.

Spivey, M. J., & Geng, J. J. (2001). Oculomotor mechanisms activated by imagery and memory: Eye movements to absent objects. *Psychological Research*, *65*(4), 235–241. Retrieved from http://www.ncbi.nlm.nih.gov/pubmed/11789427.

Sulpizio, V., Committeri, G., Lambrey, S., Berthoz, A., & Galati, G. (2013). Selective role of lingual/parahippocampal gyrus and retrosplenial complex in spatial memory across viewpoint changes relative to the environmental reference frame. *Behavioural Brain Research*, *242*, 62–75. Available from http://dx.doi.org/10.1016/j.bbr.2012.12.031.

Tseng, Y. C., & Lleras, A. (2013). Rewarding context accelerates implicit guidance in visual search. *Attention, Perception, & Psychophysics*, *75*(2), 287–298. Available from http://dx.doi.org/10.3758/s13414-012-0400-2.

van Asselen, M., Almeida, I., Andre, R., Januario, C., Goncalves, A. F., & Castelo-Branco, M. (2009). The role of the basal ganglia in implicit contextual learning: A study of Parkinson's disease. *Neuropsychologia*, *47*(5), 1269–1273. Available from http://dx.doi.org/10.1016/j.neuropsychologia.2009.01.008.

van Asselen, M., Almeida, I., Julio, F., Januario, C., Campos, E. B., Simoes, M., & Castelo-Branco, M. (2012). Implicit contextual learning in prodromal and early stage Huntington's disease patients. *Journal of the International Neuropsychological Society: JINS*, *18*(4), 689–696. Available from http://dx.doi.org/10.1017/S1355617712000288.

van Asselen, M., Kessels, R. P., Frijns, C. J., Kappelle, L. J., Neggers, S. F., & Postma, A. (2009). Object-location memory: A lesion-behavior mapping study in stroke patients. *Brain and Cognition*, *71*(3), 287–294. Available from http://dx.doi.org/10.1016/j.bandc.2009.07.012.

van Asselen, M., Kessels, R. P., Kappelle, L. J., & Postma, A. (2008). Categorical and coordinate spatial representations within object-location memory. *Cortex*, *44*(3), 249–256. Available from http://dx.doi.org/10.1016/j.cortex.2006.05.005.

van Asselen, M., Kessels, R. P., Neggers, S. F., Kappelle, L. J., Frijns, C. J., & Postma, A. (2006). Brain areas involved in spatial working memory. *Neuropsychologia*, *44*(7), 1185–1194. Available from http://dx.doi.org/10.1016/j.neuropsychologia.2005.10.005.

van Asselen, M., Kessels, R. P., Wester, A. J., & Postma, A. (2005). Spatial working memory and contextual cueing in patients with Korsakoff amnesia. *Journal of Clinical and Experimental Neuropsychology*, *27*(6), 645–655. Available from http://dx.doi.org/10.1081/13803390490919281.

van Asselen, M., Sampaio, J., Pina, A., & Castelo-Branco, M. (2011). Object based implicit contextual learning: A study of eye movements. *Attention, Perception, & Psychophysics*, *73*(2), 297–302. Available from http://dx.doi.org/10.3758/s13414-010-0047-9.

van der Ham, I. J., Postma, A., & Laeng, B. (2014). Lateralized perception: The role of attention in spatial relation processing. *Neuroscience and Biobehavioral Reviews*, *45*, 142–148. Available from http://dx.doi.org/10.1016/j.neubiorev.2014.05.006.

Wang, R. F., & Simons, D. J. (1999). Active and passive scene recognition across views. *Cognition*, *70*(2), 191–210. Retrieved from http://www.ncbi.nlm.nih.gov/pubmed/10349763.

Wansard, M., Bartolomeo, P., Bastin, C., Segovia, F., Gillet, S., Duret, C., & Meulemans, T. (2015). Support for distinct subcomponents of spatial working memory: a double dissociation between spatial-simultaneous and spatial-sequential performance in unilateral neglect. *Cognitve Neuropsychology*, *32*(1), 14–28. Available from http://dx.doi.org/10.1080/02643294.2014.995075.

Zimmer, H. (2012). Visual imagery in the brain: Modality-specifc and spatial, but perhaps without space. In V. Gyselinck, & F. Pazzaglia (Eds.), *From mental imagery to spatial cognition and lanugage: Essays in honour of Michel Denis*. London and New York: Psychology Press.

Zimmer, H. D. (2008). Visual and spatial working memory: From boxes to networks. *Neuroscience and Biobehavioral Reviews*, *32*(8), 1373–1395. Available from http://dx.doi.org/10.1016/j.neubiorev.2008.05.016.

Zimmermann, K., & Eschen, A. (in press). Brain regions involved in subprocesses of small-space episodic object-location memory: A systematic review of lesion and functional neuroimaging studies. *Memory*.

Zimmer, H. D., Speiser, H. R., & Seidler, B. (2003). Spatio-temporal working-memory and short-term object-location tasks use different memory mechanisms. *Acta Psychologica*, *114*(1), 41–65. Retrieved from http://www.ncbi.nlm.nih.gov/pubmed/12927342.

CHAPTER 8
Navigation Ability

Ineke J.M. van der Ham[1,2] and Michiel H.G. Claessen[1,3]
[1]Experimental Psychology, Helmholtz Institute, Utrecht University, Utrecht, The Netherlands
[2]Department of Health, Medical and Neuropsychology Leiden University, Leiden, The Netherlands
[3]Rudolf Magnus Institute of Neuroscience and Center of Excellence for Rehabilitation Medicine, University Medical Center Utrecht and Rehabilitation Center De Hoogstraat, Utrecht, The Netherlands

> *I have these moments when I do not know where to go next to get to where I am heading. It happens suddenly, I cannot predict when it will happen again. I can be driving on the highway with my three children in the back of the car and when it happens I have no idea of where I should be going. Then I get scared; all of a sudden I do not know which exit to take, but I am driving 120 km/hour and I have to make a decision.*
>
> ***Patient AC***

> *I am afraid to go out by myself, as I get lost very easily. Especially the speed at which I move is important. I cannot go by bike anymore, as biking is too fast for me to make decisions about turns I have to take. Walking speed is okay, and I can stop to think if I need to. I am always thinking about possible construction work on my way, even on routes I know very well, I may be forced to cross the street or take a detour. Then I doubt whether I am able to continue my way.*
>
> ***Patient WJ***

Patient AC and WJ both suffer from navigation impairment, or topographical disorientation. This type of impairment can have severe consequences on daily life activities; not only anxiety plays an important role, but also the ability to travel independently. Apart from the severity of the impact, the frequency at which we rely on our navigation skills is very high: whether we find our way to the kitchen in our house or travel to a foreign country, intact navigation ability is essential.

Navigation may well be the most complex skill within the domain of spatial cognition. Not only does it entail an elaborate range of cognitive abilities, there is quite some ambiguity about its definition in literature. To explain what is meant by navigation, it can be helpful to think about situations in which our navigation ability fails us. For instance when a traffic situation is very complicated, as in Fig. 8.1. The traffic sign can be helpful, but the good luck wishes are a clear indication that many people will have some trouble figuring out this particular situation.

Neuropsychology of Space.
DOI: http://dx.doi.org/10.1016/B978-0-12-801638-1.00008-2

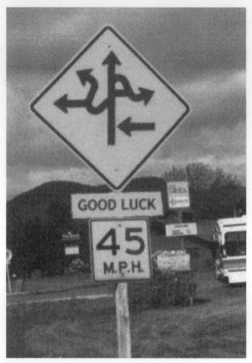

Figure 8.1 Navigation in daily life is not always easy.

Especially when we have to find our way around locations we have not visited before; when we are on holiday for instance, we are confronted with the limitations of our navigation ability and resort to different types of navigation aids, like maps, GPS support, or the help of locals we may meet on our way. So, navigation entails all processes involved when we try to reach a certain goal location. This goal location does not have to be at a substantial distance, but can be as nearby as the kitchen in our own house. Any goal that requires us to physically move around to reach it falls within the territory of navigation ability.

This chapter covers human navigation behavior. This complex spatial ability encompasses many of the spatial processes discussed in the previous chapters, like spatial perception, attention, and geometrical knowledge. In this chapter we will first cover the concept of navigation and provide an overview of navigation research carried out in the past decades. The first studies on navigation were performed in animals, and later on these findings were translated to human studies, with a steep increase in behavioral as well as neuroanatomical studies over the past two decades. We will provide an overview of these experimental and theoretical developments. This will be followed by a discussion of current perspectives on navigation. This overview will be complemented by a discussion of current methods used to measure navigation behavior and how novel technological advances can be used to stimulate experimental developments. In the second part of the chapter we will place navigation ability in a clinical context, with an overview of methods to diagnose navigation impairments and a discussion of diagnostic tools and treatment of this type of neuropsychological impairment. In the third part, the latest theoretical developments and clinical findings are brought together and lead to a discussion of future directions in navigation research. The main strategy we take in this chapter is to combine the contemporary theoretical views on navigation with current clinical insights. We consider it worthwhile to explore possibilities for mutual exchange of these views and insights to reach a more in-depth understanding of navigation ability as a whole.

PART 1: NAVIGATION RESEARCH

8.1 BASIC SPATIAL BEHAVIOR

Most animals master some form of navigation ability, albeit very basic in some cases. Three general levels of complexity can be distinguished here: route following, piloting, and dead reckoning. Route following refers to the very simple skill of identifying cues in the environment and following their spatial location. Ants do this for instance, when finding food sources near their nests. They create pheromone trails to their target locations that can be detected and followed by other ants (eg, Van der Meer, 1986). Humans also apply this type of simple navigation, for instance when following route markers when hiking, for example, taking the "red trail."

Slightly more advanced is piloting. This behavior entails the intentional exploration of an environment to reach a certain target item or location. The Morris Water Maze (Morris, 1984) is the perfect experimental example of this behavior. This maze consists of a circular pool filled with opaque water, with a small platform hidden somewhere in the pool just below the water surface. A mouse or rat is then placed in the pool and will start to swim around. Mice and rats are typically skilled swimmers, but will avoid swimming when possible, as being in the water lowers their body temperature. They will swim and explore the environment until they have detected the platform and can rest on it. When repeating this procedure with the same animal, the accumulation of some form of spatial location memory becomes evident: there is a steep learning curve as the animals take into account their environment and memorize the platform location in relation to the environment, which indicates the ability to perform basic mapping of an environment. Humans display this kind of behavior when searching for items on a scavenger hunt for instance.

Dead reckoning concerns spatial behavior in which detailed geometric calculations take place: an animal can infer its starting location based on the path it has taken from that location. Such path integration is associated with the right temporal lobe in humans (Worsley et al., 2001). Not only distance, but also directional information is taken into account to perform this calculation (eg, McNaughton, Chen, & Markus, 1991). Sailors mimic this process with mechanical measures when insufficient visual input is available. Then the ship's movement, speed, and direction are used to calculate positions.

These three types of spatial behavior fall within the realm of human navigation ability, but are complemented by a range of more complex cognitive activities that concern the processing of information derived from landmarks, routes taken, and the layout of the environment.

8.2 CELLS IN THE HIPPOCAMPAL FORMATION

In 2014, the Nobel Prize for Medicine was awarded to John O'Keefe and Edvard and May-Britt Moser. They received this award for the discovery of two different cell types within the hippocampal formation: place cells and grid cells. These discoveries have proven to be highly influential in cognitive neuroscience and in the field of spatial cognition in particular.

The first report on place cells dates back to 1971, when John O'Keefe reported about hippocampal cells that fire when the animal is at a specific location in an environment, regardless of motor or motivational aspects of the task at hand (see also Morris, Garrud, Rawlins, & O'Keefe, 1982). These cells are termed place cells, as they provide information about a specific location. Later on, grid cells, boundary vector cells, and head direction cells were also found in the hippocampal formation in the rat brain (Burgess, Recce, & O'Keefe, 1994; Fyhn, Molden, Witter, Moser, & Moser, 2004; Sargolini et al., 2006). Grid cells fire at regularly spaced intervals and therefore provide an indication of the layout of an environment. Boundary vector cells show activity when an animal is in the vicinity of a specific edge of an environment, providing further information about the animal's relative position in its surroundings. The orientation of the animal's head is indicated by the head direction cells, which is explicitly liked to the head itself, not the eyes or the rest of the body. In Fig. 8.2 a visual illustration of the activity of place cells, head direction cells, and grid cells is provided. The combination of these cells, coding for location, layout, boundaries, and head orientation, respectively, allows for the creation of a mental map of an environment, which is essential for many navigation tasks. This mental map provides a representation of the spatial layout of an environment, not bound by a specific viewpoint.

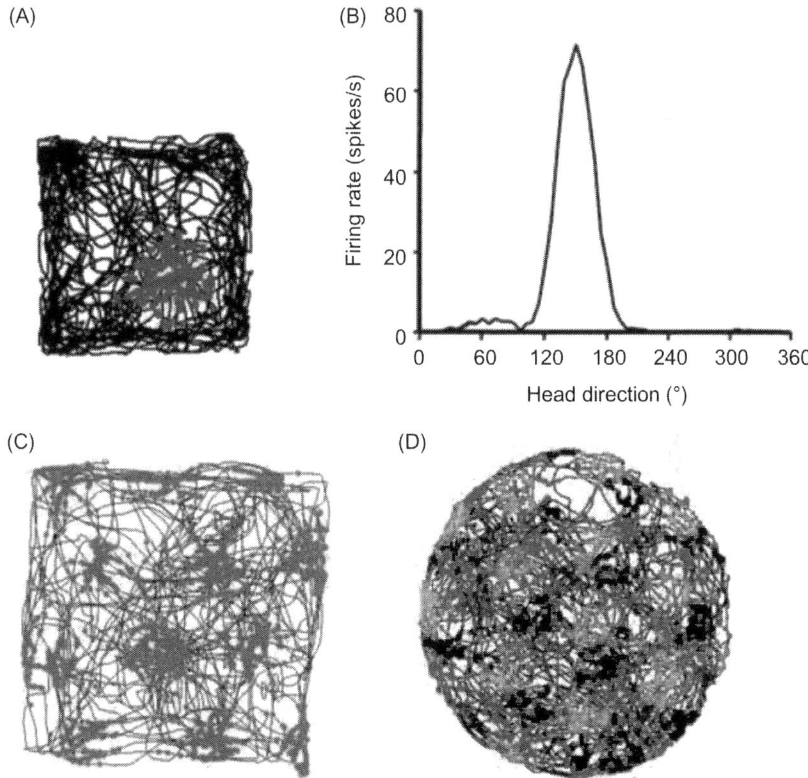

Figure 8.2 Single cell recordings of place cells, head direction cells, and grid cells. (A) Place cells: the black line indicates the rat's path in exploring a square enclosure, red squares highlight the locations at which a neuron fired. (B) Head direction cell activity: firing rate as a function of head direction. (C) Grid cell activity: firing at an array of locations in a regular triangular grid across the environment (same color scheme as A). (D) Example of three grid cells recorded on the same tetrode, firing in the three cells is highlighted in red, blue, and green. *Adapted from Jeffery, K. J., & Burgess, N. (2006). A metric for the cognitive map: found at last? Trends in Cognitive Sciences, 10(1), 1–3.*

Important parallels have been found between the rat and human brain in mental map creation, suggesting this process is highly similar in both species (eg, Burgess, Jackson, Hartley, & O'Keefe, 2000; Maguire, Burgess, & O'Keefe, 1999). In the following section on perspective taking we further discuss the use of such viewpoint-independent mental maps.

Apart from these specifically spatial cells, cells coding for time have also been detected in the hippocampus. While navigation is an obviously spatial process, mainly involving spatial distances, directions, and spatial maps, such temporal information may also play a significant role. When someone is asked how far away the train station is, they most likely will say something like "10 minutes away," instead of "850 meters away." This shows that in some instances we have a natural tendency to approach navigation from a temporal perspective. Some studies suggest that in rodents, time cells are another important cell type within the hippocampus, in addition to place cells. It has been proposed that coding of time and space coexist in the hippocampus and that temporal input may be of significant value to navigation (Bird & Burgess, 2008; Eichenbaum, 2013). Some researchers have suggested that distance and time may even be integrated in another class of cell types (MacDonald, Lepage, Eden, & Eichenbaum, 2011; Rowland & Moser, 2013), thus allowing for richer memories, including both space and time (Eichenbaum, 2014).

8.3 SPATIAL PERSPECTIVES

The mental map created based on the input from the different cell types found in the hippocampus is viewpoint independent, or based on an allocentric perspective. The use of various spatial perspectives is a central theme within navigation literature. Navigation-related input can be processed from this allocentric, environment-based, as well as from an egocentric, observer-based perspective. The location of a specific landmark can be coded as being either "north of city hall" (allocentric) or "to my left" (egocentric). The use of these two perspectives is clearly dissociated, behaviorally as well as neurologically.

A very elegant task design that has been used to assess such allocentric and egocentric processes is the Starmaze (Burguière et al., 2005; see Fig. 8.3). This task design has been used in a number of publications, with both rodent and human subjects and in a real world and virtual setting (eg, Fouquet, Tobin, & Rondi-Reig, 2010). This maze consists of five equally spaced arms, which are connected by a pentangular corridor.

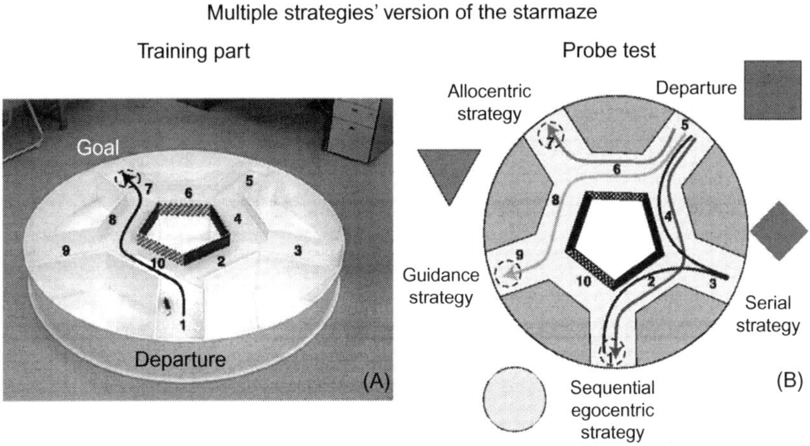

Figure 8.3 Layout of the starmaze. (A) The shortest route between a departure and goal arm. (B) Four different strategies that can be used to perform this task. When the participant is placed in a different arm, the different strategies lead to different selection of goal arm. If a participant is trained to find the goal arm from the departure arm as depicted in Figure A, then a change in departure arm can bring to light the use of different strategies. Serial strategy: visiting each arm sequentially; Sequential egocentric strategy: using the same sequence of turns; Guidance strategy: using proximal cues on the inner walls; Allocentric strategy: determining the goal location based on external landmarks (adapted from Burguière et al., 2005).

The regular shape of the maze allows for a clear assessment of egocentric and allocentric strategies. A participant is always placed at the end of one arm, and is instructed or motivated to find a specific target. This target is placed at the end of another arm. First, a participant is trained in a number of trials to find this target from a fixed starting position. After training, the participant is placed at a different starting position. When the participant searches for the target from this new starting point, several options are possible, as also shown in Fig. 8.3B. The two most prominent approaches make use of an egocentric or allocentric strategy. As the maze looks exactly the same from each possible starting point, the same geometric route can be followed. In Fig. 8.3 this is left turn-right turn-left turn. This is an egocentric strategy: the turns are based on the observer's position and do not take into account any features of the environment. The opposite is also possible; the allocentric strategy. Then, the participant will only take into account the environment and will use external cues (landmarks visible outside the maze) to find the target. A major advantage of the starmaze setup is that it allows the assessment of both strategy and ability. This is achieved by manipulating the target position. If the actual target is hidden in either the allocentrically or egocentrically correct target location, participants are forced to switch between the respective strategies in order to solve the task. This allows for assessment of a specific spatial ability; if forced to apply either an egocentric or allocentric strategy, does the participant succeed? In contrast, preferred strategy can be measured using multiple target locations, if the target is present at both the egocentrically and allocentrically correct goal location, the participant will be rewarded for either strategy. We thus can measure spontaneous preferences for a spatial strategy at an individual level.

The adoption of an egocentric perspective is generally easier and only requires exposure to an environment from one particular viewing angle. An allocentric perspective on the other hand, relies on the mental map of an environment, in which viewing angle is disregarded. In terms of neural correlates the two types of perspectives are also dissociated. Allocentric perspective taking is typically linked to hippocampal activation, whereas egocentric perspective use correlates strongly with parietal cortex activation (eg, Ciaramelli, Rosenbaum, Solcz, Levine, & Moscovitch, 2010; Vogeley & Fink, 2003).

The implementation of egocentric and allocentric perspective use has evolved over the years. A striking example of this process is the experimental setup to test spatial memory as first developed by Wang and Simons (1999) and later adjusted by Burgess, Spiers, and Paleologou (2004). Instead of only focusing on egocentric versus allocentric processes, Burgess and colleagues address a process called "egocentric updating." This process entails the adjustment of an egocentric viewpoint based on the body's own movements, which is highly relevant to spatial navigation. In their experiment, egocentric updating could be measured by having participants actively move to a different position between memorizing spatial positions and retrieving them from memory (see also chapter: Keeping Track of Where Things Are in Space: The Neuropsychology of Object Location Memory).

8.4 ROUTE AND SURVEY KNOWLEDGE

Apart from the matter of egocentric versus allocentric perspective taking, a similar distinction is also prominent in navigation literature. Spatial knowledge used to navigate can be considered either route knowledge or survey knowledge (eg, Siegel & White, 1975). Roughly, these two types of knowledge overlap with the egocentric–allocentric distinction. Route knowledge concerns information about which turns to take at which points in an environment to reach a given goal location. Such information typically engages the application of egocentric perspective. However, egocentric updating can be used and route information from a different angle than the viewpoint of the observer is possible. Survey knowledge uses spatial information from a bird's eye viewpoint, closely linked to the representation of an allocentric perspective. Later views on route and survey knowledge point out that the distinction between the two is not very strict. Ishikawa and Montello (2006), for instance, argue that earlier claims that landmark and route knowledge precede survey knowledge are false. They show that from the first exposure onward, metric configurational information can be obtained.

An elegant example of an experiment tapping into route and survey knowledge is the task performed by Noordzij, Zuidhoek, and Postma (2006). In this task knowledge of an environment (a zoo and a mall) is described verbally in either a route or survey fashion. In a route description, the participant is taken through the environment as if they were walking through it, with descriptions like "You walk towards the toy store and in front of the toy store you turn to the right with an angle of 90 degrees, and then you walk straight." In contrast, the survey description uses the cardinal directions to portray the layout of the environment, such as: "The toy store is in the northwest corner of the first part. To the east of the toy store is the furniture shop, in the northeast corner of this part." After participants study descriptions like these, their memory about the layout of the environment can be tested in various ways, as a measure of the quality of the mental map they have constructed. Noordzij et al. (2006) have used a distance comparison task, in which participants were asked to compare two pairs of locations based on the distance between the two locations within each pair. Healthy individuals perform better on such distance comparisons after a survey knowledge description, and data from blind individuals show that this is most likely linked to visual experience, as they perform better after a route knowledge description (see also chapter: Tell Me Where to Go: On the Language of Space).

8.5 STRUCTURING NAVIGATION

One of the largest challenges in navigation research is to capture this complex ability in a single model. The common denominator in the existing lines of navigation research is that navigation ability is considered a cognitive function consisting of multiple components. Most studies focus on one particular component, such as perspective taking. In contrast, other studies show dissociations between different components, such as between spatial and temporal coding of route information (eg, van der Ham et al., 2010). In literature, only a relatively small number of approaches to structure navigation components have been reported. However, they are typically limited to lists of navigation attributes, based on literature review, in which separate studies are brought together. They lack the essential combination of both thorough literature review and direct empirical evidence to compose a comprehensive neurocognitive model of navigation. Wolbers and Hegarty (2010) have provided one of the most commonly cited overviews of navigation. In their paper they organize most processes involved in navigation according to their link to the perception, processing, and representation of information relevant to navigation (see Fig. 8.4). They have listed the different types of cues that are used to navigate, the different mechanisms in which these cues are processed and the representations that are constructed based on the outcome of these mechanisms.

Although listing many of the processes of interest in these three categories is informative and useful, this approach focuses primarily on the

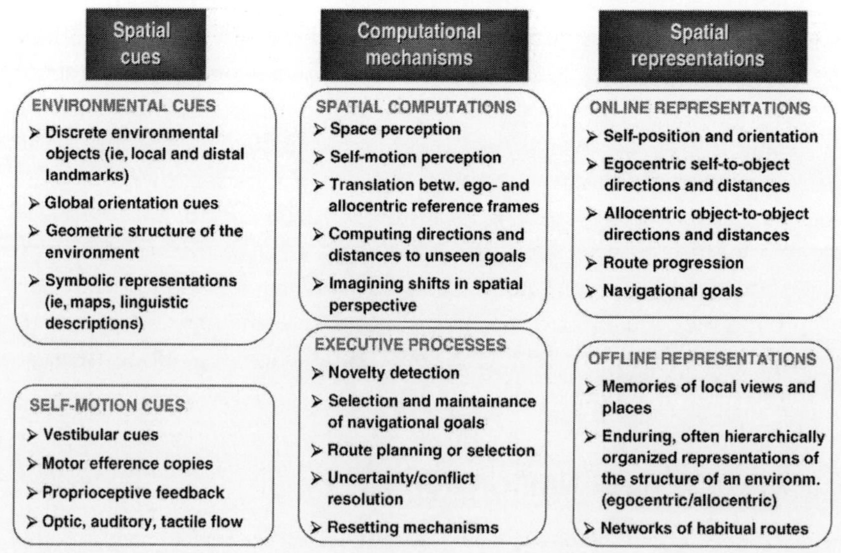

Figure 8.4 The structure of navigation as proposed by Wolbers and Hegarty (2010).

order of these processes, not their functional characteristics. For example, landmark identity memory is present in all three phases; landmarks function as environmental cues, are perceived spatially, and are used in offline memories of a certain spatial situation. However, landmark memory is most likely a unitary function, as illustrated by landmark agnosia for instance (eg, Aguirre & d'Esposito, 1999; Mendez & Cherrier, 2003). Therefore, it might be more useful to think of navigation ability in terms of the separate cognitive functions involved and group the processes involved accordingly. That would mean that landmark identity memory is one of the components of navigation ability, instead of a feature that is present in multiple phases.

Other authors have presented alternative ways to structure navigation ability. Wiener et al. (2009) offer a taxonomy of wayfinding tasks (see Fig. 8.5). In this taxonomy, the focus lies with the cognitive properties of wayfinding aspects. An important feature of this taxonomy is that it offers a structure by which the properties of many different wayfinding tasks can be dissected. It is however, only a taxonomy of wayfinding, not

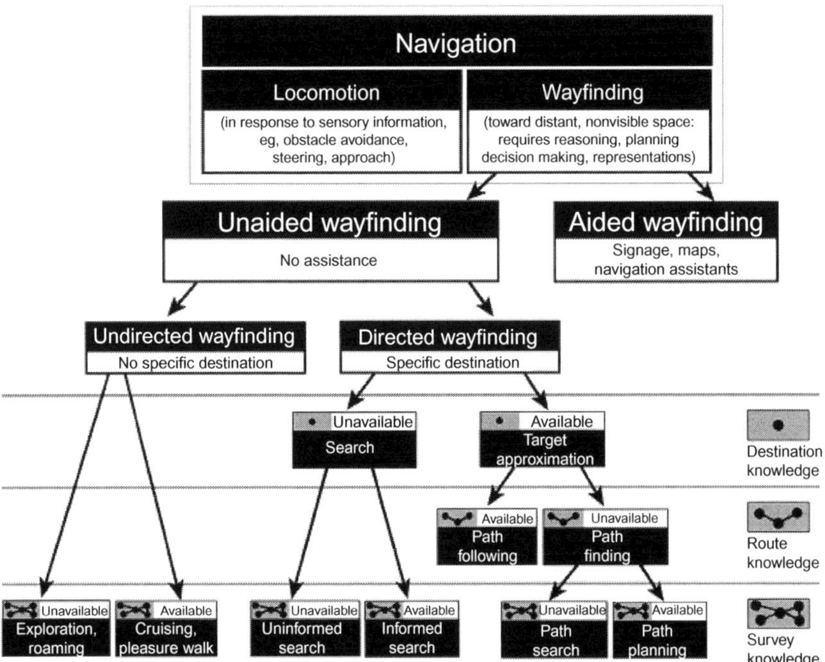

Figure 8.5 A taxonomy of wayfinding tasks as presented by Wiener, Büchner, and Hölscher (2009).

navigation ability as a whole. It described the various ways in which people follow a specific path between two points. Other important aspects of navigation, such as perspective taking ability or sense of direction are not addressed by this taxonomy. Nonetheless, it offers a useful method to carefully characterize this spatial behavior, which could possibly be extended to include such other aspects of navigation as well.

In contrast to this focus on behavioral properties of wayfinding, Chrastil (2013) presents a framework of navigation, based on neural evidence. This taxonomy (see Table 8.1) describes seven different cognitive processes across four categories of spatial knowledge. This taxonomy builds on the distinction between route and survey knowledge. Although, there is abundant behavioral documentation of this distinction, neural support for this dissociation is not as clear. As a solution, Chrastil (2013) adds graph knowledge as distinct subtypes of knowledge used for navigation. Graph knowledge serves as a hybrid between route and survey knowledge. Such graph knowledge is proposed to be used when survey knowledge is consulted to provide route information between two given locations. For instance, when someone is asked to generate a route description between the city hall and the library, they use their mental map of the city to reconstruct route information they have not necessarily experienced themselves. One important drawback to the models presented by Wiener and colleagues (2009) and Chrastil (2013) is that they are based on existing literature, and that to date, no experiments have been specifically designed to directly address the viability of these models. These models can be considered viable if at a (neuro)cognitive level, these different processes are indeed separated and represent fundamentally different functions. Therefore, an important next step is to perform large-scale, within subject, individual differences studies that incorporate a collection of tasks representing the different processes. Not only performance

Table 8.1 A taxonomy of spatial knowledge, as presented by Chrastil (2013)

	Landmark	Route	Graph	Survey
Place recognition	x	x	x	x
Sequence learning		x	x	
Identifying decision points	x	x	x	
Response learning		x		
Forming associations		x	x	
Locating the goal			x	x
Path integration				x

patterns within the healthy population can be informative for this matter. As will be discussed in the second part of this chapter, clinical cases can also provide valuable insight into identifying and isolating these processes.

8.6 INDIVIDUAL DIFFERENCES

A particularly fruitful approach within navigation research is that of individual differences. Navigation shows very high variation between otherwise comparable individuals. Everyone knows that particular person who always gets lost; typically this person is not any less intelligent than people who can find their way around just fine. Apart from the fundamental interest in understanding why people can vary in their navigation ability, it also can be very informative to study performance patterns of groups of individuals. It can show us how good and bad navigators differ in brain activation and how they approach navigation problems (see eg, Etchamendy & Bohbot, 2007). Moreover, variation across navigation subtasks can indicate which aspects of navigation are dissociated from others. For instance, when there is very little correlation between landmark recognition and memory for landmark order, these two aspects are likely to be functionally dissociated. Three domains are of particular interest in explaining such individual variations.

First of all, gender is a popular variable to take into account. Commonly, males are thought of as being superior in spatial cognition in general. However, when more detail is paid to the precise nature of the tasks used, some nuance is in order. Males outperform females when it comes to basic, metric tasks like mental rotation (eg, Collins & Kimura, 1997), although some argue that this effect is due to strategic differences (eg, Hugdahl, Thomsen, & Ersland, 2006). The opposite pattern is often found when space is categorized or put into a meaningful context (eg, Alexander, Packard, & Peterson, 2002). When it comes to navigation, males tend to outperform females when it comes to wayfinding and pointing tasks, and performance of both genders is equal in map drawing and distance estimation tasks (for a review see Coluccia & Louse, 2004). Explanations for these differences range from biological (eg, hemispheric lateralization patterns are stronger in men; Annett, 1992) to environmental (eg, boys participate more in high-spatial activities; see eg, Baenninger & Newcombe, 1989).

Second, age can have a strong impact on navigation performance. In particular, when it comes to more difficult tasks, such as the use of an allocentric perspective, clear patterns of development and aging are found. Although children are able to use an allocentric perspective from a very young age, they start to use it as a preferred strategy between the ages of 7 and 10 (Bullens, Iglói, Berthoz, Postma, & Rondi-Reig, 2010). This later increase in allocentric performance is mirrored by an earlier decrease with older age (eg, Moffat & Resnick, 2002). Several studies have shown that with older age in particular, there is a relationship between age-related volumetric changes in the brain and allocentric task performance (eg, Wiener, de Condappa, Harris, & Wolbers, 2013).

Third, strategy use and particularly strategy flexibility is predictive of navigation success. Typically, those who can use different strategies, like an egocentric and allocentric perspective approach, and can identify which strategy fits best with a given task, perform best (eg, Etchamendy & Bohbot, 2007; Janzen, Jansen, & van Turennout, 2008; Jordan, Schadow, Wuestenberg, Heinze, & Jäncke, 2004). Therefore it is crucial to be very specific about what is measured in a given task: does a task force participants to use a particular strategy and does performance reflect that strategy, or does it allow for multiple strategies and does performance reflect whether the most efficient strategy was selected. This is where experiments like the star-maze task are of use, as task properties can be controlled to select whether the ability or preference for a specific strategy is measured (Box 8.1).

BOX 8.1 Navigation Ability and Aging

Human life expectancy has notably increased over the past century thanks to major advancements in health care, sanitation, nutrition, and education. For 33 countries, life expectancy at birth nowadays exceeds 80 years of age (United Nations Population Fund, 2012). Longer life expectancy, in combination with decreased birth rate, will continue to lead to increases in the proportion of older adults around the world. Given this influential trend, it is no wonder that cognitive researchers have intensified their interest in age-related cognitive changes in the healthy elderly population.

Although individual differences in cognitive aging occur (Lindenberger, 2014), common consensus exists that the physiological changes in the brain associated with aging go hand in hand with cognitive changes (Drag & Bieliauskas, 2010). Cross-sectional studies have identified two general patterns of age-cognition relations. Whereas experience-based or crystallized abilities, such as vocabulary and general information, tend to improve until around 60 years of age, a notably different pattern has been described for fluid abilities,

(*Continued*)

BOX 8.1 Navigation Ability and Aging—cont'd

such as reasoning and working memory. People show nearly linear decreases in this latter type of abilities from early adulthood and probably as early as in their 20s and 30s (Salthouse, 2010).

Obviously, navigation ability as being a complex cognitive structure does not escape from the effects of cognitive aging. Older adults report experiencing difficulties with wayfinding and therefore tend to avoid driving in unfamiliar environments (Burns, 1999). This might in turn lead to impaired mobility and reduced involvement in daily activities with negative implications for their well-being. Direct assessment of navigation skills in healthy older adults, whether based on real-world or virtual environments, has provided extensive evidence for these self-reported difficulties with navigation (Moffat, 2009). Moreover, the finding that these difficulties are more pronounced in new rather than familiar environments accords with the self-reported coping strategy of seniors to avoid driving unfamiliar routes and places (Devlin, 2001).

Researchers are now having a closer look at the specific components of navigation ability that are susceptible to the effects of normal aging. Special attention has been devoted to the hippocampus which is among the most prominent brain structures to be affected by the normal aging process (Raz et al., 2005). As discussed in Section 8.3 of this chapter, the hippocampus is involved in the formation of cognitive maps, which holds viewpoint-independent information on the relationships between environmental landmarks. Evidence is now accumulating that older adults have particular difficulties with navigation tasks that depend on allocentric strategies. Wiener, Kmecova, and de Condappa (2012) have supported this notion using a new paradigm that differentiates between the ability to repeat and to retrace a learned route. They argue that a series of stimulus–response associations between landmarks and directions (eg, "turn left at the railway station") is sufficient for successful repetition of a previously encountered route. During learning of the route, these stimulus–response associations have been encoded from an egocentric frame of reference. While retracing a route, however, landmarks are approached from a different viewpoint than during the first exposure. Viewpoint-independent, allocentric representations are thus required for being able to accurately retrace a route. The results of their study revealed specific age-related deficits in route retracing ability. Older participants performed remarkably lower than their younger counterparts when asked to indicate the travel direction and to identify the next movement of direction in route retracing but not in route repeating trials. Several studies have now coupled the deficient performance of older adults in allocentric navigation tasks to both structural and functional age-related changes in the hippocampal formation (eg, Head & Isom, 2010; Moffat, Elkins, & Resnick, 2006). Given that older adults

(*Continued*)

BOX 8.1 Navigation Ability and Aging—cont'd

have difficulties with switching to and using an allocentric navigation strategy (Harris, Wiener, & Wolbers, 2012), they tend to rely more heavily on egocentric navigation strategies (Rodgers, Sindone, & Moffat, 2012).

With the notion in mind that the cognitive structure underlying navigation ability is of a complex nature, it is unlikely that the age-related navigation deficits can be explained by changes in the hippocampus and allocentric navigation alone. Indeed, two extra-hippocampal areas have been identified as playing critical roles in spatial navigation: the prefrontal areas and the caudate nucleus. Age-related changes in the prefrontal cortex might be related to poorer strategy selection for navigation purposes in older adults (Moffat, 2009). The caudate nucleus, on the other hand, contributes to egocentric navigation and nonspatial response strategies (Iaria, Petrides, Dagher, Pike, & Bohbot, 2003). Both of these brain areas are, as is the hippocampal formation, among the neural systems that are affected in an early stage by normal aging.

8.7 SUMMARY AND CONCLUSION

Navigation is a complex feature in human cognition. In short, there are roughly three levels of navigation behavior present in both animals and humans. Route following is simply following cues in an environment. Piloting is slightly more advanced and concerns the exploration of an environment in search of a specific target. Dead reckoning entails a certain level of calculation to find back a starting point. These navigation behaviors have a strong link to cell activity in the hippocampus: place, head direction, and grid cells allow for coding of specific locations, orientations, and layouts of environments, respectively. A novel addition to these hippocampal functions is the coding of temporal features of event by so-called times cells. The coexistence of spatial and temporal cells in the hippocampus highlights its importance for episodic memory and suggests a more important role of temporal processes in navigation than previously assumed.

A particularly well-studied theme in navigation research is that of using different perspectives. The main distinction lies between egocentric/observer-based and allocentric/environment-based. Depending on the situation, each of these perspectives can be effective. Typically, those who are able to use both perspectives and are able to switch between them according to task demands are the best navigators. A distinction closely related to egocentric versus allocentric is that of route versus survey knowledge. These types of knowledge indicate how spatial information concerning an environment is represented, either based on how it is experienced on a specific route, or based on the layout of the environment.

A clear structural description of human navigation that entails the more complex processes, such as perspective taking and refers to the different types of knowledge still needs to be developed. In recent literature, three suggestions have been presented to model human navigation. They report the various types of input, processing mechanisms, and output involved in navigation, the distinctions between the different tasks to measure wayfinding behavior, and expand on the typical landmark, route and survey knowledge distinction to specify different elements of navigation. The next step in navigation research should be to present the empirical evidence for these theoretical models, in order to create this clear structural description of human navigation. Large-scale individual differences studies are highly suitable for this purpose, as potential (neuro) cognitive dissociations between elements of navigation can easily be detected. Not only studies in healthy participants can be meaningful here, studying patients with specific lesions or behavioral impairments can be highly informative. Therefore, the next part of this chapter will cover the neuropsychological viewpoint on navigation.

PART 2: A NEUROPSYCHOLOGICAL PERSPECTIVE ON NAVIGATION BEHAVIOR

In the first part of this chapter, we have discussed the cognitive neuroscience approach to investigate navigation behavior in healthy people. In a somewhat different approach, researchers have attempted to contribute to our knowledge of navigation by studying people who experience navigation difficulties as a consequence of brain damage. Here, we will describe why this cognitive neuropsychological approach is essential in understanding the cognitive deficits that can cause someone to experience difficulties in navigation. Furthermore, it provides valuable input to the discussion on how to define and classify navigation behavior. First we will show, on the basis of a case study with two patients, that the inability to navigate can have negative consequences to daily life functioning of the patients. We will provide a brief historical overview of the earliest patient studies on navigation ability and describe what is currently known about the factors responsible for navigation impairment in neurological patients. Then, we will point out some limitations of the current approach and provide suggestions for future neuropsychological research into navigation (dis)ability.

8.8 INTRODUCTION TO THE NEUROPSYCHOLOGICAL APPROACH

The neuropsychological approach contributes to our knowledge of spatial navigation by way of investigating the associations between navigation performance and brain damage in clinical groups. Neuropsychological researchers have been doing so (and still do) by investigating single cases or a small number of brain-damaged patients with navigation difficulties. An important advantage of such a single case approach is that it enables the researcher to extensively investigate the association between the cognitive or behavioral deficit—navigation impairment—and damage on the neural level. Moreover, a careful description of the patient's daily life functioning can provide important insights in the relationship between the navigation problems and daily life effects as well.

The possible daily life impact of the inability to navigate was demonstrated in a study entailing two case descriptions (Van der Ham et al., 2010). The first patient was a 36-year-old woman (AC), who was diagnosed with an ischemic stroke involving the superior region of the right parietal cortex. As described at the beginning of this chapter, she reported to experience sudden periods of disorientation on a regular basis, also while navigating in familiar environments. Even more strikingly, these episodes of "not knowing where to go" were accompanied by intense feelings of anxiety. It is no wonder that her navigation problems were initially mistaken as resulting from an anxiety disorder. The second case description involves a 44-year-old woman (WJ) suffering from a brain tumor. As a consequence of multiple attempts to operate the tumor, the posterior areas of the right hemisphere were severely damaged. In daily life, she experienced notable navigation difficulties with route planning and remembering locations. She would specifically indicate to have problems with the speed of movement, finding her way while walking was manageable whereas riding a bicycle would be too fast to process all spatial information necessary. As might be evident from these two case descriptions, an inability to navigate can inflict far-reaching negative consequences to the level of independent daily life functioning of the patient.

Further evidence for a close relationship between navigation ability and daily life functioning comes from a more systematic study in mild stroke patients (Van der Ham, Kant, Postma, & Visser-Meily, 2013). This study showed positive correlations between self-reported navigation ability and measures of quality of life, suggesting that navigation impairment will lead to a lower quality of life, mobility, and autonomy after stroke. Van der Ham and colleagues (2013) also reported that nearly 30% of the stroke patients participating in their study complained about navigation difficulties after their stroke event. Yet, navigation impairment is not only commonly present after stroke, but others have shown that this type of deficit can be found in patients suffering from other neuropsychological disorders, such as mild cognitive impairment (Hort et al., 2007), Alzheimer's disease (topographical disorientation was found in 61 out of 112 patients; Pai & Jacobs, 2004), and Korsakoff's syndrome (Oudman et al., 2014). Hence, the above studies emphasize the importance of closely investigating impairments in the ability to navigate in brain-damaged patients.

8.9 HISTORICAL OVERVIEW

The first neuropsychological report on a brain-damaged patient suffering from navigation impairment was published by Jackson in 1876 (1958; in Barrash, 1998). In this case study report, he described a female patient with extensive damage to the right posterior lobe as a result of a large glioma. Jackson characterized her problems with navigation, or "topographical orientation," as difficulties with finding her way around in familiar environments. For example, she got lost during a visit to a park she knew well. Although the entrance was within her visual field, she was still unable to find it. On the other hand, she was found to be relatively accurate in recalling topographical knowledge, such as describing routes between two places. It thus seemed that her navigation problems were the result of a failure to recognize topographical scenes that had previously been familiar to her. Another important case study, concerning three individual patient cases, was published by Meyer in 1900 (in Barrash, 1998). He first describes the case of a 49-year-old male suffering from a right-sided vascular lesion who experiences, like Jackson's patient, notable difficulties in finding his way around in his home town. Testing revealed that, on the one hand, the patient was accurate in naming the streets belonging to several important buildings in his hometown. In contrast, when asked to indicate how to reach these buildings from his own home, he failed to provide sufficient descriptions or drawings. In a more ecologically valid test, the patient was requested to walk to his home from the hospital. Although he managed to reach his home in the end, he felt highly uncertain and got lost multiple times. In addition to his navigation difficulties in familiar places, he was also found unable to learn the layout of new environments such as that of the hospital he was staying in.

These and other case studies published at that time commonly shared the view that navigation impairment is a nonspecific consequence of brain damage (Barrash, 1998). In most of the investigated cases, the inability to navigate was one cognitive deficit among many others. In fact, researchers commonly interpreted navigation inability as a direct consequence of these other cognitive deficits such as visuospatial problems at the perceptual level. Furthermore, there often was confusion about the key deficits underlying navigation impairment as well. This uncertainty resulted from the fact that assessments of patients with navigation difficulties tended to be incomplete in these studies. For example, investigation of perceptual and cognitive abilities was mainly focused on spatial characteristics, while other important capacities other than of spatial nature, such as visual recognition, were not assessed in most cases (Barrash, 1998; Farrell, 1996).

Two influential papers were able to initiate a broader view on navigation impairment in neurological patients. In previous case studies, the condition of topographical disorientation was usually discussed in the light of other syndromes or conditions, such as visuospatial disturbances and aphasia. Brain (1941), however, was the first to note that navigation impairment could be functionally independent from these other cognitive deficits. He thus suggested that the inability to navigate might be a specific type of impairment that would be worth closer investigation in its own right. In his study, he assessed six patients on a range of visual and spatial tasks. He found that four out of these six patients suffered from topographical disorientation, but he also noted that this condition could be the result of different types of underlying disturbances. Rather than just observing that a patient is being disoriented in space, he argued that looking for the functional impairment that causes the disorientation is of key importance. In another important paper, Paterson and Zangwill (1945) referred to their patient as having a "specific topographical agnosia." Their patient suffered from focal damage to the right posterior areas as a consequence of a mortar fragment ($2 \times 1 \times 1$ cm) penetrating his head. Although this patient presented with several cognitive problems, the most prominent impairment was of a topographical nature.

Paterson and Zangwill (1945) identified that, apart from the fact that their patient's object recognition ability was intact, he faced serious difficulties with recognizing specific places, such as distinct landmarks and scenes. Moreover, the paper by these two authors was also important in another sense. Previous authors were selectively focusing on the role of the left hemisphere in topographical ability. For the time being, it was thought that everyone uses a "dominant" hemisphere, usually the left side of the brain, because of its relationship to speech. Paterson and Zangwill (1945), however, emphasized that the role of the right hemisphere in navigation had been largely ignored at that time. Indeed, later studies soon began to provide support for the notion that the ability to navigate was highly dependent on the integrity of the occipital and parietal areas in the right hemisphere.

Already in 1950, three authors (McFie, Piercy, & Zangwill, 1950) pointed to the importance of controlled group studies as opposed to single case studies in order to facilitate the acquisition of knowledge on neural correlates of the condition of topographical disorientation. Their call for such studies was indeed followed by several papers focusing on (small) groups of neurological patients in the following two decades. Apart from several substantial methodological limitations of these early group studies (such as a lack of comprehensiveness and standardization in the assessment procedures of topographical disorientation), they provided consistent support for the notion that the condition of topographical disorientation can be present in patients with both left or right unilateral lesions, but tends to be more prevalent in those with right-sided brain damage.

After 1962, the literature on topographical disorientation moved to a long-lasting discussion of the "essential nature" of the deficit (Barrash, 1998). Several authors, including Hécaen, DeRenzi, and Warrington, posited different conceptualizations of the central deficit underlying the condition of topographical disorientation. As an example, researchers have distinguished between topographical agnosia and topographical amnesia, without providing clear theoretical definitions of these aspects (Aguirre & D'Esposito, 1999). The inconsistent use and conceptualization of terms have seriously hindered the theoretical progress in the literature about topographical disorientation over a long period of time (Barrash, 1998; Brunsdon, Nickels, & Coltheart, 2007).

Another significant development in the study of topographical disorientation is also worth mentioning here. Authors began, from the end of the 1970s, to notice the correspondence between findings of animal and human lesion studies (Barrash, 1998), for example, with regard to the role of the medial temporal structures in learning and memory (O'Keefe & Nadel, 1978) and the importance of the occipital lobes for visual recognition (Humphrey, 1970). Therefore, the influence of the animal literature on the investigation of topographical disorientation started to become stronger, mainly by shifting the attention to unravel the neural correlates of the ability to navigate (Barrash, 1998). This tendency was, for example, reflected in a study by Levine and colleagues (1985) who hypothesized that patients with topographical disorientation can be subdivided in two groups. On the one hand, patients may show impaired ability to represent information of visuospatial nature, whereas others have impairment in the ability to represent visual object information. This distinction was analogous to Ungerleider and Mishkin's (1982) theory about two different visual processing systems that work in parallel: a ventral pathway for object identity processing and a dorsal stream with the aim to process object location. In 1995, Milner and Goodale (1995) presented an alternative model posing that both the dorsal and the ventral stream are responsible for processing object identity *and* location information, but for different purposes. Whereas the dorsal pathway was thought to be involved in the production of actions, the ventral stream was argued to be of importance to object identification. Both the original and the alternative model have been of importance in guiding the study of topographical disorientation.

8.10 THE TAXONOMY OF "TOPOGRAPHICAL DISORIENTATION"

A few years later, Aguirre and D'Esposito (1999) published a paper that would become highly influential in the neuropsychological literature devoted to human spatial navigation. At the time, their goal was to develop a parsimonious taxonomy based on the several dozens of (multiple) case studies that had been published over the years. While these case studies provided important insights in the (neuro)cognitive mechanisms of spatial navigation, no previous attempts had been undertaken to rigorously classify the findings of this line of studies. In their paper, Aguirre and D'Esposito classified all available case studies according to both the types of navigational impairment on the behavioral level and the associated damage on the neural level. This resulted in a taxonomy of four distinct patterns of navigation impairment and underlying brain damage (see Table 8.2).

Table 8.2 Taxonomy of topographical disorientation as proposed by Aguirre and D'Esposito (1999)

Disorder	Proposed impairment	Lesion site
Egocentric disorientation	Unable to represent the location of objects with respect to self	Posterior parietal
Heading disorientation	Unable to represent direction of orientation with respect to external environment	Posterior cingulate
Landmark agnosia	Unable to represent the appearance of salient environmental stimuli (landmarks)	Lingual gyrus
Anterograde disorientation	Unable to create new representations of environmental information	Parahippocampus

The patients who fall in the first category of the taxonomy—egocentric disorientation—are said to suffer from deficits in the ability to represent "the relative location of objects with respect to the self" (p. 1619) in the absence of visual recognition impairment. On the behavioral level, these patients experience notable difficulties in finding their way around in previously familiar as well as novel environments. However, their inability to egocentrically represent the location of objects seems not to be constricted to large-scale, environmental space alone. Usually, these patients have difficulties with small-scale spatial tasks as well, such as mental rotation and visuospatial span tasks. The concordance of patients showing this type of behavioral deficit lies in the fact that they all suffered from unilateral or bilateral lesions to the posterior parietal area of the right hemisphere.

Patients in the second category of the taxonomy—heading disorientation—suffer from the inability to derive directional information from landmarks without the global egocentric disorientation that is characterizing patients in the egocentric disorientation category. While they are accurate in recognizing landmarks and their current location, they seem unable to determine the direction in which to continue. Their navigation difficulties are thus likely to be the result of a disturbance in the ability to form or recall associations between specific landmarks and directional information. The few patients who have been reported as suffering this type of navigational deficit had damage to the posterior region of the cingulate.

The third section of the taxonomy regards patients that suffer from a condition that has been named "landmark agnosia." The inability that these patients share lies in their difficulties to use highly salient environmental features for orientation purposes. Aguirre and D'Esposito argue that both perceptual and mnemonic aspects are damaged in these patients, which leads to disorientation in novel as well as previously familiar environments. Interestingly, several authors have described a specific strategy that these patients tend to use to compensate for their inability to use landmarks, by relying on details in the environment or complex scenes. For example, JC (a patient described by Whiteley & Warrington, 1978) recognizes his house by way of the number or by his car in case it is parked in front of the door. Despite their problems with landmarks, patients with this type of disorder usually perform at an adequate level on spatial representation tasks, such as providing route descriptions or drawing maps of known environments. Lesions of the lingual gyrus are thought to underlie the navigation impairment of the landmark agnosia type.

Lastly, the shared characteristic of the patients in the fourth category of the taxonomy concerns their selective impairment to navigate in novel environments. As these patients tend to be relatively intact in the ability to find their way around in familiar environments, this condition has been called "anterograde disorientation." Aguirre and D'Esposito hypothesized that this type of navigation impairment is most likely the result of parahippocampal damage.

After the taxonomy of topographical disorientation had been published in 1999, researchers continued to add new case descriptions to the literature. Some of these studies have suggested the existence of other types of navigation impairment in addition to the ones described in the taxonomy. An example of such a recent case study was published by Ciaramelli (2008). She describes the case of patient LG, a 56-year-old male, who experiences severe navigational difficulties after ventromedial damage to the prefrontal cortex as caused by an event of subarachnoid hemorrhage (see Fig. 8.6 for the localization of the lesion). The ruptured aneurysm was clipped immediately following hospitalization and after a 3-month period of recovery, the patient was discharged to home. For several years, he was unable to return to work as a consequence of his severe memory and executive problems as well as spontaneous confabulations. However, after 5 years, as the confabulations diminished, he returned to his daily activities and started off with a new job as well. Whereas he did so almost fully independently, his wife noticed that he regularly lost his

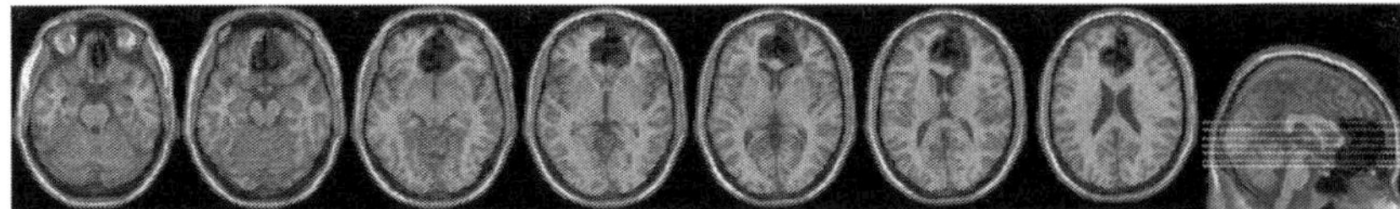

Figure 8.6 Extent of the brain lesion in LG. Brodmann's areas (BA) affected were areas BA 10, 11, 12, 24, and 32. *Image taken from Ciaramelli, E. (2008). The role of ventromedial prefrontal cortex in navigation: A case of impaired wayfinding and rehabilitation.* Neuropsychologia, 46, *2099–2105.*

way when going to work on his own. Ciaramelli (2008) observed him on his way to the office and found out that he initially followed the correct route but then took a wrong turn and ended up at his former office. This observation led her to believe that LG experiences difficulties in maintaining the goal destination active in working memory. Laboratory and ecological testing revealed that LG indeed frequently lost his way, mainly as a consequence of the fact that he was attracted toward goal destinations that were more familiar to him than the actual goal destinations. Spiers (2008) has interpreted Ciaramelli's findings (2008) as showing that LG fails "to maintain the *intention* to reach the destination in working memory and a reduced suppression of previously learned information (in this case routes)." The case of LG teaches us that intact functioning of the ventromedial prefrontal cortex is not only involved but required for successful navigation behavior.

In another case study, Aradillas, Libon, and Schwartzman (2011) also present a different type of navigation impairment that is not yet covered in the taxonomy. Their patient concerns a 70-year-old male who suffered from an ischemic stroke in the posterior circulation resulting in selective damage to the right hippocampus and the dentate gyrus. He presented to the emergency room complaining about an acute loss of the ability to navigate. Indeed, he even got lost on the way from home to the ER in the hospital, a route he had taken for over 20 years as he used to work at the same hospital as a psychologist. Navigation assessment revealed difficulties in several processes allowing cognitive mapping, that is, its formation, storage, and retrieval. These findings led the authors to conclude that the integrity of the right hippocampus plays a crucial role in enabling the usage of mental representations of the environment, which is in line with a wide range of neuroimaging studies in healthy participants (eg, Maguire et al., 1998).

The influence of the hippocampus on navigation behavior has also been pointed out in a totally different line of neuropsychological studies.

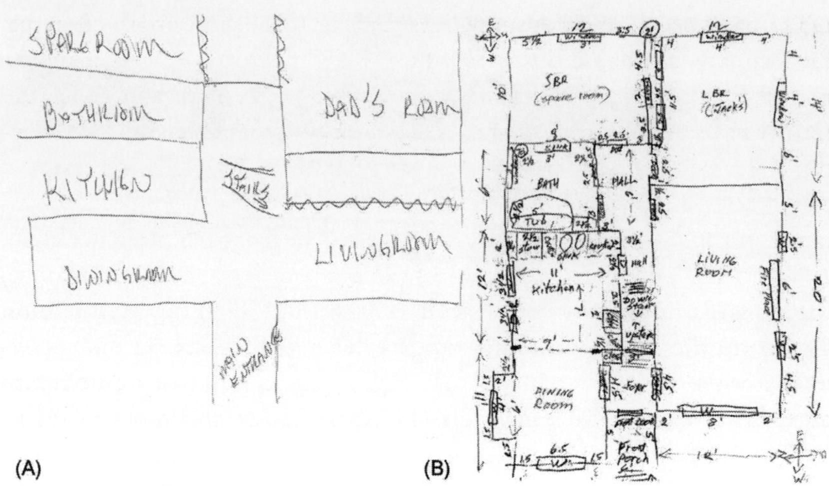

Figure 8.7 Comparison of Pt1's map drawing of her home (A) to an actual map as provided by her father (B). While she correctly represented the number of rooms, the spatial scaling of her map is clearly distorted (Iaria, Bogod, Fox & Barton, 2009).

These studies have shown that navigation deficits not only do occur in brain-damaged patients, but might also be present in individuals without any signs of brain damage or malformation, or intellectual dysfunction. The first case study of "developmental topographical disorientation" or DTD, a term introduced by Iaria and Barton (2010), was reported by Iaria, Bogod, Fox, and Barton in 2009. In their paper, they report on a 43-year-old woman (Pt1) whose cognitive development followed normal paths but, remarkably, she never mastered the ability to navigate. In her younger years, she would only leave her parents' home when accompanied by others. At the moment of testing, she lived with her father. The only route that she could find relatively independently was from home to her work by relying on a specific set of directions. However, she would get lost every time she tried to reach other destinations, such as stores or theaters. Extensive testing revealed a highly specific deficit confined to the ability to generate a cognitive map of the environment (see Fig. 8.7). After this first case report, additional cases involving individuals with DTD have been published by several other authors (Bianchini et al., 2010, 2014; Palermo, Foti, Ferlazzo, Guariglia, & Petrosini, 2014; Palermo, Piccardi et al., 2014). At first glance, it might be unclear in what way this study approach would lead to a better understanding of the neural correlates of navigation behavior. But, as several individuals with

DTD have been described now, it is starting to become more clear that the primary deficit of this condition lies in the formation of a mental representation of the environment (cognitive map). Iaria and colleagues (2014) have hypothesized that this deficit arises from an ineffective functional connectivity between the hippocampus and other brain areas that play a role in spatial navigation. The hippocampus itself has been consistently linked to the ability to generate cognitive maps (eg, Maguire et al., 1998). Iaria and colleagues (2014) conducted resting-state functional MRI scans in individuals with DTD and control participants. Comparison of these groups pointed to a decreased functional connectivity between the right hippocampus and the prefrontal cortex, whereas differences on the structural level were absent. In this way, Iaria et al. (2014) confirmed that the condition of DTD is indeed not the result of neural differences on the structural (ie, volumetric) level. Moreover, important evidence is provided for the notion that the functional integrity of the connection between these two brain areas is crucial in generating mental environmental representations. As such, the study of DTD has gained in importance in the neuropsychological approach of investigating the neural correlates of navigation ability.

It should be noted that the taxonomy by Aguirre and D'Esposito is still cited in many neuropsychological studies on spatial navigation nowadays. However, when using the taxonomy as guidance, it seems difficult to interpret recent findings, such as reported in the case studies by Ciaramelli (2008) and Aradillas and colleagues (2011). Firstly, Aguirre and D'Esposito (1999) do not mention the role of the prefrontal areas in navigation. With respect to the contribution of the hippocampus to navigation behavior, they (Aguirre & D'Esposito, 1999) argue that, in humans, this brain structure is not specifically devoted to navigation alone but other aspects of memory as well. Therefore, they did not include a distinct category in order to separate hippocampus-damaged patients and their type of behavioral navigation deficit from patients in the other four categories. Furthermore, some of the categories were initially based on a limited set of patients, such as the condition referred to as "heading direction." This category is primarily supported by the cases of three patients reported in a single study (Takahashi, Kawamura, Shiota, Kasahata, & Hirayama, 1997). Given the above it appears to be reasonable to work toward an extended or updated taxonomy of topographical disorientation, or navigation impairment.

8.11 GROUP STUDIES INVESTIGATING NAVIGATION IN NEUROLOGICAL PATIENTS

Above, we have mostly described findings that are the result of investigating the relationship between the cognitive abilities relevant to navigation and their neural correlates *in single patients*. However, there also exist a small number of studies that have investigated navigation impairments more systematically in larger groups of neurological patients. This type of approach has, due to the large-scale, systematic setup, great potential to contribute to our knowledge about the cognitive and neural complexity underlying navigation behavior.

Maguire, Burke, Phillips, and Staunton (1996) were among the first to report on the findings of such a systematic and large-scale patient study into navigation disability. Their study was of importance to the neuropsychological investigation of navigation ability in two ways. Firstly, 20 patients who had undergone unilateral temporal lobe surgery because of intractable epileptic seizures participated in the study. But, even more importantly, Maguire and colleagues also assessed the navigation abilities of these patients in a rigorous and systematic way. Patients were first shown movies of two partly overlapping routes in order to stimulate the integration of the two routes into an allocentric representation of the environment. Each of the navigation tasks was only started after the patient reached the criterion score on a task assessing their ability to discriminate between scenes that were and were not part of the presented routes. If the patient did not satisfy the criterion on the scene recognition task, they were again exposed to the route movies. This allowed the authors to be sure that any confirmed impairment on the navigational tasks could not be explained by an inability to visually perceive or recognize scenes. The navigation assessment was relatively extensive and included six tasks. Patients were asked to make proximity and distance judgments, were assessed on route knowledge and their ability to order a set of landmarks according to their occurrence, and had to draw a map of the environment. In the last task, patients were asked to indicate the position of several landmarks on a map of the environment. The main analysis in this study concerned a group comparison of patients with left and right temporal lobe damage on the six navigation tasks. The results showed that both the left and right temporal lobe groups were impaired relative to the control group on almost all of the navigation tasks. Only on the proximity judgment task was the right temporal lobe group performance impaired as compared to controls, whereas accuracy of the left temporal lobe group did not differ significantly with the accuracy reached by the control participants. Given their exclusion criteria and study design, Maguire and colleagues showed that impairments on the navigation tasks could not be explained by either general neuropsychological deficits or an inability to identify specific landmarks and scenes from the route. In general, their study emphasized the importance of both temporal lobes for the purpose of remembering information that is relevant to navigation.

With their paper, Maguire and colleagues (1996) cleared the way for further systematic, large-scale investigation of navigation ability in neurological patient groups. Indeed, their study was followed by a number of well-conducted studies mostly investigating small to medium patient groups (eg, Barrash, Damasio, Adolphs, & Tranel, 2000; Bell, 2012; Busigny et al., 2014; Livingstone & Skelton, 2007; Spiers et al., 2001; Van Asselen et al., 2006). These studies can be roughly divided in two categories in terms of their specific approach of assessing navigation ability. Some regard navigation ability as a relatively unitary process, whereas others approach navigation, like in the study by Maguire and colleagues, as a cognitive function that is of a highly complex nature.

For example, Barrash et al. (2000) tested navigation ability as a unitary cognitive ability in 127 patients with focal lesions using their Route Learning Test (RLT). In this test, participants learn a one-third mile route through the medical center at which Barrash and colleagues performed their study. Participants were instructed to pay careful attention to the route, as they would have to walk the route themselves for three consecutive trials after the examiner had guided them through the route the first time. During the testing phase, the examiner would follow the participant and immediately correct each error by indicating the correct direction. Performance on the test was expressed in terms of the number of errors in the testing trials. Navigation disability was found to be highly prevalent in patients with lesions in different brain areas, including the medial occipital and posterior parahippocampal areas of either hemisphere, the right hippocampus as well as the inferotemporal regions of the right hemisphere.

Nowadays a small number of studies have investigated navigation impairment in neurological patients using a rather multidimensional approach to navigation ability. Two studies are specifically worth mentioning in this respect. Firstly, Van Asselen and colleagues (2006) provided an interesting report on a study in which they investigated navigation ability in 31 stroke patients. In this study, the examiner first showed the participant a route through the university building. After a 30-minute delay, navigation ability was measured by way of four subtasks: a landmark recognition task, a landmark-ordering task, a route reversal task (in which participants were asked to navigate from the end back to the beginning of the route), and a route-drawing task. Rather than comparing performance of different lesion groups like in Maguire and colleagues' study (1996), Van Asselen and her coworkers (2006) correlated performance on each of the four subtasks with the lesion locations of the patients. They found evidence for an association between right hippocampal damage and impairment on the scene recognition task. Furthermore, weak correlations were found between landmark-ordering performance and damage to the dorsolateral areas of the prefrontal cortex, suggesting that this brain area is engaged in processing of temporal information. Route reversal ability was related to damage in several brain areas of the right hemisphere, such as the hippocampus, temporal cortex, posterior areas of the parietal cortex as well as the dorsolateral prefrontal areas, indicating that performance on this task relies on the integrity of multiple abilities. Lastly, damage to the right temporal cortex was associated with difficulties in drawing an accurate map of the learned route. Clearly, by differentiating several subabilities underlying navigation behavior and correlating them with the patients' lesions, the study approach taken by Van Asselen and colleagues, leads to a more fine-grained understanding of the neural substrates of navigation.

A recent study by Busigny and colleagues (2014) specifically focused on the navigation abilities of patients suffering from posterior cerebral artery (PCA) infarctions. Navigation was tested using five computerized subtasks and four ecological subtasks (the latter being highly similar to the four subtasks used by Van Asselen and colleagues, 2006) in 15 PCA patients. Busigny and colleagues (2014) followed a similar statistical approach as Maguire and colleagues did in their study in 1996. Firstly, they found that, on group level, patients have more difficulties with the navigation tasks than controls. Another group analysis comparing patients with left- and right-sided damage did not show clear differences. However, when carefully addressing the individual profiles corrected for the effects of age and gender, patients with right PCA infarctions were found to be more severely impaired on the behavioral level as compared to patients with left-sided brain damage. Attempts to investigate associations between lesion location and behavioral performance showed significant correlations between right-sided damage in the cuneus and calcarine sulcus and navigation task performance. Their findings indicate that navigation impairment might be highly prevalent after PCA (8 out of 15 patients), specifically when assessing navigation ability with sensitive, ecologically valid tasks. Furthermore, their finding that right cuneus and calcarine sulcus damage is related to behavioral performance is in line with earlier neurocognitive studies. That is, the cuneus has shown to become active in navigation tasks as well as for the purpose of scene recognition and retrieval of object locations.

8.12 FUTURE PERSPECTIVE: WORKING TOWARD SYSTEMATIC ASSESSMENT OF NAVIGATION ABILITY

In this part of the chapter, we have shown that neuropsychological case studies investigating navigation impairment in brain-damaged patients have contributed in a considerable way to our knowledge about the cognitive structure of navigation ability. Without doubt navigation impairment can lead to lower levels of independent daily life functioning. But, more importantly, neuropsychological studies have suggested that the inability to navigate might actually result from different types of underlying impairments. The taxonomy by Aguirre and D'Esposito (1999) described four different causes of navigation impairment, for example, as resulting from an inability to recognize landmarks or to derive directional information from landmarks. Moreover, recent case studies have demonstrated the existence of additional types of navigation disabilities (Aradillas et al., 2011; Ciaramelli, 2008). All of these findings clearly point to navigation ability as a multidimensional cognitive structure rather than being a unitary function, which is also in congruence with findings of neurocognitive studies in healthy participants (Wolbers & Hegarty, 2010).

We think that the neuropsychological approach can continue to be helpful in furthering our knowledge about navigation ability in the future in two ways. Firstly, by shifting toward the conductance of large-scale studies investigating groups of brain-damaged patients rather than single cases, and secondly, by addressing navigation ability as a complex cognitive function. Conducting large-scale patient studies measuring multiple aspects of navigation ability would enable the neuropsychological researcher to correlate (subabilities of) behavioral navigation performance and neural damage in a more systematic way.

As described previously, we have seen that a small number of large-scale patient studies already exist. Still, the cognitive complexity of spatial navigation is usually not or only marginally assessed in these studies. For example, in the study by Barrash and colleagues (2000), the RLT was used to assess navigation capacity. An important limitation of the RLT concerns the fact that it measures navigation only in terms of the number of errors when retracing the learned route. It does, however, not explain what factors underlie the navigation problems of these patients (eg, inability to recognize landmarks, inability to form associations between decision points and directional information, inability to generate an allocentric representation of the environment). The same comment applies to two studies (Bell, 2012; Pereira et al., 2011) investigating navigation impairment in patients with temporal lobe epilepsy using similar assessment procedures as Barrash' RLT. We feel that investigating navigation ability in terms of an error score when retracing a learned route is too restrictive and does not cover the cognitive complexity that has been shown to characterize this important daily life capacity. Furthermore, most of the reported test procedures depend on real-world routes that are specific to a particular building of a university or hospital. It is very hard to create routes in other buildings that resemble the reported ones in terms of route length, landmarks, number of decision points, etc. This is a matter of concern, as all of these factors are shown to influence performance on such tasks.

As a consequence of lacking standardized test procedures to assess navigation ability, this capacity has not yet gained the attention it deserves in neuropsychological practice. In clinical neuropsychological practice, assessment of navigation ability is mostly not part of the assessment procedures in brain-damaged patients at all. This is specifically striking as several studies have shown that navigation impairment and getting lost behavior is prevalent after stroke (Van der Ham et al., 2013), mild cognitive impairment (Hort et al., 2007), Alzheimer's disease (Pai & Jacobs, 2004), and Korsakoff's syndrome (Oudman et al., 2014). This means that the presence of navigation disability in neurological patients must therefore be structurally overlooked.

In our own laboratory, we therefore developed a systematic test procedure to measure navigation ability on a range of 12 subtasks in both healthy and clinical groups (eg, Claessen, van der Ham, Jagersma, & Visser-Meily, in press; Van der Ham et al., 2010). In this test, the Virtual Tübingen task battery, we make use of a large, realistic virtual rendition of the German city Tübingen (see Fig. 8.8, Van Veen, Distler, Braun, &

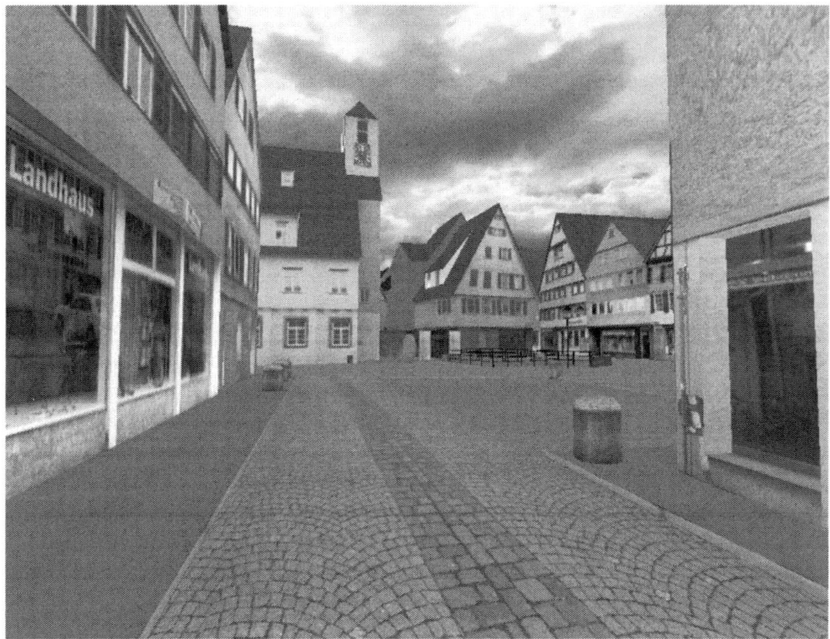

Figure 8.8 An image taken from the Virtual Tübingen environment.

Bülthoff, 1998). After the participant has watched a movie of a route through the virtual environment, different aspects of knowledge about the learned route are systematically assessed by way of 12 subtasks (see Table 8.3). The test starts off with a scene recognition task and, after that, addresses various aspects of route knowledge, for example, associations between scenes and directional information and memory for relative and absolute scene order. Abstract knowledge of the route is tested in two pointing tasks as well as in the map drawing task. Moreover, participants are also asked to indicate distances between several scenes as encountered during the route. The advantage of using virtual reality in this case is that assessment of this test does not depend on a specific building or route, but can be applied basically everywhere. Furthermore, the 12 subtasks do cover an important range of abilities that have previously been shown to be important for navigation purposes. In this way, the Virtual Tübingen test incorporates a standardized assessment procedure that covers the cognitive complexity underlying navigation ability to a large extent.

A systematic approach to navigation ability might, however, not only be valuable for diagnostic purposes, but also be helpful in guiding treatment of this condition. In a recent study, Claessen et al. (in press),

Table 8.3 Description of the 12 subtasks of the Virtual Tübingen test battery

Subtask	Task description
1. Scene recognition	Participants are shown, one-by-one, 22 scenes taken from Virtual Tübingen. Their task is to indicate whether each scene was part of the studied route (target) or not (distractor)
2. Route continuation	Participants are randomly presented with 11 decision points and requested to indicate in which direction the route continued from each of these decision points
3. Route sequence	Participants are asked to indicate the sequence of turns by using a set of printed arrows
4. Route order	Participants are presented with a set of 11 scenes taken from the route. They are instructed to arrange the scenes according to the order in which they encountered them along the route
5. Route progression	For each of 11 scenes, participants are asked to indicate its position in the route on a line representing the total route distance
6. Route distance	For each of nine trials, participants are presented with two scenes taken from the studied route. Their task is to indicate the distance between these scenes on a line representing the total route distance
7. Distance estimation	Participants are requested to provide a distance estimate of the studied route
8. Duration estimation	Participants are asked to provide a duration estimation of the studied route
9. Pointing to start	For each of 11 scenes, participants have to point to the start point of the route using a rotational device
10. Pointing to end	For each of 11 scenes, participants are asked to point to the end point of the route using a rotational device
11. Route drawing	Participants have to reproduce the studied route on a map representing Virtual Tübingen
12. Map recognition	Participants are presented with four different routes on maps of Virtual Tübingen. Their task is to indicate the map that correctly depicts the studied route

developed a virtual reality-based navigation training for six stroke patients. Whereas all six patients experienced navigation difficulties in daily life after their stroke event, the underlying causes were found to be different for each individual patient. More specifically, patients were assessed in their navigation ability pretraining by way of the Virtual Tübingen test battery. Each patient showed a different pattern of navigational strengths and weaknesses. For this reason, the content of the training was different for each patient and closely matched to their individual needs. This study suggests that addressing the cognitive nature of navigation ability might be important not only in the context of diagnosis, but for treatment purposes as well (Box 8.2).

BOX 8.2 Virtual Reality in Navigation Research

A number of recent technological developments are very relevant for navigation research, both for experimental and for clinical applications. Virtual reality, or the digital rendering of artificial environments is one of the most important developments. Although -"virtual reality" was first described in 1860, it was first applied in a computer game no earlier than 1991 (SEGA). In the past two decades the quality of publicly available virtual reality software has increased tremendously and commercial devices like the Oculus rift (2014) benefit from this development.

The majority of navigation studies make use of such virtual worlds, which are usually presented on simple flat screens (eg, Maguire et al., 1999; Waller, Loomis, & Steck, 2003) and sometimes allow for more physical interaction (see eg, Bülthoff, Campos, & Meilinger, 2008). Some advantages of using virtual reality are that they allow for complete control over what is presented and every participant will be presented with the exact same input, factors like weather and traffic can be avoided, and potential familiarity with the environment is not an obstacle. Moreover, assessment can be performed in much more detail, precise tracking of a participant's movement through an environment is possible, as well as additional measures such as eye tracking (eg, Gillner & Mallot, 1998; Rey & Alcañiz, 2010). However, these virtual worlds are not perfect. They remain artificial, and they still look artificial, although visual quality is rapidly increasing. Also, especially for navigation research, physical involvement in an environment affects navigation performance (eg, Chrastil & Warren, 2013; Klatzky, Loomis, Beall, Chance, & Golledge, 1998). Therefore, findings in virtual worlds cannot be automatically generalized to real world navigation. Yet, task designs like the one used by van der Ham and colleagues (2015) may provide a solution here, by integrating virtual elements into the real world; by presenting experimental stimuli on a tablet computer, while participants are physically walking around in the real world, the disadvantage of no physical involvement is overcome, while the advantage of control of experimental input is preserved. As technical aspects like GPS tracking are quickly gaining in speed and accuracy, we expect a rapid increase in such experimental tools and their quality.

(*Continued*)

BOX 8.2 Virtual Reality in Navigation Research—cont'd

In a clinical sense, these developments also provide useful tools. Given the fact that a substantial proportion of stroke patients report navigation problems (van der Ham et al., 2013), a brief measurement tool of their navigation ability would be useful. A virtual reality experiment, to be performed on a regular computer in a hospital or rehabilitation clinic is highly suitable for this purpose. Moreover, not only diagnosis but also treatment of navigation impairment could benefit. In training navigation skills, repetition and precise task properties are important. By introducing digital training, factors like physical fatigue, restricted physical mobility, and that specific spatial situations may not be available in the vicinity can be avoided. In return, experimental researchers could benefit from such an approach as well. Patients' performance can be easily registered this way and it allows for in depth analyses due to the potential level of detail in the data.

So in short, depending on the experimental or clinical purpose of a given task, implementing virtual reality could well be beneficial. An eye should be kept on the rapidly advancing field of technology concerning virtual reality, as disadvantages like the lack of physical involvement may soon be reduced.

8.13 SUMMARY AND CONCLUSION

In this part of the chapter, we have reviewed the cognitive neuropsychological (case) study approach that aims to reveal the neural correlates of our capacity to navigate. We have argued that these numerous case studies have been informative in generating an initial taxonomy of navigation impairment (Aguirre & D'Esposito, 1999). However, recent case studies as well as group studies of neurological patients have been published that proposed that other types of deficits, in addition to the four types as described in the taxonomy, can result in an inability to navigate. Moreover, the conductance of large-scale patient studies addressing navigation ability in its full cognitive complexity are an important prerequisite for developing valuable knowledge about the brain areas that allow for the capacity to navigate. We introduced the Virtual Tübingen test battery, developed in our own laboratory over the years, as an example of how standardized and systematic assessment of navigation ability in both healthy and brain-damaged patient groups could be accomplished. Therefore, the Virtual Tübingen test is suitable for use in neuropsychological practice and could be helpful in diagnosis of navigation impairment and in guiding treatment of this condition.

8.14 GENERAL DISCUSSION

In this chapter we have discussed the neurocognitive characteristics of navigation ability. The complexity of this ability is visible at different levels. At a cellular level, different cell types underlie different functions, within the hippocampus. Behaviorally, people are shown to differ substantially in their preferred approach of navigation and use different perspectives for a given task, for instance. This complexity is substantiated further by clinical findings. Many different cases of navigation impairment, or topographical disorientation, have been combined into a taxonomy. Given the increasing amount of neuropsychological case and patient group studies, there is a need to update and possibly expand this taxonomy. We advocate a multidisciplinary approach in which both neurocognitive and clinical findings are consulted to accurately reflect the complexity of navigation. This should ultimately result into a uniform definition in which all key components of navigation are identified. Novel tools such as virtual and immersive reality and serious game designs can be particularly helpful for this approach.

REFERENCES

Aguirre, G. K., & D'Esposito, M. (1999). Topographical disorientation: A synthesis and taxonomy. *Brain, 122*, 1613–1628.

Alexander, G., Packard, M., & Peterson, B. (2002). Sex and spatial position effects on object location memory following intentional learning of object identities. *Neuropsychologia, 40*(8), 1516–1522.

Annett, M. (1992). Spatial ability in subgroups of left- and right-handers. *British Journal of Psychology, 83*(4), 493–515.

Aradillas, E., Libon, D. J., & Schwartzman, R. J. (2011). Acute loss of spatial navigational skills in a case of right posterior hippocampus stroke. *Journal of the Neurological Sciences, 308*(1–2), 144–146.

Baenninger, M., & Newcombe, N. (1989). The role of experience in spatial test performance: A meta-analysis. *Sex Roles, 20*(5–6), 327–344.

Barrash, J. (1998). A historical review of topographical disorientation and its neuroanatomical correlates. *Journal of Clinical and Experimental Neuropsychology, 20*(6), 807–827.

Barrash, J., Damasio, H., Adolphs, R., & Tranel, D. (2000). The neuroanatomical correlates of route learning impairment. *Neuropsychologia, 38*, 820–836.

Bell, B. D. (2012). Route learning impairment in temporal lobe epilepsy. *Epilepsy & Behavior, 25*(2), 256–262.

Bianchini, F., Incoccia, C., Palermo, L., Piccardi, L., Zompati, L., Sabatini, U., ... Guariglia, C. (2010). Developmental topographical disorientation in a healthy subject. *Neuropsychologia, 48*(6), 1563–1573.

Bianchini, F., Palermo, L., Piccardi, L., Incoccia, C., Nemmi, F., Sabatini, U., & Guariglia, C. (2014). Where am I? A new case of developmental topographical disorientation. *Journal of Neuropsychology, 8*(1), 107–124.

Bird, C. M., & Burgess, N. (2008). Insights from spatial processing into the hippocampal role in memory. *Nature Reviews Neuroscience*, *9*, 182–194.

Brain, W. R. (1941). Visual disorientation with special reference to lesions of the right cerebral hemisphere. *Brain*, *64*, 244–272.

Brunsdon, R., Nickels, L., & Coltheart, M. (2007). Topographical disorientation: Towards an integrated framework for assessment. *Neuropsychological Rehabilitation*, *17*(1), 34–52. Available from http://dx.doi.org/10.1080/09602010500505021.

Bullens, J., Iglói, K., Berthoz, A., Postma, A., & Rondi-Reig, L. (2010). Developmental time course of the acquisition of sequential egocentric and allocentric navigation strategies. *Journal of Experimental Child Psychology*, *107*(3), 337–350.

Bülthoff, H. H., Campos, J. L., & Meilinger, T. (2008). Virtual reality as a valuable research tool for investigating different aspects of spatial cognition. Spatial Cognition VI. Learning, Reasoning, and Talking about Space. *Lecture Notes in Computer Science*, *5248*, 1–3.

Burgess, N., Jackson, A., Hartley, T., & O'Keefe, J. (2000). Predictions derived from modelling the hippocampal role in navigation. *Biological Cybernetics*, *83*, 301–312.

Burgess, N., Recce, M., & O'Keefe, J. (1994). A model of hippocampal function. *Neural Networks*, 7(6/7), 1065–1081.

Burgess, N., Spiers, H. J., & Paleologou, E. (2004). Orientational manœuvres in the dark: Dissociating allocentric and egocentric influences on spatial memory. *Cognition*, *94*(2), 149–166.

Burguière, E., Arleo, A., Hojjati, M. R., Elgersma, Y., de Zeeuw, C. I., Berthoz, A., & Rondi-Reig, L. (2005). Spatial navigation impairment in mice lacking cerebellar LTD: A motor adaptation deficit? *Nature Neuroscience*, *8*(10), 1292–1294.

Burns, P. C. (1999). Navigation and the mobility of older drivers. *Journal of Gerontology: Social Sciences*, *54B*, S49–S55.

Busigny, T., Pagès, B., Barbeau, E. J., Bled, C., Montaut, E., Raposo, N., & Pariente, J. (2014). A systematic study of topographical memory and posterior cerebral artery infarctions. *Neurology*, *83*(11), 996–1003.

Chrastil, E. R. (2013). Neural evidence supports a novel framework for spatial navigation. *Psychonomic Bulletin and Review*, *20*, 208–227.

Chrastil, E. R., & Warren, W. H. (2013). Active and passive spatial learning in human navigation: Acquisition of survey knowledge. *Journal of Experimental Psychology: Learning, Memory, and Cognition*, *39*(5), 1520–1537.

Ciaramelli, E. (2008). The role of ventromedial prefrontal cortex in navigation: A case of impaired wayfinding and rehabilitation. *Neuropsychologia*, *46*, 2099–2105.

Ciaramelli, E., Rosenbaum, R. S., Solcz, S., Levine, B., & Moscovitch, M. (2010). Mental space travel: Damage to posterior parietal cortex prevents egocentric navigation and reexperiencing of remote spatial memories. *Journal of Experimental Psychology: Learning, Memory, and Cognition*, *36*(3), 619–634.

Claessen, M. H. G., van der Ham, I. J. M., Jagersma, E., & Visser-Meily, J. M. A. (2015). Navigation strategy training using virtual reality in six chronic stroke patients: A novel and explorative approach to the rehabilitation of navigation impairment. *Neuropsychological Rehabilitation*, 1–25.

Collins, D. W., & Kimura, D. (1997). A large sex difference on a two-dimensional mental rotation task. *Behavioral Neuroscience*, *111*(4), 845–849.

Coluccia, E., & Louse, G. (2004). Gender differences in spatial orientation: A review. *Journal of Environmental Psychology*, *24*, 329–340.

Devlin, A. S. (2001). *Mind and maze: Spatial cognition and environmental behavior.* Westport, CT: Greenwood Press.

Drag, L. L., & Bieliauskas, L. A. (2010). Contemporary review 2009: Cognitive aging. *Journal of Geriatric Psychiatry and Neurology*, *23*, 75–93.

Eichenbaum, H. (2013). Memory on time. *Trends in Cognitive Sciences*, *17*, 81–88.

Eichenbaum, H. (2014). Time cells in the hippocampus: A new dimension for mapping memories. *Nature Reviews Neuroscience*, *15*, 732–744.

Etchamendy, N., & Bohbot, V. D. (2007). Spontaneous navigational strategies and performance in the virtual town. *Hippocampus*, *17*, 595–599.

Farrell, M. J. (1996). Topographical disorientation. *Neurocase*, *2*, 509–520.

Fouquet, C., Tobin, C., & Rondi-Reig, L. (2010). A new approach for modelling episodic memory from rodents to humans: The temporal order memory. *Behavioural Brain Research*, *215*, 172–179.

Fyhn, M., Molden, S., Witter, M. P., Moser, E. I., & Moser, M.-B. (2004). Spatial representation in the entorhinal cortex. *Science*, *305*, 1258–1264.

Gillner, S., & Mallot, H. A. (1998). Navigation and acquisition of spatial knowledge in a virtual maze. *Journal of Cognitive Neuroscience*, *10*(4), 445–463.

Harris, M. A., Wiener, J. M., & Wolbers, T. (2012). Aging specifically impairs switching to an allocentric navigational strategy. *Frontiers in Aging Neuroscience*, *4*, article 29.

Head, D., & Isom, M. (2010). Age effects on wayfinding and route learning skills. *Behavioural Brain Research*, *209*, 49–58.

Hort, J., Laczó, J., Vyhnálek, M., Bojar, M., Bureš, J., & Vlček, K. (2007). Spatial navigation deficit in amnestic mild cognitive impairment. *Proceedings of the National Academy of Sciences of the United States of America*, *104*(10), 4042–4047.

Hugdahl, K., Thomsen, T., & Ersland, L. (2006). Sex differences in visuo-spatial processing: An fMRI study of mental rotation. *Neuropsychologia*, *44*(9), 1575–1583.

Humphrey, N. K. (1970). What the frog's eye tells to the monkey's brain. *Brain and Behavioral Evolution*, *2*, 324–337.

Iaria, G., Arnold, A. E. G. F., Burles, F., Liu, I., Slone, E., Barclay, S., & Levy, R. M. (2014). Developmental topographical disorientation and decreased hippocampal functional connectivity. *Hippocampus*, *24*(11), 1364–1374.

Iaria, G., & Barton, J. J. S. (2010). Developmental topographical disorientation: A newly discovered cognitive disorder. *Experimental Brain Research*, *206*(2), 189–196.

Iaria, G., Bogod, N., Fox, C. J., & Barton, J. J. S. (2009). Developmental topographical disorientation: Case one. *Neuropsychologia*, *47*(1), 30–40.

Iaria, G., Petrides, M., Dagher, A., Pike, B., & Bohbot, V. D. (2003). Cognitive strategies dependent on the hippocampus and caudate nucleus in human navigation: Variability and change with practice. *The Journal of Neuroscience*, *23*, 5945–5952.

Ishikawa, T., & Montello, D. R. (2006). Spatial knowledge acquisition from direct experience in the environment: Individual differences in the development of metric knowledge and the integration of separately learned places. *Cognitive Psychology*, *52*(2), 93–129.

Jackson, H. (1958). Case of large cerebral tumor without optic neuritis and with left hemiplegia and imperception. In J. Taylor (Ed.), *Selected writings of John Hughlings Jackson* (pp. 146–152). New York, NY: Basic Books (Reprinted from *Royal London Ophthalmologic Hospital Reports*, *8*, 434–439, 1876).

Janzen, G., Jansen, C., & van Turennout, M. (2008). Memory consolidation of landmarks in good navigators. *Hippocampus*, *18*, 40–447.

Jordan, K., Schadow, J., Wuestenberg, T., Heinze, H.-J., & Jäncke, L. (2004). Different cortical activations for subjects using allocentric or egocentric strategies in a virtual navigation task. *Neuroreport*, *15*(1), 135–140.

Jeffery, K. J., & Burgess, N. (2006). A metric for the cognitive map: found at last? *Trends in Cognitive Sciences*, *10*(1), 1–3.

Klatzky, R. L., Loomis, J. M., Beall, A. C., Chance, S. S., & Golledge, R. G. (1998). Spatial updating of self-position and orientation during real, imagined and virtual locomotion. *Psychological Science*, *9*(4), 293–298.

Levine, D. N., Warach, J., & Farah, M. J. (1985). Two visual systems in mental imagery: dissociation of 'what' and 'where' in imagery disorders due to bilateral posterior cerebral lesions. *Neurology, 35*, 1010–1018.
Lindenberger, U. (2014). Human cognitive aging: Corriger la fortune? *Science, 346*(6209), 572–578.
Livingstone, S. A., & Skelton, R. W. (2007). Virtual environment navigation tasks and the assessment of cognitive deficits in individuals with brain injury. *Behavioural Brain Research, 185*(1), 21–31.
MacDonald, C. J., Lepage, K. Q., Eden, U. T., & Eichenbaum (2011). Hippocampal "time cells" bridge the gap in memory for discontiguous events. *Neuron, 71*, 737–749.
Maguire, E. A., Burgess, N., & O'Keefe, J. (1999). Human spatial navigation: Cognitive maps, sexual dimorphism, and neural substrates. *Current Opinion in Neurobiology, 9*, 171–177.
Maguire, E. A., Burgess, N., Donnett, J. G., Frackowiak, R. S., Frith, C. D., & O'Keefe, J. (1998). Knowing where and getting there: A human navigation network. *Science, 280*(5365), 921–924.
Maguire, E. A., Burke, T., Phillips, J., & Staunton, H. (1996). Topographical disorientation following unilateral temporal lobe lesions in humans. *Neuropsychologia, 34*(10), 993–1001.
McFie, J., Piercy, M. F., & Zangwill, O. L. (1950). Visual-spatial agnosia associated with lesions of the right cerebral hemisphere. *Brain, 73*, 167–190.
McNaughton, B., Chen, L., & Markus, E. (1991). "Dead reckoning," landmark learning, and the sense of direction: A neurophysiological and computational hypothesis. *Journal of Cognitive Neuroscience, 3*(2), 190–202.
Mendez, M. F., & Cherrier, M. M. (2003). Agnosia for scenes in topographagnosia. *Neuropsychologia, 41*, 1387–1395.
Milner, A. D., & Goodale, M. A. (1995). *The visual brain in action*. Oxford: Oxford University Press.
Moffat, S. D. (2009). Aging and spatial navigation: What do we know and where do we go? *Neuropsychology Review, 19*, 478–489.
Moffat, S. D., Elkins, W., & Resnick, S. M. (2006). Age differences in the neural systems supporting human allocentric spatial navigation. *Neurobiology of Aging, 27*, 965–972.
Moffat, S. D., & Resnick, S. M. (2002). Effects of age on virtual environment place naivgation and allocentric cognitive mapping. *Behavioral Neuroscience, 116*(5), 851–859.
Morris, R. (1984). Developments of a water-maze procedure for studying spatial learning in the rat. *Journal of Neuroscience Methods, 11*, 47–60.
Morris, R. G. M., Garrud, P., Rawlins, J. N. P., & O'Keefe, J. (1982). Place navigation impaired in rats with hippocampal lesions. *Nature, 297*, 681–683.
Noordzij, M. L., Zuidhoek, S., & Postma, A. (2006). The influence of visual experience on the ability to form spatial mental models based on route and survey descriptions. *Cognition, 100*, 321–342.
O'Keefe, J., & Nadel, L. (1978). *The hippocampus as a cognitive map*. Oxford: Clarendon Press.
Oudman, E., Van der Stigchel, S., Nijboer, T. C. W., Wijnia, J. W., Seekles, M. L., & Postma, A. (2014). Route learning in Korsakoff's syndrome: Residual acquisition of spatial memory despite profound amnesia. *Journal of Neuropsychology*. Available from http://dx.doi.org/10.1111/jnp.12058.
Pai, M.-C., & Jacobs, W. J. (2004). Topographical disorientation in community-residing patients with Alzheimer's disease. *International Journal of Geriatric Psychiatry, 19*(3), 250–255.

Palermo, L., Foti, F., Ferlazzo, F., Guariglia, C., & Petrosini, L. (2014). I find my way in a maze but not in my own territory! Navigational processing in developmental topographical disorientation. *Neuropsychology, 28*(1), 135–146.

Palermo, L., Piccardi, L., Bianchini, F., Nemmi, F., Giorgio, V., Incoccia, C., ... Guariglia, C. (2014). Looking for the compass in a case of developmental topographical disorientation: A behavioral and neuroimaging study. *Journal of Clinical and Experimental Neuropsychology, 36*(5), 464–481.

Paterson, A., & Zangwill, O. L. (1945). A case of topographical disorientation associated with unilateral cerebral lesion. *Brain, 68*, 188–221.

Pereira, A. G., Portuguez, M. W., Da Costa, D. I., Azambuja, L. S., Marroni, S. P., Da Costa, J. C., & Pereira-Filho, A. A. (2011). Route learning performance: Is it a hippocampus function? *Cognitive & Behavioral Neurology, 24*(1), 4–10.

Raz, N., Lindenberger, U., Rodrigue, K. M., Kennedy, K. M., Head, D., Williamson, A., ... Acker, J. D. (2005). Regional brain changes in aging healthy adults: General trends, individual differences and modifiers. *Cerebral Cortex, 15*, 1676–1689.

Rey, B., & Alcañiz, M. (2010). *Research in neuroscience and virtual reality.* InTech.

Rodgers, M. K., Sindone, J. A., & Moffat, S. D. (2012). Effects of age on navigation strategy. *Neurobiology of Aging, 33*, 15–22.

Rowland, D. C., & Moser, M.-B. (2013). Time finds its place in the hippocampus. *Neuron, 78*, 953–954.

Salthouse, T. A. (2010). Selective review of cognitive aging. *Journal of the International Neuropsychological Society, 16*, 754–760.

Sargolini, F., Fyhn, M., McNaughton, B. L., Witter, M. P., Moser, M.-B., & Moser, E. I. (2006). Conjunctive representation of position, direction, and velocity in entorhinal cortex. *Science, 312*, 758–762.

Siegel, A. W., & White, S. H. (1975). The development of spatial representations of large environments. In H. W. Reese (Ed.), *Advances in child development and behavior* (pp. 9–55). New York, NY: Academic Press.

Spiers, H. J. (2008). Keeping the goal in mind: Prefrontal contributions to spatial navigation. *Neuropsychologia, 46*(7), 2106–2108.

Spiers, H. J., Burgess, N., Maguire, E. A., Baxendale, S. A., Hartley, T., Thompson, P. J., & O'Keefe, J. (2001). Unilateral temporal lobectomy patients show lateralized topographical and episodic memory deficits in a virtual town. *Brain, 124*, 2476–2489.

Takahashi, N., Kawamura, M., Shiota, J., Kasahata, N., & Hirayama, K. (1997). Pure topographical disorientation due to right retrosplenial lesion. *Neurology, 49*, 464–469.

Ungerleider, L. G., & Mishkin, M. (1982). Two corticalvisual systems. In D. J. Ingle, M. A. Goodale, & R. J. W. Mansfield (Eds.), *Analysis of visual behavior* (pp. 549–586). Cambridge, MA: MIT Press.

United Nations Population Fund (2012). *Ageing in the twenty-first century: A celebration and a challenge.* New York, NY and London: The United Nations Population Fund (UNFPA) and HelpAge International.

Van Asselen, M., Kessels, R. P. C., Kappelle, L. J., Neggers, S. F. W., Frijns, C. J. M., & Postma, A. (2006). Neural correlates of human wayfinding in stroke patients. *Brain Research, 1067*(1), 229–238.

Van der Ham, I. J. M., Faber, A. M. E., Venselaar, M., Van Kreveld, M. J., & Löffler, M. (2015). Ecological validity of virtual environments to assess human navigation ability. *Frontiers in Psychology, 6*, 637.

Van der Ham, I. J. M., Kant, N., Postma, A., & Visser-Meily, J. M. A. (2013). Is navigation ability a problem in mild stroke patients? Insights from self-reported navigation measures. *Journal of Rehabilitation Medicine, 45*, 429–433.

Van der Ham, I. J. M., Van Zandvoort, M. J. E., Meilinger, T., Bosch, S. E., Kant, N., & Postma, A. (2010). Spatial and temporal aspects of navigation in two neurological patients. *NeuroReport, 21*, 685–689.

Van der Meer, R. K. (1986). The trail pheromone complex of Solenopsis invicta and Solenopsis richteri. In C. S. Lofgren, & R. K. Vander Meer (Eds.), *Fire ants and leaf-cutting ants: Biology and management*. Boulder, CO: Westview Press.

Van Veen, H. J., Distler, H. K., Braun, S., & Bülthoff, H. H. (1998). Navigating through a virtual city: Using virtual reality technology to study human action and perception. *Future Generation Computer Systems, 14*, 231–242.

Vogeley, K., & Fink, G. R. (2003). Neural correlates of the first-person-perspective. *Trends in Cognitive Sciences*, 7(1), 38–42.

Waller, D., Loomis, J. M., & Steck, S. D. (2003). Inertial cues do not enhance knowledge of environmental layout. *Psychonomic Bulletin & Review, 10*(4), 987–993.

Wang, R. F., & Simons, D. J. (1999). Active and passive scene recognition across views. *Cognition, 70*, 191–210.

Whiteley, A. M., & Warrington, E. K. (1978). Selective impairment of topographical memory: A single case study. *Journal of Neurology, Neurosurgery, and Psychiatry, 41*, 575–578.

Wiener, J. M., Büchner, S. J., & Hölscher, C. (2009). Taxonomy of human wayfinding tasks: A knowledge-based approach. *Spatial Cognition and Computation, 9*, 152–165.

Wiener, J. M., de Condappa, O., Harris, M. A., & Wolbers, T. (2013). Maladaptive bias for extrahippocampal navigation strategies in aging humans. *The Journal of Neuroscience, 33*(14), 6012–6017.

Wiener, J. M., Kmecova, H., & de Condappa, O. (2012). Route repetition and route retracing: Effects of cognitive aging. *Frontiers in Aging Neuroscience, 4*, article 7.

Wolbers, T., & Hegarty, M. (2010). What determines our navigational abilities? *Trends in Cognitive Sciences, 14*(3), 138–146.

Worsley, C. L., Recce, M., Spiers, H. J., Marley, J., Polkey, C. E., & Morris, R. G. (2001). Path integration following temporal lobectomy in humans. *Neuropsychologia, 39*(5), 452–464.

CHAPTER 9

How Children Learn to Discover Their Environment: An Embodied Dynamic Systems Perspective on the Development of Spatial Cognition

Hanna Mulder, Ora Oudgenoeg-Paz, Annika Hellendoorn and Marian J. Jongmans
Department of Education & Pedagogy, Utrecht University, Utrecht, The Netherlands

In the first few years of life, human infants evolve from helpless creatures that are totally dependent on others around them into walking and talking preschoolers. Just after birth, infants have merely relatively immature perception and action systems to learn about the world around them. Yet, by the time they enter school, children have mastered many important skills within the domain of spatial cognition already. They have a good understanding of spatial relations between objects and, between objects and people; they can use spatial language, such as the words "in," "under," and "above"; they can navigate and remember the routes they most frequently use in their neighborhood; and they can remember where they have hidden their favorite toy in their bedroom. The speed at which these functions develop, only in a couple of years' time, has amazed cognitive psychologists, parents, and professionals working with children for a long time. In one of his books, the Flemish author Bernard Dewulf (2011, p. 7) wrote an almost poetic description of the development of his own baby son in this regard (loosely translated here):

> *He is not able to sit yet. Not completely. For a little while longer, he prefers to sit inside himself, which is easier than on that chair. But on that chair he can do things that he is unable to do otherwise. That's why he sits inside himself on that chair. With his arms, which he found on himself yesterday, he can reach twenty centimetres further into his expanding room-universe. And if his rubber back allows, he manages to get twice as far. Whatever is beyond, the milky way of the milk bottle, he cries towards himself.*

Neuropsychology of Space.
DOI: http://dx.doi.org/10.1016/B978-0-12-801638-1.00009-4

Knowingly or unknowingly, Dewulf's accurate description touches upon some of the grand theories that developmental psychologists have been working on in the past decades to try and explain the mysteries of child development, including the development of spatial cognition. These theories do not just ask which developmental milestones occur at which age, but rather, they ask *how* development proceeds. What are the driving forces behind all these major developmental changes that we observe in the first few years of life? One of these theories is known as the theory of embodied cognition, which is part of the larger group of dynamic systems theories and the perception–action approach to development. One of their major premises, touched upon by Dewulf, is that advances in children's motor development lead to changes in the way children can explore the world. Through exploration, children get new information about the world around them, which in turn elicits new actions and allows them to learn about objects, people, language, and places. These ongoing perception–action cycles are what drives development (see Gibson, 1988; Thelen & Smith, 1996). This chapter first provides an overview of dynamic systems theory, before moving on to a focus on the embodied cognition and perception–action theories. Subsequently, we discuss studies into the development of spatial cognition, which are based on these theories, with a specific focus on mental rotation and spatial memory (including memory for object locations, orientation, and navigation). A number of important questions are addressed such as if, and if so, how, motor development and exploration are related to these different aspects of spatial cognition. Furthermore, if motor development and exploration are indeed related to mental rotation and spatial memory, are such relations restricted to infancy? Is there any evidence that such relations may be causal? To illustrate the challenges associated with developmental research in this area, a section on methods is included. Moreover, sections on clinical groups are presented to describe selected aspects of the development of spatial cognition in children with autism spectrum disorder (ASD), cerebral palsy (CP), and Nonverbal Learning Disability (NLD). The chapter ends with challenges and future directions in this field of research.

9.1 DYNAMIC SYSTEMS THEORY

We begin with an overview of the dynamic systems theory, which is the broader theory under which the embodied cognition approach falls.

Dynamic systems theory, which originally stems from physics, chemistry, and mathematics, was taken over by biology researchers studying the complex dynamics that occur in the natural world, and has found its application in developmental psychology toward the end of the 20th century (Thelen & Smith, 1996). Its major premise is that the developing infant and child can be seen as a complex dynamic system, in which multiple internal and external influences continuously interact (Smith & Thelen, 2003). Within this model, no specific factor, such as biological maturation, is seen as the single cause for driving developmental change. Rather, development is thought to occur as a function of a process called "self-organization." In the process of self-organization, new structures form and previous ones dissolve through the continuous interactions between the individual parts of the system. Resulting new structures may seem to follow complex rules, but, according to dynamic systems theorists, there are no such higher order organizational principles. In his book on dynamic systems, Kelso (1997, p. 8) describes the concept of self-organization as follows: "(. . .) spontaneous pattern formation is exactly what we mean by *self-organization*: the system organizes itself, but there is no 'self', no agent inside the system doing the organizing." Thus, the individual parts of the system together make up a larger, more complex, and coherent whole. As Thelen and Smith (1996) describe it: "These emergent organizations are totally different from the elements that constitute the system, and the patterns cannot be predicted solely from the characteristics of the individual elements" (p. 54). What, then, does this tell us about the developing infant? If we view the infant as the system itself, which shows complex behavior, how do changes in this behavior come about?

The answer to this question is that changes in the systems' complexity occur as a function of any small change in the individual components that the system is made up of. An often-used example to illustrate this principle is the following. Consider a campus with paved paths and green fields in between university buildings. If the shortest path between two buildings is cutting directly through the grass, then likely, over time, a new path will appear. At first one student will cross along the shortest route, then a few more, and suddenly all students will take this route which is now visible as a clear path. This is the principle of self-organization at work: something seemingly complex emerges through a single small change in the system (the one student taking the shortest route), which leads to a cascade of effects (all the other students who follow his or her path which becomes increasingly visible). Another example, from the field of spatial development, is the way behavior comes about in infants during a visuospatial working memory task. In this task, the classical A-not-B task (Piaget, 1954), infants are presented with two identical wells that are carved out in the table in front of them. In one of these wells, a toy is hidden while the infant is watching, and subsequently both wells are covered with a cloth. The infant is then distracted from looking at the wells for a few seconds, before being asked to find the toy (see Fig. 9.1). If the infant reaches correctly toward the hiding location, the toy is hidden there again. This first hiding location is called the "A" location. After two correct reaches to this location, the toy is hidden in the other, "B" location. Despite the fact that the infant has seen how the object was hidden in the new location, B, after a short delay infants often reach back to the first location, A. This effect occurs because the infant has formed a habit of reaching to A, and this habit is a stronger determinant of their subsequent action than the new visual input they received when watching the toy being hidden at B (Thelen, Schöner, Scheier, & Smith, 2001). Infants make this error until they reach the age of about 12 months, after which they can normally pass this task in its classical form (Wellman, Cross, & Bartsch, 1986). However, this story is much more complex than it may

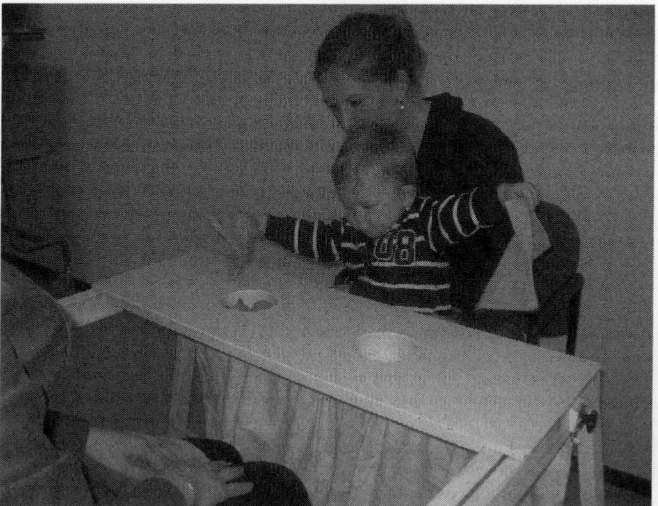

Figure 9.1 A-not-B task setup, in which the infant has to remember in which of two wells a toy is hidden. *Reprinted from Van de Weijer-Bergsma, E. (2009).* Developmental trajectories of attention and executive functioning in infants born preterm: The influence of perinatal risk factors and maternal interactive styles *(PhD thesis). Available from NARCIS.*

seem at first. Decades of experimental research have shown that there is actually no set age at which infants can pass this task; rather, passing or failing is a function of all specifics of the perceptual input generated by the task environment and the child's previous experiences (Thelen et al., 2001). For example, Smith, Thelen, Titzer, and McLin (1999) have shown that the child's position is one of the many determinants influencing task performance. They altered the child's position between the last reach toward the A location and hiding the toy at the B location for the first time, by moving the child out of a seated position to a standing position on their parents' lap. In this experimental condition, 10-month-old infants suddenly no longer make the A-not-B error. Thus, the new position somehow disrupts the strong tendency, or habit, to reach toward the A location, illustrating how any small change in the interaction between child and environment can generate novel, seemingly complex, behavior, namely passing the visuospatial working memory task.

In addition to the concept of self-organization, the notion that development occurs across multiple nested timescales is central to dynamic systems theory. The changes that can be observed across, for example, the first few years of life, are ultimately the result of much smaller changes occurring during second-by-second interactions between the child and its environment that take place every day. This focus on nested timescales and microgenetic changes leading to larger developmental changes over time in dynamic systems theory, provides a different view on a typical and widely discussed problem occurring with more traditional so-called "stage theories" of child development. In the traditional stage theories, development is viewed as a succession of stages of increasing complexity. Novel behaviors are acquired quite abruptly; they emerge at once because the child has suddenly grasped a new understanding or skill. However, this suddenness of development is rarely seen in real life. For example, there is a point in the first 2 years of life when all healthy infants learn to walk. From a stage-like view of child development, the infant either can walk already or does not walk yet; there is no in-between. However, when very detailed observations of infant's behavior are conducted, it becomes clear that this is not how development actually occurs. True, most infants will take their first steps at some point, but this does not mean they will walk wherever they want to go thereafter. Rather, after they have taken their first steps, most infants will revert back to crawling, before they again take a few steps, and then a few more, and so onward, until they use walking as their main way of self-locomotion (Adolph, Robinson, Young, & Gill-Alvarez, 2008; for a detailed review of the huge amount of natural variability occurring in the acquisition of independent mobility, see also Adolph & Robinson, 2013). These temporary regressions to a previous "stage" accompanied with temporary progressions to a more advanced "stage" are seen as noise in traditional theories. However, in reality, this intraindividual variability is the rule rather than the exception. Dynamic systems theory offers an alternative perspective on this issue. Development across stages occurs only when one looks at the bigger scale of time (Adolph & Robinson, 2013; Thelen & Smith, 1996). At the microscale temporary regressions and progressions are perfectly logical, and stem from the ever-changing conditions in children and their environment. For example, Corbetta and Bojczyk (2002) investigated infants' reaching responses before, while, and after they had learned to walk. In particular, the authors assessed whether infants reached to objects with one or two hands. During the first year of life, children usually progress from reaching with two hands without adapting to the properties of the objects to more adaptive reaching using one hand for small objects and two hands for larger objects. In the study of Corbetta and Bojczyk, before the onset of walking, infants indeed tended to reach adaptively as would be expected. However, in the process of learning to walk, infants started to reach with two hands to smaller objects as well, thus showing a temporary regression in their reaching skill. After having gained sufficient experience with walking and balance control, infants' increasingly reached to smaller objects with one hand again, showing the same adaptive behavioral pattern that they had already shown before learning to walk. Thus, the developing system is constantly reorganizing, and development is infinitely more complex than stage theories suggest. It is this complexity and variability that is seen as one of the major characteristics of child development in dynamic systems theory.

To summarize, in dynamic systems theory, development is seen as a process of self-organization in which, as Smith and Thelen (2003, p. 344) put it, "no single element has causal priority." Rather, new behaviors and skills emerge as a function of the interactions between the child and its environment, and relatively small changes in these interactions can offset reorganization of the developing system, leading to developmental change over time (Smith & Thelen, 2003).

9.2 EMBODIED COGNITION THEORY

Within the broad theory of dynamic systems, embodied cognition theory is particularly important to consider for understanding the development of spatial cognition in infants and children. Previous theories of human cognition have focused on abstract mental representations, in which sensory and motor systems serve the purpose of delivering input and output to and from the cognitive system (Wilson, 2002). In this approach to human cognition, the computer metaphor is often used: the human mind functions just like a computer, with input, output, and a set of computations in between. In contrast, in the embodied cognition approach, sensory and motor systems are seen as fundamentally integrated with cognitive processing. The philosopher Larry Shapiro gives a good example of the distinction between the traditional approach, which uses the computer analogy to cognition, and the embodied cognition approach. In this example, a psychologist is depicted who gives a particular sensory code as input to an organisms' nervous system in the laboratory, resulting in a given set of cognitive processes. Had the psychologist given the same code to the same organism walking about in the outside world, would the cognitive processes be the same? From the traditional cognitive psychology approach, the answer would be "yes"; as the input to the neural system is the same, so will be the output. From the embodied cognition approach, the answer would clearly be "no," because cognition in this account is viewed as occurring in constant and direct interaction with the environment (Shapiro, 2007). Thelen (2000, adapted from Chiel & Beer, 1997) provides a clear schematic overview of this theoretical account and the way it contrasts to the view of a decoupled environment, body, and brain, which is shown in Fig. 9.2.

What does embodied cognition theory tell us about the process through which children acquire spatial knowledge and understanding? The answers given by the embodied cognition approach are rooted in the ecological psychology approach to development. The ecological psychologist Eleanor Gibson proposed that infants learn increasingly more about the world around them through active exploration. Through exploration, infants learn about "affordances" which are the possibilities for action that occur in the environment (Gibson, 1988; Gibson, 1979). For example, a cup offers the affordance of drinking, a bike offers the affordance of cycling. Clearly, these affordances are not the same for all organisms: for a bird, a bike does not offer the affordance of cycling, but instead may offer the affordance of sitting on (the seat or handlebars) instead. Affordances thus exist in the interaction between agent and environment. Gibson (1988) describes three phases of infant exploration that occur in the first year of life as follows:

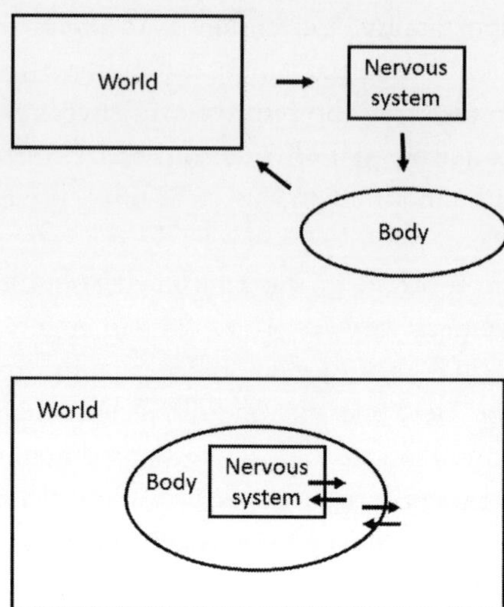

Figure 9.2 Thelen's (2000) schematic overview of the contrast between an "input–output" model of human cognitive processing (top panel) and an integrated embodied dynamic systems model (bottom panel). *Reproduced from Thelen, E. (2000). Grounded in the world: Developmental origins of the embodied mind.* Infancy, 1*(1), 3–28. Copyright 2000, reprinted with permission from John Wiley and Sons. Based on: Chiel, H. J., & Beer, R. D. (1997). The brain has a body: Adaptive behavior emerges from interactions of nervous system, body, and environment.* Trends in Neuroscience, 20, *553–557.*

1. From birth through 4 months of age, infants explore whatever is nearby enough for them to see, mouth, or touch.
2. Around the age of 5 months, on average, infants learn to reach to objects in their vicinity and manipulate them. This brings about new opportunities for exploration, such as turning, banging, and shaking objects.
3. Around the age of 9 months, on average, infants learn to crawl. With this new skill comes the opportunity to explore a much larger world around them. Not only can infants now seek out objects for exploration which are beyond reaching distance, they also learn to navigate through space independently, allowing them to learn about basic spatial relations between themselves, others, and objects, as well as gain understanding about distance and depth.

Subsequently, in the first half of the second year of life, most infants learn to walk, which again brings about many new opportunities for exploring what is around them. For example, they may learn the affordance of "transportability" when they start exploring carrying objects from place to place (Gibson, 1988). Subsequently, new phases in exploration may occur through which children can discover other, even more complex affordances (Gibson, 1988). Think, for example, of learning to angle a mirror in such a way that you can see yourself in it or someone standing on the other side of the room, and, a relatively new affordance to learn for children growing up in modern day society, the act of swiping used with technological devices such as smart phones and tablets. Following Eleanor Gibson's theory, exploration takes a central place in the development of cognition. The way children can explore their environment, in turn, changes with development as a function of advances in visual perception and increasing motor skill, among other factors. For example, with the acquisition of new gross motor skills, such as sitting upright, infants gain access to a whole new array of opportunities to elicit perceptual information from the world around them and discover novel affordances (see also Bernard Dewulfs' description of his son at the outset of this chapter). Thus, through exploration, infants learn about the properties of the physical and social world around them. With respect to visuospatial cognition, achievement of motor milestones for self-locomotion (i.e., crawling, walking) seems especially important. We will turn to this issue in section 9.3.1

9.3 INTERIM SUMMARY

To summarize, dynamic systems and embodied cognition theory suggest that developmental changes in (spatial) cognition come about through the child's interactions with his or her environment that occur second-by-second and day-by-day through ongoing perception–action cycles. As infants grow older and learn to sit, crawl, and walk, they are increasingly able to explore the world around them, allowing them to discover new affordances and gain insight in spatial relations. Having briefly explained the general ideas behind dynamic systems and embodied cognition theory, we now turn to the application of these theories to studies of the development of spatial cognition. Landau (2002) defined spatial cognition as "the capacity to discover, mentally transform, and use spatial information about the world to achieve a variety of goals, including navigating through the world, identifying and acting on objects, talking about objects and events, and using explicit symbolic representations such as maps and diagrams to communicate about space" (p. 395). Here, we focus on the role of infant motor development and exploration in the development of two central aspects of spatial cognition touched upon by Landau, which first emerge in the first years of life: mental rotation and spatial memory (including memory for object locations, orientation, and navigation). Although many studies have also investigated other aspects of spatial cognition from an embodied dynamic systems perspective, such as spatial language, for reasons of space limitations this is not the focus of the current chapter (for further information on the topic of spatial language, see, eg, Oudgenoeg-Paz, Leseman, & Volman, 2015). For each of the domains of mental rotation and spatial memory, first, examples of current methods used with infants and older children are described, followed by a review of studies looking into how motor development and exploration are related to these key aspects of spatial cognition.

9.3.1 Mental Rotation

Assessment methods and developmental change. Mental rotation is "the imagined movement of an object (or array of objects) in 2- or 3-dimensional space" (Frick, Ferrara, & Newcombe, 2013, p. 117). Various paradigms exist to assess mental rotation ability in infants and children. In infants, the violation-of-expectation paradigm is often used in which look duration toward a stimulus is measured. The central tenet of this paradigm is that infants will look longer at what is unexpected and novel than to what is familiar to them. Thus, by familiarizing infants with the stimulus first and then showing another stimulus that is subtly different, infants' sensitivity to these differences can be tested. For example, in studies of mental rotation, as shown in Fig. 9.3, infants are shown an object which has a different colored front and back and is asymmetrical in shape (familiarization phase). Subsequently, the object is rotated behind an occluder and then presented again (test phase). In the test phase, the object is either the same as the object in the familiarization phase, but rotated in angle (congruent condition) or its own mirror image presented at an angle (incongruent condition). If infants look longer toward the incongruent compared to the congruent condition, this is taken as evidence for their understanding that the former is impossible, implying they would have had to use mental rotation to match the objects between the familiarization and test phase (but see Box 9.1 on methodology). Möhring and Frick (2013) used this paradigm with 6-month-old infants and showed that under certain conditions,

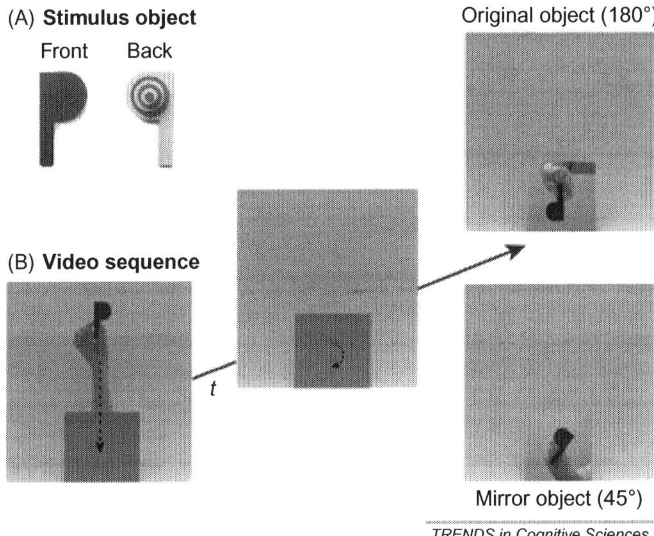

Figure 9.3 Illustration of infant violation-to-expectation paradigm to test mental rotation. *Reprinted from Frick, A., Möhring, W., & Newcombe, N. S. (2014). Development of mental transformation abilities.* Trends in Cognitive Sciences, 18*(10), 536–542 (Adapted from Frick & Möhring, 2013, and Möhring & Frick, 2013—permission obtained from John Wiley and Sons).*

BOX 9.1 Methodology

Studying Cognitive Development—Methodology Matters

The present chapter is, very deliberately, not focused at describing age-related trends in the development of spatial cognition. In fact, we have tried to stay away from general claims that children at a certain age are able to do X or Y—instead we have aimed to discuss children's task performance in particular experimental setups at particular ages. The reason behind this choice of focus is not that we do not believe infants and children make large progress in spatial cognitive skills, such as mental rotation, navigation, and memory, over time—clearly, large developmental advances are observed. Instead, in our point of view, such developmental improvements can only be accurately described when different age groups are given exactly the same task, which is only rarely the case across different studies.

To illustrate, consider the section on mental rotation in which we describe how 6-month-old infants seem capable of mentally rotating an object, at least after having been allowed to manually explore the object prior to the task

(*Continued*)

BOX 9.1 Methodology—cont'd

(Möhring & Frick, 2013). In contrast, when Frick et al. (2013) assessed mental rotation using the touch screen task shown in Fig. 9.4 in 3.5- to 5.5-year-old-children, they observed that the younger age group (ie, 3.5–4.5 years) performed quite poorly. How might these differences come about? A close look at the two tasks administered reveals marked differences. First, the response mode is different: whereas infants only had to look at the screen, the preschoolers in the study by Frick et al. (2013) had to integrate looking at the screen while pointing to indicate their response. Keen (2003) studied these differences in task demand between different age groups in another field of cognitive development: children's knowledge of physical laws of solidity and continuity. The title of her paper nicely summarizes the problem at hand: "Representations of objects and events: Why do infants look so smart and toddlers look so dumb?" Keen describes the exact same phenomena of contradictory results between infant and toddler studies: whereas infants showed signs of having at least rudimentary understanding about object solidity and continuity, as evidenced by their looking behavior in a violation-to-expectation paradigm, toddlers failed to demonstrate such knowledge in a reaching task. However, when toddlers were also given a looking-time task, like infants, they looked longer at the unexpected outcome (Mash, Novak, Berthier, & Keen, 2006). The question as to why pointing and looking responses may produce such different behavioral patterns in young children has been much debated (see, eg, Thelen et al., 2001). One potential explanation which has received

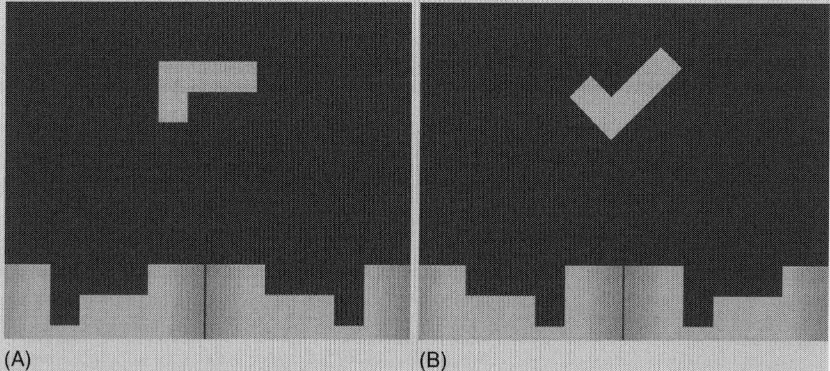

Figure 9.4 Mental rotation task example used with 3.5- to 5.5-year-olds. In this task, children had to indicate in which of the two holes the figure would fit. *Reprinted from Frick, A., Ferrara, K., & Newcombe, N. S. (2013). Using a touch screen paradigm to assess the development of mental rotation between 3½ and 5½ years of age.* Cognitive Processing, *14, 117–127. Copyright 2013, reprinted with permission from Springer.*

(Continued)

BOX 9.1 Methodology—cont'd

some support is that, in addition to the apparent difference in terms of response mode, there is a more "hidden" difference in requirements between the expectation-to-novelty and reaching tasks: whereas the former present infants with an end-state which they have to judge as either correct or incorrect, the latter asks children to actively predict the outcome themselves (Frick, Möhring, & Newcombe, 2014; Keen, 2003). However, the difference between predicting action outcomes and solely having to judge outcomes that are given does not fully seem to explain the different results obtained from violation-to-expectation paradigms administered to infants and reaching tasks administered to older children. For example, Lee and Kuhlmeier (2013) studied the difference in looking and pointing behavior in 2-year-olds in a physical reasoning task. When asked to predict the task outcome, children's looking behavior was more frequently correct than their reaching. Similar effects have been observed in the A-not-B task: infants' correct looking seems to precede correct reaching (Cuevas & Bell, 2010; Diamond, 1985). Thelen et al. (2001) argue for a dynamic systems' interpretation of these findings, in which looking and reaching behavior should not be seen as separate clues as to what the infant "really" knows or not, but rather, as the result of the complex interaction between the different perceptual inputs and the child's previous experiences with the task.

To summarize, children's cognitive task performance relies so strongly on the exact task demands that outcomes of studies that used different paradigms to assess the same cognitive "skill" are very difficult to compare. This general finding fully fits with a dynamic systems theory of cognitive development (Smith & Thelen, 2003). Along these same lines, Acredolo (1990) cautions in her review on spatial orientation in infancy that the fact that infants of a particular age seem to use a nonegocentric strategy to solve a particular orientation task, should not be taken as evidence that infants at that age switch from using egocentric to nonegocentric strategies *in general*. Rather, as Acredolo states, the (behavioral) patterns "were obtained in a particular paradigm, with a particular environment, and with particular training procedures" (p. 603). For example, as discussed in the section on spatial orientation and navigation in this chapter, the familiarity of the testing environment may strongly influence infants' response pattern (Acredolo, 1979). What is it that we can learn from these studies then? We can learn about the nature of developmental change within studies using exactly the same paradigm across different age groups, and we can learn that children are able to use strategy X under condition Y at a certain age; this does not mean they will always do so, but it shows something about the expanding behavioral repertoire that they have available from which they may increasingly select the most efficient

(*Continued*)

BOX 9.1 Methodology—cont'd

strategy, or the strategy with the most proof of success (Siegler, 1996). The developmental picture, then, is far from black and white.

Novel Techniques to Assess Spatial Cognition in Infants and Children

In the past decade, novel techniques have facilitated the study of spatial cognition in infants and children, such as the use of eye tracking and virtual reality tasks. Very recently, the technique of head-mounted eye tracking has been added to researchers' repertoires for studying development in this domain (Franchak, Kretch, Soska, & Adolph, 2011). A head-mounted eye tracker consists of two very small cameras connected to a lightweight cap, which is placed on the infants' head (see Fig. 9.5). The first camera points outward and captures what is in the infants' field of view. The second camera points

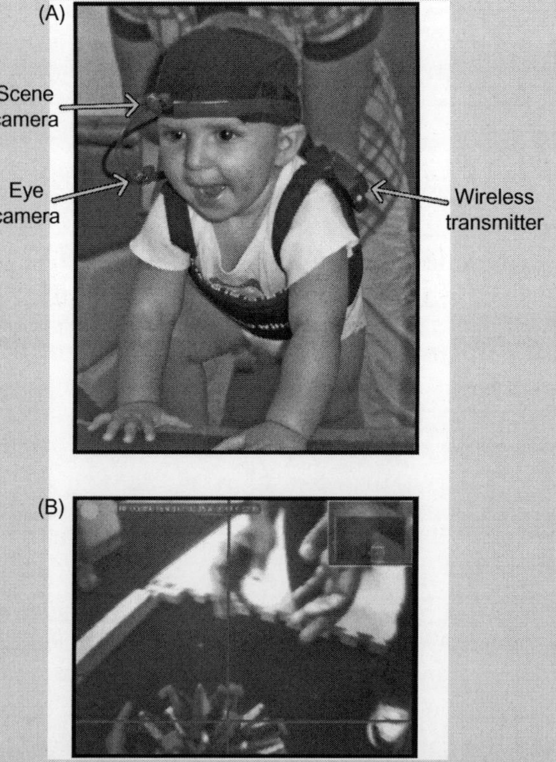

Figure 9.5 Image of child wearing head-mounted eye tracker. *Reprinted from Franchak, J. M., Kretch, K. S., Soska, K. C., & Adolph, K. E. (2011). Head-mounted eye tracking: A new method to describe infant looking.* Child Development, 82, *1738–1750. Copyright 2011, reprinted with permission from John Wiley and Sons.*

(Continued)

BOX 9.1 Methodology—cont'd

toward the infants' eye and records their eye movements. By integrating the information obtained from both sources, a precise measure can be gained of where the infant is looking within the visual scene. The advantage of this technique over screen-based eye tracking is clear: because the eye tracking equipment is fitted to the infants' head, looking data can be obtained while the infant is moving in the real 3D world. As such, questions regarding, for example, the actual use of landmarks can be addressed as infants crawl or walk as they naturally would, thus increasing ecological validity.

The first studies using head-mounted eye tracking have revealed that the acquisition of self-locomotion milestones radically changes the way that infants interact with the world around them (eg, also Karasik, Tamis-Lemonda, & Adolph, 2011; Kretch, Franchak, & Adolph, 2014). For example, Kretch et al. (2014) studied 13-month-old crawlers' and walkers' visual experiences as they moved along a walkway toward their caregiver. Clear differences were observed between the two different modes of self-locomotion: the highest point visible, as assessed with the scene camera, was twice as high for walkers compared to crawlers. In addition, walkers looked at their caregiver more often than crawlers as they moved, while crawlers looked at the floor more often. Thus, the visual input available by infants as they self-locomote is very different for crawlers and walkers. As walking infants have more of the larger environment in view while they are moving compared to crawlers, Kretch et al. (2014) suggest this may facilitate the use of landmarks for spatial memory and navigation in walkers. Thus, the technique of head-mounted eye tracking can be used to provide new information about infants' interactions with the world around them, opening up new avenues of research in the study of the development of spatial cognition.

detailed further below, infants this young already looked longer at the incongruent outcome compared to the congruent outcome.

In older children, a different task setup to assess mental rotation is often used (eg, Frick et al., 2013; Örnkloo & Von Hofsten, 2007). Frick et al. (2013) used a touch screen design to asses 3.5- to 5.5-year-olds' mental rotation abilities. Children were shown a display with a figure and two different holes on the screen, and asked to indicate in which of the two holes the figure would fit, as shown in Fig. 9.4. After dividing the sample into two age groups (ie, 3.5–4.5 years and 4.5–5.5 years), Frick et al. (2013) showed that 27% of children in the youngest age group performed well on the task, compared to 46% in the older age group. Good performance was defined as pointing to the correct hole in more than 10 out of 16 trials. Furthermore, they studied the effect of disparity, or the degree of rotation necessary to fit the figure into the hole, on task performance. Interestingly, both error rates and response times significantly increased with increasing disparity in the older, but not the younger age group. These findings suggest that the children in the older age group used mental rotation as a strategy to solve the task, whereas the younger age group failed to do so effectively. As such, results seem to conflict with those observed by Frick and colleagues in infants, who showed signs of being able to mentally rotate an object at a much younger age. To understand these contradictory results, the specific methods used and what they exactly require of children should be considered—an issue further discussed in Box 9.1.

Motor development and exploration in relation to mental rotation. Embodied dynamic systems theory poses that both motor development and exploration may be important factors in the development of (spatial) cognition. Thus, having described a number of frequently used measures to assess mental rotation in infants and children and developmental change in performance on those, we turn to the following question next: is there any evidence for an association between motor development, exploration, and mental rotation? In their study using the violation-of-expectation paradigm with 6-month-old infants, Möhring and Frick (2013) divided infants into two conditions: those in the manual exploration condition were given the opportunity to manually explore the object at the outset of the experiment, in an encoding phase, while those in the observation condition were only allowed to watch the object during this time. A clear difference between groups emerged: infants in the manual exploration condition looked significantly longer at the objects in the incongruent compared to the congruent condition, while this difference was not apparent in the observation condition. Thus, the authors conclude that infants as young as 6 months of age are capable of rudimentary forms of mental rotation, but only when given the opportunity to manually explore the object first. This finding fits in well with the dynamic embodied cognition view described above: exploration experience plays a crucial role in spatial cognition, mental rotation in this case.

These findings raise the question at what age manual experience with an object is no longer a prerequisite for mental rotation. Using the same experimental setup, Frick and Möhring (2013) addressed this question in 8- and 10-month-old infants. Infants were given only visual experience with the stimulus prior to the experiment. Eight-month-olds showed the same behavioral pattern as the 6-month-olds without manual exploration experience in the study by Möhring and Frick (2013): they did not look longer at the incongruent compared to congruent condition, thus showing no signs of being able to mentally rotate the object. However, 10-month-olds clearly distinguished between the two stimulus types in the test phase. The difference was large: whereas only 45% of 8-month-olds looked longer at the incongruent compared to congruent trials in the test phase, this was the case for 90% of the 10-month-olds. These findings may be taken to suggest that manual experience is no longer a prerequisite for mental rotation in 10-month-old infants. However, in order to better understand this effect, we must consider what happens between the age of 8 and 10 months in development: major advances in gross motor development occur during this time, as many infants learn to self-locomote. When studying performance on the mental rotation task in relation to infants' motor development, a clear pattern emerged: after statistically controlling for age, infant mental rotation ability was significantly related to a number of aspects of gross motor development, such as standing and walking with assistance (note however, that no association with crawling was found after controlling for age) (Frick & Möhring, 2013). The authors conclude that, with increasing experience with self-locomotion, infants' "reasoning about spatial relations between objects (or objects and agents) may become increasingly independent from their own location and perspective" (Frick & Möhring, 2013, p. 717).

Further evidence for the role of motor development and exploration experience on mental rotation in infants comes from the work of Schwarzer, Freitag, Buckel, and Lofruthe (2013). Schwarzer and colleagues investigated mental rotation abilities in 9-month-old infants with and without crawling experience. After letting infants habituate to a rotating shape, infants were shown six test trials of rotating stimuli: three with the same shape as was used during the habituation phase, and three with its mirror image. The authors showed that infants with crawling experience looked significantly longer toward the unexpected test outcome (ie, the mirror image shape) than toward the expected test outcome, whereas infant who could not yet crawl, did not. An important question is whether the associations observed between motor development, exploration, and mental rotation ability are restricted to infancy. Recent studies show that this is not the case. For example, Jansen and Heil (2010) found that specific aspects of motor development in 5- to 6-year-olds were associated with mental rotation ability at this age. They included a standardized motor test (the motor development test (MOT),

Zimmer & Volkermar, 1987) to assess coordination ability, fine-motor skills, balance, catching, jumping, speed of movements, and motor control. Their results showed that, after statistically controlling for nonverbal intelligence, motor control was significantly related to mental rotation ability, as assessed using a paper-and-pencil test.

Thus, in infants, having experience with the object itself and manipulating it (ie, exploration), facilitates mental rotation. Also, advances in gross motor development, in particular self-locomotion, allow infants to learn about object properties and spatial relations, facilitating mental rotation. In older children, links between motor control and mental rotation are also observed. Do these findings also fit in with the embodied dynamic systems framework? And if so, how? The answer, we believe, is yes if mental rotation itself is—at least in part—seen as the making of a motor plan which is not executed. This assumption was put to the test by Wexler, Kosslyn, and Berthoz (1998). Wexler and colleagues asked a group of adults to perform a mental rotation task *while* turning a joystick with their hand. The direction of the joystick turn was either compatible or incompatible with the mental rotation task (ie, clockwise mental and motor rotation or clockwise mental rotation and counterclockwise motor rotation). Mental rotation was faster and more accurate in the compatible condition, providing support for the suggestion that mental rotation is closely tied to motor processes. Thus, if children practice making and executing motor plans in general this might facilitate making motor plans which are purely "mental" (and thus not executed) too. From this perspective, it is noteworthy that in the study by Jansen and Heil (2010), many aspects of motor development were studied in relation to mental rotation and only one of them was found to be a significant predictor over and above nonverbal intelligence: motor control. Thus, the precision with which motor plans are practiced may make a difference. Further evidence for this suggestion comes from studies with adults. Moreau, Mansy-Dannay, Clerc, and Guerrién (2011) studied mental rotation ability in athletes with various levels of experience: novices and experts. They showed mental rotation ability was better in expert athletes, but whether this effect was observed depended on the number of hours spent in training and the type of sport assessed. Specifically, the difference in mental rotation ability between novices and experts was apparent in combat sports (fencing, judo, and wrestling) but not in roadrunners. Whereas practicing combat sports requires very precise motor plans in terms of directionality, timing, and force, which need to be adapted all the time to the specific situation, this is not as much the case for roadrunners.

In summary, there is evidence for the relation between motor skill and mental rotation ability, which would be expected based on an embodied cognition perspective. Moreover, this relation is observed throughout development, from infancy through to adulthood. It seems that in particular practice with making and executing precise coordinated motor plans relates to the ability to solve mental rotation tasks. This suggests that, when mentally rotating an object, this may not be much different from imagining *the act* of rotating the object—something which may not so much be an abstract representation in the brain, but rather much more closely aligned to the act of rotation itself, even if that act is not executed (see Wexler et al., 1998). Studies of the role of exploration on mental rotation to date appear to be restricted to infancy; further research is needed to study if and how exploration relates to mental rotation ability in older children. Next, we turn to another important aspect of spatial cognition: spatial memory.

9.3.2 Spatial Memory: Remembering Locations and Finding One's Way in the World

Studies of the development of spatial memory ask at what age infants and children are able to memorize nearby and distant (object) locations, and which information infants and children use to guide their memory. A complete literature review of this broad research area falls outside of the scope of this chapter (for comprehensive reviews, see, eg, Cornell & Heth, 2006 for a review on children's way finding; Campos et al., 2000; Newcombe & Huttenlocher, 2003; Newcombe, Uttal, & Sauter, 2013). Instead, we focus on the key questions raised above, namely how changes in the development of spatial memory relate to motor development and exploration in infants and children, after having described a number of frequently used assessment methods and developmental changes in performance on those. In doing so, we distinguish between studies that have investigated spatial memory in task situations where children remain stationary, from studies in which children move or are moved before they respond.

9.4 SPATIAL MEMORY ON THE MOVE: ORIENTATION AND NAVIGATION

Assessment methods and developmental change. The study of the development of navigation skills to date has focused on the question as to how infants and children are able to orient themselves in the environment. Which cues do children use to reorient themselves after having been moved (younger children) and how do they find their way (older children)? Studies in this area have addressed developmental changes in the use of egocentric versus allocentric reference systems, and related the use of landmarks. Piaget (1954) already observed that young infants tend not to have an "objective" notion of space, but rather, code object locations only in relation to themselves and their own location. A series of early experimental studies have indeed confirmed that young infants tend to rely strongly on egocentric, rather than allocentric, referencing, while marked changes occur over the first years of life (Acredolo, 1978; Acredolo and Evans, 1980; Newcombe, Huttenlocher, Dummey, & Wiley, 1998).

The paradigm often used in infant studies is the reorientation task designed by Acredolo (1978). In this task, infants were placed in a chair attached to a round table in the middle of a testing room (see Fig. 9.6). Windows, labeled X and Y, were present on either side of the infant. In the first phase of the experiment, the infant learned that following the sound of a buzzer, an experimenter would appear at window X. After infants demonstrated proof of this principle, as evidenced by their anticipatory looks to window X before the experimenter appeared, he or she was moved to the other side of the table. The buzzer was then rung again, but no one appeared at the window. If the infant used an egocentric referencing strategy, they would be expected to look at window Y; if they did not respond egocentrically, they would be expected to look at window X (see Acredolo, 1978). Using this measure, Acredolo (1978) tested 24 infants longitudinally at age 6, 11, and 16 months, showing clear age-related differences in

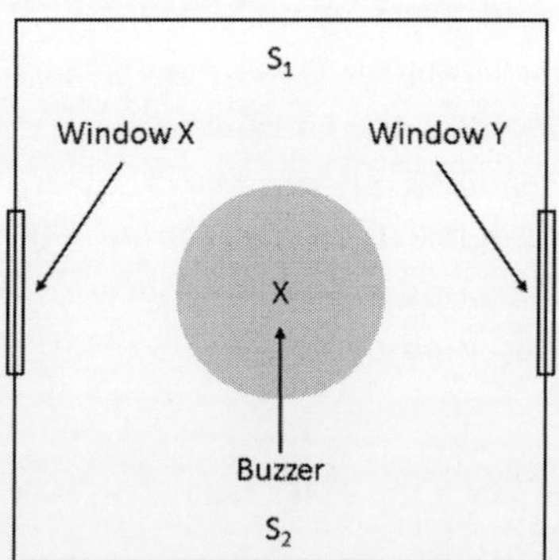

Figure 9.6 The infant reorientation experiment used by Acredolo (1978). S_1 and S_2 mark the infants' location during the training and test phase, respectively. *Reproduced from Acredolo, L. P. (1978). Development of spatial orientation in infancy.* Developmental Psychology, *14, 224–234. Reprinted with permission from the American Psychological Association.*

performance: whereas only 8% of 6-month-olds responded nonegocentrically, this was the case for 33% of 11-month-olds, and 75% of 16-month-olds (the difference between 6 and 16, and 11 and 16 months was significant, the difference between 6 and 11 months was not). In a follow-up study using the same experimental setup, Acredolo and Evans (1980) studied the effect of landmarks and landmark salience on test performance in 6-, 9-, and 11-month-old infants. In a condition with no landmark, the large majority of infants in all age groups responded egocentrically, as in the study by Acredolo (1978). However, infants greatly benefited from the introduction of a salient landmark close to the goal location (ie, a beacon). Whereas a large percentage of the 9- and 11-month-olds responded correctly in this condition, 6-month-olds gave a much more mixed pattern of results, and were seemingly undecided about which information to use.

One point of critique that has been raised in response to these findings is that there is an alternative likely explanation for the results: the role of motor habit formation (see, eg, the discussion by various experts in Acredolo's book chapter, 1990). As evidenced by the many studies on the A-not-B task, young infants tend to form strong motor habits when they are asked to repeat a specific action (ie, reach to the A location) multiple times and this habit is hard to overcome. In the Acredolo studies, infants were trained to look toward window X (say X is on their left hand side) multiple times before they were turned around the table. After rotation, their motor habit would still be to look toward their left—which is where window Y is now located. To test this alternative explanation, Acredolo (1979) repeated her experiment with two bowls on the table in front of the infant. Infants saw how an object was hidden in the bowl on their left, and were then—without establishing any prior motor habit to reach to either bowl—turned around the table. Crucially, infants—aged 9 months—still mostly responded egocentrically, but only in two of three conditions: egocentric responding dominated when infants were tested in a landmark-free laboratory and in a landmark-filled office, but correct responding dominated when infants were tested in the familiar surroundings of their own home. Thus, these findings confirm that very young infants in a lab situation indeed code object locations in relation to their own location, and the effects in the Acredolo (1978) and Acredolo and Evans (1980) studies cannot be explained by an effect of motor habit only. The role of context (home, lab, office) should not be ignored though—given that both the home and the office contained many landmarks in Acredolo's experiment (1979), yet infants' response patterns were very different, suggests that it may be something to do with the familiarity of the home that facilitates performance. As Acredolo (1979) suggests, perhaps infants are more easily oriented in their own home because they know the spatial layout, or familiar objects are more easily used as landmarks than unfamiliar ones.

To summarize, infants in the first year of life seem to have difficulty to reorient themselves in an unfamiliar environment after they have been moved, although they become increasingly able to use salient landmarks. In her review of spatial orientation in infants, Acredolo (1990) nicely summarizes this finding of the use of predominantly egocentric strategies in early infancy as (infants) "behave as if their body is the pivotal center of space" (p. 597). As they grow older, children become increasingly able to use various types of information for navigation. For example, van den Brink and Janzen (2013) presented children aged 30 and 35 months with a virtual reality scene on a screen where a bird was flying and hiding behind one of two identical trees. Once the bird had disappeared, the camera's perspective moved to change perspective by 90 degrees. The movement of the camera followed a path mimicking self-motion. Children then had to indicate where the bird was hiding. In order to do this, children had to maintain their perspective during the movement of the camera. This could be done by using the visual spatial cues provided by the optic flow and the objects present in the scene. However, as children were sitting during the task, they could not use cues generated by their own movement (proprioceptive information). Results showed 35-months-olds were able to use these selective visual cues to find the bird, while 30-months-olds were not yet able to do so. In a different study, Newcombe et al. (1998) showed toddlers aged 16–24 months and 28–34 months how a toy was hidden in a sandbox. Subsequently, they walked around the sandbox and were asked to search. The advantage of the sandbox setup is that it allows very fine calibration of children's errors, as performance can be coded in terms of the distance between the search location and the hiding location, rather than as a cruder pass/fail score. Newcombe and colleagues found that the introduction of distal landmarks improved search performance compared to a condition in which no such landmarks were present in children aged 22 months and older, but not in younger children. Subsequent studies, using a range of different methods, such as the use of touch screens, real mazes, and virtual reality tasks, have confirmed that with increasing age, children become increasingly skilled at using landmarks (Bullens, Iglói, Berthoz, Postma, & Rondi-Reig,

2010; Sutton, 2006; Van Hoogmoed, van den Brink, & Janzen, under review). However, this does not imply that a stage-like developmental shift occurs in the use of allocentric over egocentric reference frames. Rather, as Nardini, Burgess, Breckenridge, and Atkinson (2006) found, the use of egocentric and nonegocentric reference frames may operate in parallel already from 3 years of age onward, as has also been found in adults (Nadel & Hardt, 2004; Wang & Spelke, 2002).

Motor development and exploration in relation to spatial orientation and navigation. Having addressed a number of measures that have frequently been used to assess spatial exploration and navigation in infancy and childhood, and developmental improvements in performance on these measures, we next turn to the question if and how motor development and exploration relate to improvements in spatial orientation and navigations skills in child development. To address this question, Acredolo, Adams, and Goodwyn (1984) investigated how self-locomotion and visual tracking during locomotion play a role in performance on a search task in 12- and 18-month-old infants. In their search task, infants were shown how a toy was hidden in one of two wells. From the infants' position, the toy could not be reached directly. Instead, infants had to move around the display to the opposite end before they could retrieve the toy. If infants relied on a purely egocentric reference system, they would not be able to find the toy in the correct well. Experimental manipulations involved asking infants to move around the display themselves, asking the parent to carry them around, and obscuring the view of the hiding wells from the side of the display, which infants passed during movement. Results showed a clear effect of condition: 12-month-olds who were carried around the display made more errors than those who moved around it themselves. This effect seemed largely due to infants' visual tracking of the toys' location during movement, which occurred much more when infants moved around the display themselves than when they were carried. When the clear sidewalls of the display were replaced with opaque ones, so that visual tracking was no longer possible, self-locomoting around the display no longer resulted in improved performance in the 12-month-olds. Interestingly, when the same infants were 18 months of age, the effect of experimental condition on performance disappeared; almost all infants of this age were able to perform the task well, irrespective of the way they moved around the display or the opportunities they had for visual tracking. Van den Brink and Janzen (2013) also demonstrated the link between exploration and spatial skill. They measured toddlers' skill to maintain orientation while perspective changes (using a paradigm described earlier) and found that toddlers who were more independent in their daily functioning performed this task better. They hypothesized that toddlers who are more independent have more opportunities for spatial exploration than their peers who are more dependent on their caretakers.

In another study, Hazen (1982) investigated both the role of quantity and mode of exploration in relation to toddlers' ability to navigate through a playhouse. She concluded that it is the mode of exploration that matters for spatial knowledge, rather than quantity of exploration. The mode of exploration was coded as the degree to which children actively (ie, they traveled along their own path) or passively (ie, they were carried by their parents, or parents led them along a certain route) explored the playhouse. These findings match well with those of Acredolo et al. (1984) in showing that locomotion and exploration are important factors in children's navigation, particularly so if the child is an active agent. Visual tracking, elicited when children self-locomote through the environment, seems to be a key factor explaining these effects. Foreman, Foreman, Cummings, and Owens (1990) found a similar effect with 4- to 6-year-olds who either were being pushed around a maze in a wheelchair or had the opportunity to walk around and actively explore the maze themselves during a training phase. In the subsequent test phase, the latter group outperformed the former at finding hidden sweets in the maze.

If self-locomotion, as opposed to passive locomotion, is such a crucial factor in spatial memory, does the experience infants have with self-locomotion matter for their performance on spatial memory tasks? The evidence indeed suggests that this is the case. Clearfield (2004) studied 8-, 12-, and 14-month-old infants' search behavior in an octagonal arena with a number of landmarks. After a number of training trials, infants' mothers were asked to hide behind one of the sidewalls, while infants were carried to another sidewall by the experimenter. Subsequently, infants were encouraged to find their mothers by moving toward them. Performance was studied in relation to the number of weeks of experience children had with crawling and walking, showing strikingly similar results: number of weeks of crawling and walking experience was positively related to task performance. The effect of crawling may be taken to mean that it is infants' first experience with self-locomotion that propels spatial memory, but the fact that a similar effect was observed for walking suggests that something more is going on: all walking infants in this study were expert crawlers and had many weeks of crawling experience. Thus, the key message from this study is that what infants learn apparently does not (or at least not fully) transfer between crawling and walking (see also Adolph, 1997). Clearfield (2004) concluded "This implies that infants' behaviors in this task may be due to the soft assembly of available perceptual inputs, memory for the spatial location, and locomotor skill" (p. 231). Her explanation comes remarkably close to Thelen and Smith's account of infant performance on the A-not-B task described at the outset of this chapter: performance comes about through the interaction between child and environment, and any larger or smaller change may drastically alter task performance.[1] In the case of Clearfield's experiment, the fact that novice walkers performed relatively poorly, despite their extensive experience with crawling, may be explained because walking still requires much attention in novices, which reduces cognitive capacity available for spatial memory. Sarah Berger (2010) tested this assumption directly in a large version of the A-not-B task in which 13-month-old infants were required to move toward their parent on the end of one of two walkways. After having moved through one of the paths a few times toward the A location, the parent moved to the other, B, location. In one of the experimental conditions, two tunnels replaced the two paths that children could take. In this demanding tunnel condition, for walking infants, the extent to which children made perseverative errors was negatively related to walking experience. This study confirms that, indeed, there is a cognition–action trade-off which can impact memory and inhibition performance in infants (Berger, 2010): when the motor demands of a task are high, novice walkers struggle because their attention is largely consumed by the effort needed to just keep walking, thereby reducing task performance.

To conclude, there is substantial evidence to suggest that motor development, in particular experience with self-locomotion, is tied to spatial memory, the use of landmarks, and navigation (see also Campos et al., 2000, for a review on this topic). In particular, children's self-locomotion through an environment aids navigation because of enhanced visual scanning during self-locomotion compared to passive locomotion (ie, when the child is carried). Further, the more experience children have with a particular form of self-locomotion, such as crawling or walking, the more skilled they become,

[1] Note that Thelen and Smith (1996) also use the term "soft assembly" to describe the dynamics of developing cognitive function.

leaving more attentional resources available for spatial memory. In this account, advances in gross motor skill in fact interfere with spatial memory, leaving open the question as to whether motor development may be *driving* advances in spatial memory. To address this question, we turn to the literature on spatial memory in stationary tasks next. Again, we describe a number of frequently used methods in this field first, as well as developmental changes in performance, before turning to the question as to how spatial memory during such stationary tasks relates to motor development and exploration.

9.5 SPATIAL MEMORY IN STATIONARY TASKS

Assessment and developmental change. One of the most influential tasks in the cognitive developmental literature which taxes children's memory for object location, among other factors, is the A-not-B task described previously (see section 9.1). Although the A-not-B task has most often been used with infants, older children still make the A-not-B error under specific task conditions. Schutte, Spencer, and Schöner (2003) presented 2-, 4-, and 6-year-olds with a sandbox version of the A-not-B task. The sandbox task requires very fine spatial precision, because no direct cues to the objects' location are available as in the typical infant version with separate hiding wells. A clear pattern of results emerged in which age effects interacted with the distance between the A and B location: at a large distance, only 2- and 4-year-olds' responses drifted toward the A location on B trials, and 6-year-olds did not make the A-not-B error. At a very small distance between the A and B location, however, 6-year-olds also made the A-not-B error. This study thus shows that the A-not-B error and its underlying processes are not confined to infancy, and the coding of object locations in spatial memory becomes increasingly precise as children grow older (Schutte et al., 2003).

Another paradigm that has been used to assess spatial memory in children is the memory for location task. In this task, children are asked to remember at which of several hiding locations a toy is hidden. For example, Pelphrey and colleagues (2004) studied 5.5–12.5-month-old-infants' memory for location in relation to the length of delay between hide and search (range 2–10 seconds) and the number of hiding locations (range two to four). Linear age-related improvements in the ability to cope with delay were observed across the age range studied, while improvements in the number of to-be-remembered locations increased from 8 months onward. In addition to studying the effects of the length of delay and the number of hiding locations present, the number of locations that children can hold in memory simultaneously has also been of interest. Alloway, Gathercole, and Pickering (2006) investigated the development of memory for location using a Dot Matrix task as part of a larger working memory assessment in children aged 4–11 years of age. Children were shown a four by four grid on the computer screen in which a red dot appeared in 1 of the 16 spaces on the grid, and the sequence of to-be-remembered locations increased as children progressed through the task, showing clear age-related improvements across the age range tested. Thus, with increasing age, children learn to retain an increasing number of locations in short-term memory, and to remember this information over increasingly longer delays and with increasing spatial precision. We next turn to the key question addressed in this chapter: how are self-locomotion, exploration, and spatial memory linked in development?

Self-locomotion, exploration, and spatial memory performance in stationary tasks. Campos and colleagues (2000) conducted a review of studies investigating the relation between motor development and A-not-B task performance in infants. Across a number of studies conducted in the 1980s, and across multiple cultures, they conclude that indeed self-locomotion is linked to advances on A-not-B task performance (see, eg, Horobin & Acredolo, 1986). A recurrent debate concerning these findings entails the question as to whether self-locomotion and advances in spatial memory are causally linked in development, or whether this association is due to a shared general developmental factor. In the latter case, children who are ahead of their peers in one developmental domain (such as the development of gross motor skills, including self-locomotion) are ahead of their peers in other domains (such as spatial memory) too, just because they are quick to develop in general. To disentangle these two alternative explanations, Kermoian and Campos (1988) divided a sample of 8.5-month-old infants into three groups: infants with no self-locomotion experience, infants with no self-locomotion experience except for walker-assisted experience, and infants with crawling experience. If the association between self-locomotion onset and spatial cognition was due to a general maturational factor, the walker-assisted group would have to cluster with the groups of infants without self-locomotion experience (ie, walker-assistance can be seen as an artificial aid unrelated to the child's developmental level). The contrary was true: the children in the walker-assisted group performed at a similar level as the children who could crawl, and both groups scored significantly better than the infants without self-locomotion experience. Thus, self-locomotion indeed seems to facilitate

A-not-B task performance. Campos and colleagues (2000) provide four potential explanations for this association: (1) infants learn to shift from using an egocentric to allocentric reference frame through experience with self-locomotion, (2) self-locomotion experience improves attentional discrimination, (3) self-locomotion experience improves goal-directed behavior and tolerance of increasing delays, and (4) self-locomotion experience improves the use of social cues. Indeed, a study by Horobin and Acredolo (1986) showed that infant attentiveness toward the correct location in the A-not-B task was predictive of task performance, and self-locomotion experience was related to better task performance and higher attentiveness. To more fully unravel if, and if so, how, infant self-locomotion changes children's interaction with the world around them, recent studies have used novel techniques to capture what infants are seeing *as they are moving*, showing that different modes of locomotion (crawling vs walking) allow children to interact with objects and people differently (eg, Clearfield, 2011; Karasik et al., 2011; Kretch et al., 2014). For a discussion of these techniques and related findings, see Box 9.1.

Whereas the finding that self-locomotion and spatial memory are linked in infancy is well established, much less research has been devoted to addressing this question in older children. There is some evidence to suggest that not so much self-locomotion, but exploration in infancy, is still linked to spatial memory later in childhood. Oudgenoeg-Paz, Leseman, and Volman (2014) studied infant self-locomotion milestone achievement and spatial exploration during the first 2 years of life in relation to spatial memory, as assessed with the Dot Matrix task at 4 and 6 years of age. Infant self-locomotion milestone achievement was related to spatial exploration, but not to spatial memory. However, spatial exploration in infancy was related to spatial memory in childhood. These findings, taken together with those from infant studies (Campos et al., 2000; Horobin & Acredolo, 1986; Kermoian & Campos, 1988; van den Brink & Janzen, 2013), suggest that the influence of self-locomotion on spatial memory may weaken as the time interval between achievement of self-locomotion milestones and the assessment of spatial memory skill increases. This may not be surprising given the fact that interindividual differences in self-locomotion milestone achievement are typically only a few months, while the time interval in the study by Oudgenoeg-Paz et al. was a few years. Yet, the extent to which children are engaged in spatial exploration in infancy, which adds up to a great number of hours over time, does have a more stable relation with spatial memory later in childhood. Further studies are needed to unravel how motor development, exploration, and spatial memory are related beyond infancy.

This is also important for research on spatial cognition in clinical groups, such as ASD (Box 9.2), CP (Box 9.3) and NLD (Box 9.4).

BOX 9.2 Spatial Cognition in ASD

ASD is characterized by deficits in social communication and interaction, and restricted, repetitive patterns of behavior, interests, or activities (APA, 2013). However, as suggested by the term *pervasive* developmental disorder, ASD is more than the diagnostic criteria described above. It has been associated with delays, deficits, and strengths, across the whole range of developmental domains, including motor development, perception, play, language, and spatial cognition (Volkmar, Lord, Bailey, Schultz, & Klin, 2004; Yirmiya & Charman, 2010).

ASD has been associated with both strengths and weaknesses in spatial cognition (Edgin & Pennington, 2005; Mùth, Hönekopp, & Falter, 2014). A meta-analysis, that included studies with both children and adults with ASD, demonstrated superior performance of children and adults with ASD compared to a typically developing group on the Embedded Figures Test (EFT) and Block Design Test (BDT; Mùth et al., 2014). In the EFT, participants are presented with cards depicting images made up of lines with embedded geometrical shapes, such as triangles or rectangles. A target shape is presented, which the participant is asked to locate as quickly as possible in the image (Mùth et al., 2014). In the BDT, participants are asked to use blocks to recreate a two-dimensional pattern that the participant is presented with on a card (Mùth et al., 2014). While superiority for the ASD group was found, effect size was small and there was a large amount of heterogeneity (Mùth et al., 2014).

Regarding spatial memory in ASD, results are also inconsistent. One study found that high-functioning adolescents with ASD made more errors than a matched group of typically developing controls on the CANTAB (Cambridge Neuropsychological Test Automated Battery) spatial working memory task, and were less likely to consistently use a specific organized search strategy to complete the task (Steele, Minshew, Lun, & Sweeney, 2007). The CANTAB task requires participants to find targets hidden in an array of boxes on a computer screen by using a touch screen to search the boxes. The task increases in difficulty from three to eight targets. To complete the task successfully, the participant must remember the spatial locations where the target has been

(*Continued*)

BOX 9.2 Spatial Cognition in ASD—cont'd

found previously, update this information as new targets are found, and inhibit incorrect responses (Edgin & Pennington, 2005). Other studies, using the same task, did not find differences between children with ASD and a matched control group in spatial working memory (Edgin & Pennington, 2005). Moreover, no differences were found when comparing 3- to 4-year-old children with ASD and a matched typically developing control group on the A-not-B task (Dawson et al., 2002; Yerys, Hepburn, Pennington, & Rogers, 2007), which also measures visuospatial working memory.

Also for another visuospatial ability, mental rotation, no clear differences in accuracy are found between the children and adults with ASD and typically developing controls (Falter, Plaisted, & Davis, 2008; Mùth et al., 2014). However, with regard to response times in mental rotation, some studies report faster processing for individuals with ASD (Falter et al., 2008), while other studies demonstrate slower processing for the ASD group (Pearson, Marsh, Hamilton, & Ropar, 2014). These differences in results have been attributed to the type of processing strategy used. Two different strategies can be used for mental rotation. In a configural processing strategy a person will use the entire object and transform it through mental rotation (performing a holistic rotation), while in a feature-based strategy, a person will try to verify the identity and location of a key feature of an object and match it with a target (Pearson et al., 2014). When adults with ASD use a local feature-based processing strategy, they are faster than typically developing participants, and when they use a configural processing strategy, they are slower (Pearson et al., 2014). The type of processing strategy may be dependent on the familiarity of the stimuli with participants with ASD using a feature-based strategy with novel stimuli and a configural processing strategy with familiar stimuli (Behrmann et al., 2006; Mùth et al., 2014).

With regard to spatial navigation, results regarding ASD are dependent upon the kind of navigation tested. Route-based navigation relies on gradually learned, inflexible, egocentric representations of specific sequences of landmarks, junctions, and so forth. This is the type of strategy that we typically rely on when following familiar routes. Routes are easily disrupted if a landmark or other information is removed. On the other hand, survey-based navigation relies on flexible, allocentric representations, or "cognitive maps" of the layout of the environment This is the type of strategy that people use when familiar route following is not possible (Lind, Williams, Raber, Peel, & Bowler, 2013). Adolescents and adults with ASD show typical performance on tasks, which only require route-based navigation (Caron, Mottron, Rainville, & Chouinard,

(*Continued*)

BOX 9.2 Spatial Cognition in ASD—cont'd

2004), but have impaired survey-based navigation skills (Lind et al., 2013). This may also explain why both children and adults with ASD insist on always taking familiar routes and feel stressed and anxious when they have to deviate from a familiar route (Lind et al., 2013).

Theories Explaining Spatial Cognition in ASD

Several theories attempt to explain spatial cognition in ASD, namely the Weak Central Coherence account (Happé & Frith, 2006), the Enhanced Perceptual Functioning theory (Mottron, Dawson, Soulières, Hubert & Burack, 2006), the Extreme Male Brain theory (Baron-Cohen, 2002), and the Executive Dysfunction Hypothesis (Ozonoff, Pennington, & Rogers, 1991). Both the Weak Central Coherence account and Enhanced Perceptual Functioning theory assume that individuals with ASD have a bias toward local processing as opposed to the global processing tendency that typically developing individuals display (Happé & Frith, 2006; Mottron et al., 2006). Both of these theories predict superior performance for the EFT and the BDT, which is consistent with empirical findings (Mùth et al., 2014). The Extreme Male Brain theory assumes that individuals with ASD represent extreme cases of the normal male (brain) profile (Baron-Cohen, 2002). One prediction from this theory would be that the ASD group performs better on the mental rotation task, because studies have shown that males perform better than females (Falter et al., 2008). However, no superiority regarding accuracy was found for the ASD group (Falter et al., 2008; Mùth et al., 2014). Regarding spatial navigation, the Extreme Male Brain theory would also predict superior performance for individuals with ASD. Results however indicate that ASD are impaired in spatial navigation when survey-based navigation skills are needed (Lind et al., 2013) and that they perform typical with route-based navigation (Caron et al., 2004). The Executive Dysfunction theory assumes that individuals with ASD are impaired in executive functions, such as planning, working memory, flexibility, and inhibition (Hill, 2004; Ozonoff et al., 1991). This theory predicts impairments on a number of visuospatial abilities, but specifically on spatial working memory tasks. Empirical findings regarding spatial working memory in ASD are inconsistent, with some studies reporting impairments (Steele et al., 2007) and other studies demonstrating intact spatial working memory in ASD (Edgin & Pennington, 2005).

(*Continued*)

BOX 9.2 Spatial Cognition in ASD—cont'd

Spatial Cognition in ASD: An Embodied Dynamic Systems Perspective

Although these four theories provide interesting and plausible explanations for spatial cognition in ASD, none of these theories is able to explain all research results and corresponding inconsistencies. Moreover, a shortcoming of these theories is that they assume a rather static impairment without taking development and the role of developmental cascades across domains into account (López, 2015; Paterson, Brown, Gsödl, Johnson, & Karmiloff-Smith, 1999). As explained in this chapter, according to an embodied dynamic systems perspective, spatial cognition emerges from the interaction of a child and its environment, and the development of spatial cognition is influenced by other skills and processes, including motor skills, exploration, perceptual skills and social skills. Various studies have demonstrated that, in addition to the diagnostic criteria for ASD, such as social-communicative impairments, delays and deficits in fine, and gross motor skills are present in young children with ASD or at risk for ASD across all ages and levels of functioning (Bhat, Landa, & Galloway, 2011; Fournier, Hass, Naik, Lodha, & Cauraugh, 2010; Gernsbacher, Sauer, Geye, Schweigert, & Goldsmith, 2008; Landa & Garret-Mayer, 2006). Children with ASD are also different in their exploratory behavior. They display more rotating, spinning, and unusual visual exploration, and stereotyped, repetitive, and restricted uses of objects (Baranek, 1999; Bruckner & Yoder, 2007; Ozonoff et al., 2008; Wetherby et al., 2004; Williams, Costall, & Reddy, 1999), and spend less time in exploration (Koterba, Leezenbaum, & Iverson, 2012; Pierce & Courchesne, 2001) than children with developmental delays and typically developing children. Studies indicate that both motor skills and exploratory behavior are related to the development of visuospatial cognition in ASD (Hellendoorn et al., 2015), that joint engagement (shared attention) with an adult (experimenter and parents) is related to visuospatial abilities in children with ASD (Carpenter, Pennington, & Rogers, 2002), and that motor demands in a task influence the speed of information processing in ASD, that is, when a task demands a lot of motor output (action) this interferes with the ability to process information in children with ASD (Kenworthy, Yerys, Weinblatt, Abrams, & Wallace, 2013). These studies demonstrate that spatial skills are influenced by other skills and processes.

Spatial cognition in turn also influences other skills in ASD. Visuospatial information processing is, for instance, related to motor coordination deficits (Salowitz et al., 2013). Since ASD is best known for the deficits in social communication and interaction, it is also interesting to examine the relationship between spatial cognition skills and social skills. Some researchers suggest that spatial

(*Continued*)

BOX 9.2 Spatial Cognition in ASD—cont'd

perspective taking is related to social skills since spatial perspective taking is necessary to perceive the affordances (the action possibilities) for others (Creem-Regehr, Gagnon, Geuss, & Stefanucci, 2013). In this way spatial perspective taking allows humans to make predictions about what another person is likely to do next. This ability to predict another's behavior enables a person to adjust his or her own actions to the behavior of their interaction partner (Creem-Regehr et al., 2013). Studies also indicate that spatial cognition is related to gaze-following (Lind et al., 2013; Trafton & Harrison, 2011). Other researchers also believe that visual perspective taking, the ability to see the world (literally) from another person's perspective, is related to the social skill of seeing another person's perspective (Pearson, Ropar, & Hamilton, 2013). If this is the case then it is expected that children with ASD not only do display social difficulties, but are also impaired in visual perspective taking. Some studies indeed indicate that children with ASD have difficulties with visual perspective taking tasks (Pearson et al., 2013). In addition, studies demonstrate that a more detail-focused processing style (ie, faster disembedding on EFT and strength in BDT) is related to more social impairments (Jarrold, Butler, Cottington, & Jimenez, 2000; Pellicano, Maybery, Durkin, & Maley, 2006) and more impaired, autism-like play (Kuschner & Bennetto, 2007) in individuals with ASD.

In conclusion, results regarding spatial cognition in ASD are inconsistent. In order to understand the development of spatial cognition in ASD, it is necessary to take into account the fact that individuals with ASD interact in a different way with their physical and social environment and to consider interrelationships across developmental domains that are present in ASD. Taking this into account may also help to explain the large heterogeneity (the interindividual variability), the occurrence of developmental regression, the inconsistency in findings and the intraindividual variability that are reported in many studies for individuals with ASD (Dinstein et al., 2012; Mùth et al., 2014; Rogers, 2004). From a dynamic systems embodied cognition account, these phenomena can be explained as emerging from minor and major changes in the individual or the environment (and the interaction between them), and from the interrelationships between developmental domains that continuously interact with each other in individuals with ASD. These phenomena are hard to explain from the aforementioned theories that explain ASD since these theories assume a static cognitive impairment as explanation for ASD and for the differences between individuals with and without ASD in spatial cognition.

BOX 9.3 Navigating "Near" and "Further" Space in Children With Cerebral Palsy

Cerebral Palsy

CP is the most common motor disability among children (Cans, 2000). CP is the general term for "a group of disorders of the development of movement and posture, causing activity limitations, which are attributed to non-progressive disturbances that occurred in the developing fetal or infant brain. The motor disorders of CP are often accompanied by disturbances of sensation, perception, cognition, communication, and behavior, by epilepsy, and by secondary musculoskeletal problems" (Rosenbaum et al., 2007, p. 9). CP can have multiple causes, which can occur in the prenatal or perinatal period, or postnatal during the first year of life. The heterogeneous nature of CP means that the population of children with CP is characterized by much variation.

According to the Surveillance of Cerebral Palsy in Europe (SCPE) guidelines (Cans, 2000), the subtypes of CP in terms of the motor disorder can be classified into three subtypes: spastic, dyskinetic, and ataxic CP. Mixed presentations also occur, in which case the dominant subtype of the presentation determines the classification. The spastic subtype of CP can be subclassified, based on anatomical distribution, into unilateral, when one side of the body is affected (often referred to as hemiplegia), and bilateral, when both sides of the body are affected (often referred to as diplegia when the legs are most affected). The most common subtype of CP is spastic CP, as around 80% of the persons with CP are classified in the spastic subtype.

CP and Spatial Cognition: Evolution of Studies From "Near" to "Further" Space

It is generally agreed upon that limitations in movement might contribute to limitations in spatial cognition among children with CP. In fact, this idea is not new. An exemplary review by Abercrombie (1964) at a time when research interest in studying consequences of CP was thriving, showed a large number of difficulties including shape copying and assembling simple jigsaw puzzles. For many years, research remained focused on unraveling and explaining performance on manual tasks challenging children with CP to move their hands and arms through a rather restricted part of space, that is, close to the child's body. A recent example of such a study showed (again) that visual navigation in this "near" space is compromised in children with CP. Adolescents (aged between 13 and 16 years; verbal IQ within the normal range) born premature (27–33 weeks of gestation) with periventricular leukomalacia, of whom 8 out of 11 were classified as bilateral spastic CP, performed more poorly on a paper-and-pencil labyrinth test compared to premature-born adolescents without brain lesions and term-born adolescents (Pavlova, Sokolov, & Krageloh-Mann, 2007). In line with

(*Continued*)

BOX 9.3 Navigating "Near" and "Further" Space in Children With Cerebral Palsy—cont'd

other studies, navigation ability on this task in "near" space was specifically linked to (frontal) lesions in the right hemisphere.

It is only by the end of the 1980s, more than 20 years on from Abercrombie's review, that studies emerged investigating the ability of children with CP to make judgments and perform actual movements in "further" space, shifting the focus more toward the role of locomotion in spatial cognition abilities. Children were asked to judge from a distance whether they were able to move through apertures (eg, curtains which could be drawn), including sometimes locomotion conditions in which children actively navigated through space (eg, Howard & Henderson, 1989; Savelsbergh, Douwes Dekker, Vermeer, & Hopkins, 1998). As such, space literally opened up for other paradigms to be studied. It was shown that typically developing children (matched for age and intellectual ability to the children with CP) outperformed the children with CP when judging the size of an aperture in relation to their own body dimensions. In addition, children suffering from dyskinetic CP performed better than children with the spastic subtype of CP in judging whether they would be able to move through apertures of varying widths and heights (Howard & Henderson, 1989). The most plausible explanation (at that time when MRI scans were not yet routinely performed) being the underlying type of brain damage suffered by children with spastic CP more likely to encompass areas that serve perceptual functions.

On a similar task, except for the addition of a condition in which children actually had to move through the aperture, it was found that when performances in passing through apertures (measured at two occasions 12 months apart in two age groups: 5–8 years old and 9–13 years old) were adjusted for differences in body width, children with CP who could stand and walk unaided (CP-Walk), children with CP who were confined to a wheelchair (CP-Wheel), and nondisabled children, irrespective of age, had similar outcomes: all children were able to match their body width with the aperture width when locomoting toward and through the apertures (Savelsbergh, Douwes Dekker, Vermeer & Hopkins, 1998). There was one exception, namely the younger group of ambulant children with CP (CP-Walk; 5–8 years old): they made the largest overestimations of aperture width relative to body width while judging the aperture from a distance, but did not differ from the other groups in using body-scaled information to actually pass through the opening. The authors suggested that control of locomotion (ie, a standing position with more variability in sway vs a relatively more stable body position while sitting in a wheelchair) might be one plausible explanation for this finding. Likewise, the

(*Continued*)

BOX 9.3 Navigating "Near" and "Further" Space in Children With Cerebral Palsy—cont'd

improved accuracy in older children may suggest an influence of extended experience.

Navigating Streets and (Magic) Carpets

Imagine the following: a busy street, cars parked on both sides, no pedestrian crossing nearby. This is a familiar scene for many children walking to, or on their way home from, school. A quite challenging task, because it requires the child to position himself in such a way as to oversee the situation given the stationary obstacles (parked cars), to accurately estimate the time of arrival of moving obstacles (oncoming traffic) and at the same time relate this information to his own body speed both in the initial phase while standing still on the pavement and during the actual dynamic crossing moments. This is a demanding situation for any child, but what if a child with CP who is independently mobile wants to cross the street (te Velde, Savelsbergh, Barela, & van der Kamp, 2003)? Are children with unilateral spastic CP (excluding those with moderate to severe intellectual disability) just as accurate as their nondisabled peers in judging whether it is safe enough to cross? Given a simplified laboratory setting (low-speed traffic, a bicycle, approaching from one direction) and compared at a group level ($n = 10$ in each group; age range 4–14 years) they were just as accurate, irrespective of whether they started from a standing condition or a locomoting position (ie, already in motion on the pavement). However, within-group differences among children with unilateral spastic CP showed greater variability than among nondisabled peers. Children with right hemisphere lesions were more inconsistent (ie, they sometimes crossed the street while there was no sufficient time to do so safely or lingered on the pavement when they could have safely crossed) in their behavior compared to children with left hemisphere lesions. In order to explain this, the authors refer to the presumed egocentric (position of objects relative to the observer) processing of visual information of the right hemisphere (Postma, Sterken, de Vries, & de Haan, 2000) and the assumption that spatial information processed through the right hemisphere is used to guide movements (Kosslyn, 1991). While in need of replication given the small sample size, extending the design to a more real-life situation (ie, high-speed traffic approaching from two directions) and to a more diverse group of children with CP, the authors argued that these results highlight the need for discriminating between different subtypes of CP when studying spatiotemporal tasks (te Velde et al., 2003). In other words, brain damage in itself does not explain all the variance in individual differences between children in their ability to navigate through space, an assumption which can sometimes still be (implicitly) detected in the literature.

(*Continued*)

BOX 9.3 Navigating "Near" and "Further" Space in Children With Cerebral Palsy—cont'd

Moving on from streets to carpets. Starting from the point that "near" space (ie, space in which children can reach such as the manual tasks described before) and "further" space (ie, navigational space in which to walk/wheel around) involve different cognitive strategies and brain networks, children with spastic CP independently walking without aids (5–12 years of age) were compared to a sample of typically developing children matched and unmatched for age and sex on two tasks (Belmonti, Fiori, Guzzetta, Cioni, & Berthoz, 2015). The first task was the classic Corsi Block-tapping Task (CBT). The second task was an adapted version of the CBT, called the Magic Carpet, in which the children were required to walk (ie, using real body motion) on tiles laid out on the floor using the same short-term memory assessment procedure as with the CBT (ie, reproducing a sequence of blocks as pointed out by an experimenter, or walking over the tiles that light up one after the other automatically). It appeared that spatial memory in children with CP was more impaired on the "near" (ie, reaching) space than the "further" (ie, navigational) space task. Three explanations were provided: (1) more complex tasks (ie, the Magic Carpet) involve more factors, but also more possible mechanisms for compensation; (2) egocentric reference frames that are mainly used in reaching space are particularly impaired in children with CP; and (3) (simply) the larger stimuli used in the Magic Carpet are better perceived and stored by children with visual deficits. As in other studies (eg, Pavlova et al., 2007) performance on both the CBT and Magic Carpet were related to global right hemisphere impairment indicating a general association with spatial functions.

In conclusion, many children continue to suffer from CP. Therefore, the question of what the possible consequences for navigating space are of motor disabilities that delay the acquisition of independent locomotion or impair the quality of locomotion once it is acquired remains topical (Anderson et al., 2013). Unfortunately (but not surprisingly), no definite answer(s) can be given since this is a complex field of investigation which few studies have yet embarked upon. Moreover, as Anderson and colleagues argue, the major problem is separating the role of brain damage from that of mobility impairment when studying deficits in children with CP. As brain damage is often the cause of the primary motor impairments, that same damage is evidently implicated in any cooccuring spatial-cognitive deficits. Having said that, most studies among children with CP "suffer" from the fact that the level of explanation for deficits (still) mainly focuses on the presence, extent and type of brain lesions despite growing evidence that experience in locomotion and exploration does matter when examining individual children's performances. Nevertheless, quality and experience of locomotion and exploration experience are until now

(*Continued*)

BOX 9.3 Navigating "Near" and "Further" Space in Children With Cerebral Palsy—cont'd

largely ignored, which potentially might harm the rise of new intervention strategies. As such, maybe the time has come to introduce new paradigms and tests for studying and, eventually, remediating spatial deficits in children with CP (Berthoz & Zaoui, 2015), such as the "locomotor trajectory" paradigm in which the shift from "near" to "further" space is seen as necessary in order to effectively deal with, and make use of, the demands of the environment.

BOX 9.4 Nonverbal Learning Disability

Nonverbal learning disability (NLD) is the term used to describe people who have normal or even high verbal skills but show weak skills in nonverbal domains, especially in the visuospatial domain. This disability has been of interest to researchers and clinicians since it was described in 1967 by Johnson and Mykelbust and later extensively studied by Rourke (for a review see Mammarella & Cornoldi, 2014; Spreen, 2011). Despite extensive research, the diagnostic criteria of NLD as well as its prevalence are still unclear. Moreover, the symptoms of NLD often resemble that of other disabilities such as Asperger's syndrome (Semrud-Clikeman, Goldenring Fine, & Bledsoe, 2014; Spreen, 2011). Mammarella and Cornoldi (2014) analyzed 35 studies on children with NLD and concluded that the factor that distinguishes children with NLD most from typically developing children (ie, effect sizes reported are the largest) is visuospatial intelligence. Other factors are: discrepancy between verbal and nonverbal intelligence, poor visuoconstructive and fine-motor skills, discrepancy between reading achievement and mathematical achievement. In the last group with smaller effect sizes, but still significant differences they list visuospatial memory and socioemotional skills. Based on this analysis, Mammarella and Cornoldi suggested five criteria for diagnosing NLD. The first criterion has to be met and at least two out of criteria 2–4 also have to be met. The fifth criterion is possibly an associated criterion. The five criteria are:

1. Poor visuospatial intelligence with a relatively good verbal intelligence;
2. Visuoconstructive and fine-motor impairments;
3. Poor mathematical achievement at school with relatively good reading decoding skills;
4. Spatial working memory deficits;
5. Emotional and social difficulties.

(*Continued*)

BOX 9.4 Nonverbal Learning Disability—cont'd

While only one of these criteria concerns academic achievement, this disability can have profound effects on the performance of children in school, as performance in many subjects requires visuospatial and fine-motor skills (Cornoldi, Venneri, Marconato, Molin, & Montinari, 2003).

NLD and Spatial Cognition

Poor spatial skills are one of the main diagnostic criteria for NLD. Multiple studies reveal difficulties for these children in spatial memory. For example, Mammarella, Lucangeli, and Cornoldi (2010) presented 7–11 years old typically developing children and children with symptoms of NLD with a series of tests designed to measure spatial memory, visual memory, and arithmetic skills. The spatial memory tasks involved recalling the location of dots presented in a matrix, lines presented in a matrix, and lightbulbs presented in a circle. The stimuli were presented either sequentially (ie, one dot, line or lightbulb at a time) or simultaneously (ie, all dots, lines or lightbulbs at once). The number of stimuli varied from two to eight. After the presentation, the children saw the stimuli again and had to judge if the locations were the same as what they had seen before. In the visual tasks children saw a series of two to eight nonsense shapes, fish or balloons in different patterns of filling. After the initial presentation of the visual stimuli, children again were presented with the stimuli and asked to judge if the shapes, fish, or balloons were the same as the ones previously presented. Results revealed that children with NLD symptoms performed worse than typically developing children on the spatial tasks but not on the visual tasks. The NLD children, interestingly, were not different on the sequential spatial task involving the lines. Mammarella et al. suggested that this might be because the children focused on the shapes created by the lines rather than on the locations, thus making this more a visual than spatial task. This study suggests that the difficulties experienced by children with NLD are highly specific to the spatial domain. In addition, the children with NLD showed poorer performance on arithmetic tasks involving a spatial component, such as carrying and aligning numbers in columns. This suggests that the difficulty with arithmetic might also be essentially a spatial difficulty.

In another study, Narimoto, Matsuura, Takezawa, Mitsuhashi, and Hiratani (2013) showed 8–11 years old children with NLD, children with verbal comprehension difficulties and typically developing children a stimuli consisting of 3, 5, or 7 green squares at random locations. Following this, a second frame with the same squares was shown and children had to judge if one of the squares (indicated by a red outline) had shifted its location. The task had two conditions, one with a minimal change in location of the target and one with a larger change (maximal change). Results showed that children with NLD performed worse than typically developing children and children with verbal comprehension difficulties

(*Continued*)

BOX 9.4 Nonverbal Learning Disability—cont'd

on the task in the condition with the minimal change in location, but not on the maximal location change. All children performed worse on the maximal change task than on the minimal change task. The authors argued that in order to succeed on the minimal change task, the relation between the individual squares have to be coded rather than their absolute location. This suggests that spatial memory deficits of children with NLD are at least partially related to a difficulty with processing spatial relations between objects.

NLD From an Embodied Cognition Approach

From an embodied cognition perspective, it is interesting that the pattern of difficulties characterizing children with NLD involves fine-motor difficulties. It is possible that due to these motor difficulties, these children explore their environment in a less optimal manner. If they are less able to successfully engage in activities including the manipulation of spatial relations such as building with blocks, stacking cups and doing puzzles, then they have less experience with exploring spatial relations in their environment. This reduced experience, in turn, might mean that their knowledge of spatial concepts is not as well-grounded in sensorimotor real-life experiences as it would be if they had gained more experience with manipulating spatial relations. Studies with typically developing children reviewed in this chapter (eg, Oudgenoeg-Paz et al., 2015) suggest that exploration of spatial relations is an important predictor of future spatial skills, including spatial memory. Therefore, reduced exploration (caused by poor fine-motor skills) seems to be one possible mechanism underlying the development of NLD. However, this is merely a hypothesis which will have to be put to an empirical test in future studies.

9.6 GENERAL DISCUSSION

In the current chapter, we have aimed to provide a review of the literature on the development of spatial cognition in young children from a dynamic systems embodied cognition perspective, in particular focusing on studies that have investigated the link between motor development, exploration, mental rotation, and spatial memory (including memory for object locations, orientation, and navigation). From the dynamic systems embodied cognition theory, the prediction is that motor development, exploration, and advances in spatial cognition are strongly intertwined. In general, the studies reviewed in this chapter provide support for this hypothesis: there is evidence that infant self-locomotion is related to advances in spatial memory and mental rotation, motor processes play a role in mental rotation from infancy through to adulthood, and infant exploration is related to spatial memory even at school age. Yet, the evidence is not as clear as it may seem upon first glance and there are several lines of investigation that need further study.

First of all, a current debate concerns how the role of motor processes in (spatial) cognitive function changes over developmental time (see Needham & Libertus, 2011). Whereas Thelen (2000) argued for an embodied view of cognition throughout the life span, others have suggested that the close ties between our body and actions on the one hand and cognition on the other becomes weaker over developmental time, as we leave the acquisition of some of the largest motor milestones (ie, sitting, crawling, walking) far behind us. To address this issue, Frick, Daum, Walser, and Mast (2009) investigated the role of motor processing in mental rotation in different age groups: 5-, 8-, and 11-year-olds, and adults. Study subjects at each age were given a similar experiment as Wexler and colleagues (1998) used (see section 9.3.1), in which they were asked to perform a manual and mental rotation task at the same time. Frick et al. (2009) found that when the direction of motor action was incompatible with the direction of mental rotation, this negatively influenced performance on the mental rotation task in 5- and 8-year-olds, but not in 11-year-olds and adults. Thus, they conclude that with development, cognitive processing may become increasingly distanced from motor processing. These findings seem to conflict with those of Wexler and colleagues (1998) and Moreau and colleagues (2011) who showed that motor processes and motor skill training were related to mental rotation performance in adults, respectively. Clearly, the changing role of embodiment in cognitive processing over developmental time requires further investigation, but this is no easy enterprise. Comparison across child and adult data is hampered by a number of factors. First, other developmental factors than the one under study may explain age-related differences (such as advances in inhibitory control, which Frick et al. (2009) suggest may contribute to explaining their age-related differences). Second, motor development is on at full speed in infancy; there is no later time when we learn such drastically new ways of moving about. As adults, we do learn new motor skills occasionally, such as ice skating or driving a car, but none of these skills offer such a thoroughly new perspective on the world as infants' first successes in self-locomotion, neither are they typically trained as extensively. As such, a fair comparison of the role of motor processes and experience in spatial cognition between adults and young children is challenging to make, to say the least. However, current evidence shows that even as adults our mental representations and cognitive functions are related to our physical body and actions, suggesting cognition remains embodied as we grow older (see, eg, Price & Harmon-Jones, 2010; Richardson, Spivey, Barsalou, & McRae, 2003).

Final, although the studies described in this chapter seem to fit in with a dynamic systems embodied cognition account of the development of spatial cognition, the evidence is not always conclusive. For example, as described in the section on mental rotation, mental rotation ability was related to the gross motor milestones standing and walking with assistance, but not to crawling in the study by Frick and Möhring (2013). In contrast, Schwarzer and colleagues (2013) reported a positive relation between crawling experience and mental rotation ability in infants of about the same age. Likewise, Campos and colleagues (2000) also describe a number of studies that fail to find support for the relation between self-locomotion and spatial memory in their review. Such discrepancies need not be ignored, and in fact may help further fine-tune the theory about the mechanism through which the development of spatial cognition occurs. In fact, given that each new mode of self-locomotion drastically alters infants' interactions with the world (see Box 9.1), their opportunities for exploration, and the affordances they can discover, the impact of these different modes of self-locomotion on spatial cognition is likely to be at least partly unique. To further put the theory to the test, it seems important to start specifying hypotheses much more precisely—rather than testing the association between a range of motor milestones and spatial cognition, more specific hypotheses could be drawn up based on what is now known about the different ways the attainment of sitting, crawling, and walking influence infants' visual perceptual experience (Kretch et al., 2014). In addition, it is worth considering whether infant self-locomotion may be *unrelated* to particular aspects of cognitive function—if such relations indeed prove to be absent, a "general" underlying developmental factor driving both self-locomotion and spatial cognition becomes a less likely explanation of study results (see also Oudgenoeg-Paz, 2014).

In relation to the latter point, the large majority of studies that report associations between motor development and spatial cognition are correlational in nature (but see Kermoian & Campos, 1988), thus not allowing conclusions about the direction of effects. In particular, infants who acquire the ability for independent locomotion earlier may interact differently with the world around them before the onset of self-locomotion already. Several studies indeed point to such an effect, calling in particular for a role for motivation in learning new actions (von Hofsten, 2004, 2007). For example, Atun-Einy, Berger, and Scher (2013) investigated infants' motivation to move, by assessing infants' persistence to move relative to difficulty, the frequency of position changes, the proportion of time infants spent in motion, the extent to which external simulation was needed to elicit movement, and the infants' preference for high or low energy activities. Infants were assessed each 3 weeks over the course of 5 months, from 7 to 12 months of age. Gross motor milestone achievement was also recorded (sitting, pulling-to-stand, crawling, and cruising). Infants with higher motivation to move at the first session were more likely to reach these milestones earlier than infants with lower motivation to move. In addition, there was evidence for a developmental cascade effect: motivation to move in each session was related to motor skill acquisition in the next session, and the opposite effect was also true. Similarly, Karasik, Tamis-LeMonda, and Adolph (2011) observed that the frequency at which crawling infants at age 11 months engaged with objects which were out of direct reach so that they had to locomote toward them, carried objects, and shared objects with their mother by moving toward her, predicted walking attainment at age 13 months. Thus, it appears that indeed, there is something different about the actions undertaken and the motivation for action in infants who achieve self-locomotion milestones earlier. In sum, through advancing motor development, infants acquire increasingly new means to explore their environment, which ultimately leads to increased understanding about the world. However, although much research has focused on the impact of motor development on exploration and spatial cognition, rather than the other way around, this is not to suggest that these relations are unidirectional. Rather, all aspects of the developing child and its environment can be seen as a clockwork with interlocking components that continuously interact.

A further aspect to consider in the development of spatial cognition is the social context in which behavior occurs. Whereas this chapter has focused on the affordances the physical world has to offer, the role of the social environment in cognition and action cannot be ignored (eg,

Tamis-Lemonda et al., 2008; Topál, Gergely, Miklósi, Erdőheyi, & Csibra, 2008). For example, Topál and colleagues (2008) have shown that infants' performance on the A-not-B task depends partly on the infant picking up social-communicative information from the assessor who hides the toy. In this experimental study, infants perseverated much more often to the A location when the assessor engaged with them in a natural way during each hiding event, than when no such social information was available (ie, the assessor looked away from the infant or was not visible at all). These findings suggest that infants interpret what the assessor is doing as a general principle they are trying to convey ("look, toys like these are hidden here at A!") rather than the idea that an object can be hidden in different locations at different time points. Thus, this study points to the crucial role of the social environment in performance on spatial cognition tasks; yet, few other studies to date have investigated the way children use social information in the area of spatial cognition, for example, when navigating.

To conclude, the studies reviewed in this chapter have shown that young infants already have rudimentary memory for object locations, and are able to orient themselves in the environment after having been moved about. Yet, these abilities further develop over the many childhood years to follow. In the current chapter, we have provided a review of the development of spatial cognition from an embodied dynamic systems view, in which cognitive "representations," such as those required for mental rotation, are embodied and construed from the child's active exploration of and interaction with the environment. Motor development is an important driving force in the opportunities children have for exploration (Gibson, 1988), yet the studies on children with physical handicaps show that motor development is not a necessary prerequisite for advances in spatial cognitive development (see Box 9.3; see also Campos et al., 2000). Mental processes, such as mental map formations used for navigation, may not become increasingly distant from the physical world over time; the crux to development and skill acquisition may rather lie in the increased flexibility with which we can use and integrate different sources of information to attain our goals (Nardini et al., 2006; Thelen, 2000; Von Hofsten, 2004), whether they are to fit a complex shape into an aperture, finding our way in the world, or remembering an objects' location.

REFERENCES

Abercrombie, M. L. J. (1964). *Perceptual and visuomotor disorders in cerebral palsy: A review of the literature.* London: Spastics Society/Heinemann.

Acredolo, L. (1990). Behavioral-approaches to spatial orientation in infancy. *Annals of the New York Academy of Sciences, 608*, 596–612.

Acredolo, L. P. (1978). Development of spatial orientation in infancy. *Developmental Psychology, 14*, 224–234.

Acredolo (1979). Laboratory versus home: The effect of environment on the 9-month-old-infants' choice of spatial reference system. *Developmental Psychology, 14*, 224–234.

Acredolo, L. P., Adams, A., & Goodwyn, S. W. (1984). The role of self-produced movement and visual tracking in infant spatial orientation. *Journal of Experimental Child Psychology, 38*(2), 312–327.

Acredolo, L. P., & Evans, D. (1980). Developmental-changes in the effects of landmarks on infant spatial-behavior. *Developmental Psychology, 16*(4), 312–318.

Adolph, K. E. (1997). Learning in the development of infant locomotion. *Monographs of the Society for Research in Child Development, 62*(3), I–VI, 1–158.

Adolph, K. E., & Robinson, S. R. (2013). The road to walking: What learning to walk tells us about development. In P. Zelazo (Ed.), *Oxford handbook of developmental psychology.* New York, NY: Oxford University Press.

Adolph, K. E., Robinson, S. R., Young, J. W., & Gill-Alvarez, F. (2008). What is the shape of developmental change? *Psychological Review, 115*, 527–543. Available from http://dx.doi.org/10.1037/0033-295X.115.3.527.

Alloway, T. P., Gathercole, S. E., & Pickering, S. J. (2006). Verbal and visuospatial short--term memory and working memory in children: Are they separable? *Child Development*, 77(6), 1698–1716

American Psychiatric Association (2013). *Diagnostic and statistical manual of mental disorders* (5th ed.).Washington, DC: American Psychiatric Association.

Anderson, D. I., Campos, J. J., Witherington, D. C., Dahl, A., Rivera, M., He, M., ... Barbu-Roth, M. (2013). The role of locomotion in psychological development. *Frontiers in Psychology, 4*, 440. Available from http://dx.doi.org/10.3389/fpsyg.2013.00440.

Atun-Einy, O., Berger, S. E., & Scher, A. (2013). Assessing motivation to move and its relationship to motor development in infancy. *Infant Behavior and Development, 36*, 457–469.

Baranek, G. T. (1999). Autism during infancy: A retrospective video analysis of sensory-motor and social behavior at 9-12 months of age. *Journal of Autism and Developmental Disorders, 29*, 213–224.

Baron-Cohen, S. (2002). The extreme male brain theory of autism. *Trends in Cognitive Sciences, 6*, 248–254.

Behrmann, M., Avidan, G., Leonard, G., Kimchi, R., Luna, B., Humphreys, K., & Minshew, N. (2006). Configural processing in autism and its relationship to face processing. *Neuropsychologia, 44*, 110–129.

Belmonti, V., Fiori, S., Guzzetta, A., Cioni, G., & Berthoz, A. (2015). Cognitive strategies for locomotor navigation in normal development and cerebral palsy. *Developmental Medicine & Child Neurology, 57*, 31–36. Available from http://dx.doi.org/10.1111/dmcn.12685.

Berger, S. E. (2010). Locomotor expertise predicts infants' perseverative errors. *Developmental Psychology, 46*, 326–336. Available from http://dx.doi.org/10.1037/a0018285.

Berthoz, A., & Zaoui, M. (2015). New paradigms and tests for evaluating and remediating visuospatial deficits in children. *Developmental Medicine & Child Neurology, 57*, 15–20. Available from http://dx.doi.org/10.1111/dmcn.12690.

Bhat, A. N., Landa, R. J., & Galloway, J. C. (2011). Current perspectives on motor functioning in infants, children and adults with autism spectrum disorders. *Physical Therapy, 91*, 1116–1129.

Bruckner, C. T., & Yoder, P. (2007). Restricted object use in young children with autism: Definition and construct validity. *Autism, 11*, 161–171.

Bullens, J., Iglói, K., Berthoz, A., Postma, A., & Rondi-Reig, L. (2010). Developmental time course of the acquisition of sequential egocentric and allocentric navigation strategies. *Journal of Experimental Child Psychology, 107*(3), 337–350.

Campos, J. J., Anderson, D. I., Barbu-Roth, M. A., Hubbard, E. M., Hertenstein, M. J., & Witherington, D. (2000). Travel broadens the mind. *Infancy, 1*, 149–219. Available from http://dx.doi.org/10.1207/S15327078IN0102_1.

Cans, C. (2000). Surveillance of cerebral palsy in Europe: A collaboration of cerebral palsy surveys and registers. *Developmental Medicine & Child Neurology, 42*(12), 816–824. Available from http://dx.doi.org/10.1111/j.1469-8749.2000.tb00695.x.

Caron, M. J., Mottron, L., Rainville, C., & Chouinard, S. (2004). Do high functioning persons with autism present superior spatial abilities? *Neuropsychologia, 42*, 467–481.

Carpenter, M., Pennington, B. F., & Rogers, S. J. (2002). Interrelations among social-cognitive skills in young children with autism. *Journal of Autism and Developmental Disorders, 32*, 91–106.

Chiel, H. J., & Beer, R. D. (1997). The brain has a body: Adaptive behavior emerges from interactions of nervous system, body, and environment. *Trends in Neuroscience, 20*, 553–557.

Clearfield, M. W. (2004). The role of crawling and walking experience in infant spatial memory. *Journal of Experimental Child Psychology, 89*, 214–241. Available from http://dx.doi.org/10.1016/j.jecp.2004.07.003.

Clearfield, M. W. (2011). Learning to walk changes infants' social interactions. *Infant Behavior and Development, 34*, 15–25. Available from http://dx.doi.org/10.1016/j.infbeh.2010.04.008.

Corbetta, D., & Bojczyk, K. E. (2002). Infants return to two-handed reaching when they are learning to walk. *Journal of Motor Behavior, 34*, 83–95. Available from http://dx.doi.org/10.1080/00222890209601933.

Cornell, E. H., & Heth, C. (2006). Home range and the development of children's way finding. *Advances in Child Development and Behavior, 34*, 173–206.

Cornoldi, C., Venneri, A., Marconato, F., Molin, A., & Montinari, C. (2003). A rapid screening measure for teacher identification of visuo-spatial learning disabilities. *Journal of Learning Disabilities, 36*, 299–306. Available from http://dx.doi.org/10.1177/00222194030360040201.

Creem-Regehr, S. H., Gagnon, K. T., Geuss, M. N., & Stefanucci, J. K. (2013). Relating spatial perspective taking to the perception of other's affordances: Providing a foundation for predicting the future behavior of others. *Frontiers in Human Neuroscience, 7*, 596. Available from http://dx.doi.org/10.3389/fnhum.2013.00596.

Cuevas, K., & Bell, M. A. (2010). Developmental progression of looking and reaching performance on the A-not-B task. *Developmental Psychology, 46*(5), 1363–1371.

Dawson, G., Munson, J., Estes, A., Osterling, J., McPartland, J., Toth, K., ... Abbot, R. (2002). Neurocognitive function and joint attention ability in young children with autism spectrum disorder versus developmental delay. *Child Development, 73*, 345–358.

Dewulf, B. (2011). *Kleine dagen* (9th ed.). Amsterdam: Uitgeverij Atlas.

Diamond, A. (1985). Development of the ability to use recall to guide action, as indicated by infants' performance on AB. *Child Development, 56*, 868–883.
Dinstein, I., Heeger, D. J., Lorenzi, L., Minshew, N. J., Malach, R., & Behrmann, M. (2012). Unreliable evoked responses in autism. *Neuron, 75*, 981–991.
Edgin, J. O., & Pennington, B. F. (2005). Spatial cognition in autism spectrum disorders: Superior, impaired, or just intact? *Journal of Autism and Developmental Disorders, 35*, 729–745.
Falter, C. M., Plaisted, K. C., & Davis, G. (2008). Visuo-spatial processing in autism—Testing the predictions of extreme male brain theory. *Journal of Autism and Developmental Disorders, 38*, 507–515.
Foreman, N., Foreman, D., Cummings, A., & Owens, S. (1990). Locomotion, active choice, and spatial memory in children. *Journal of General Psychology, 117*, 215–232.
Fournier, K. A., Hass, C. J., Naik, S. K., Lodha, N., & Cauraugh, J. H. (2010). Motor coordination in autism spectrum disorders: A synthesis and meta-analysis. *Journal of Autism and Developmental Disorders, 40*, 1227–1240.
Franchak, J. M., Kretch, K. S., Soska, K. C., & Adolph, K. E. (2011). Head-mounted eye tracking: A new method to describe infant looking. *Child Development, 82*, 1738–1750. Available from http://dx.doi.org/10.1111/j.1467-8624.2011.01670.x.
Frick, A., Daum, M. M., Walser, S., & Mast, F. W. (2009). Motor processes in children's mental rotation. *Journal of Cognition and Development, 10*(1–2), 18–40.
Frick, A., Ferrara, K., & Newcombe, N. S. (2013). Using a touch screen paradigm to assess the development of mental rotation between 3½ and 5½ years of age. *Cognitive Processing, 14*, 117–127.
Frick, A., & Möhring, W. (2013). Mental object rotation and motor development in 8- and 10-month-old infants. *Journal of Experimental Child Psychology, 115*, 708–720. Available from http://dx.doi.org/10.1016/j.jecp.2013.04.001.
Frick, A., Möhring, W., & Newcombe, N. S. (2014). Development of mental transformation abilities. *Trends in Cognitive Sciences, 18*(10), 536–542.
Gernsbacher, M. A., Sauer, E. A., Geye, H. M., Schweigert, E. K., & Goldsmith, H. H. (2008). Infant and toddler oral-and manual-motor skills predict later speech fluency in autism. *Journal of Child Psychology and Psychiatry, 49*, 43–50.
Gibson, E. J. (1988). Exploratory behavior in the development of perceiving, acting, and the acquiring of knowledge. *Annual Review in Psychology, 39*, 1–41.
Gibson, J. J. (1979). *The ecological approach to visual perception*. Boston, MA: Houghton Mifflin, Reprinted 1986, Erlbaum.
Happé, F., & Frith, U. (2006). The weak central coherence account: Detail-focused cognitive style in autism spectrum disorders. *Journal of Autism and Developmental Disorders, 36*, 5–25.
Hazen, N. L. (1982). Spatial exploration and spatial knowledge: Individual and developmental differences in very young children. *Child Development, 53*, 826–833.
Hellendoorn, A., Wijnroks, L., van Daalen, E., Dietz, C., Buitelaar, J. K., & Leseman, P. P. M. (2015). Motor functioning, exploration, visuospatial cognition and language development in preschool children with autism. *Research in Developmental Disabilities, 39*, 32–42.
Hill, E. (2004). Executive dysfunction in autism. *Trends in Cognitive Sciences, 8*, 26–32.
Horobin, K., & Acredolo, L. P. (1986). The role of attentiveness, mobility history, and separation of hiding stages on Stage IV search behaviour. *Journal of Experimental Child Psychology, 41*, 114–127.
Howard, E. M., & Henderson, S. E. (1989). Perceptual problems in cerebral-palsied children: A real world example. *Human Movement Science, 8*(2), 141–160. Available from http://dx.doi.org/10.1016/0167-9457(89)90014-6.

Jansen, P., & Heil, M. (2010). The relation between motor development and mental rotation ability in 5–6 years old children. *European Journal of Developmental Science, 6*, 67–75.

Jarrold, C., Butler, D. W., Cottington, E. M., & Jimenez, F. (2000). Linking theory of mind and central coherence bias in autism and in the general population. *Developmental Psychology, 36*, 126–138.

Karasik, L. B., Tamis-LeMonda, C. S., & Adolph, K. E. (2011). Transition from crawling to walking and infant's actions with objects and people. *Child Development, 82*, 1199–1209. Available from http://dx.doi.org/10.1111/j.1467-8624.2011.01595.x.

Keen, R. (2003). Representation of objects and event: Why do infants look so smart and toddlers look so dumb? *Current Directions in Psychological Science, 12*(3), 79–83.

Kelso, S. (1997). *Dynamic patterns: The self-organization of brain and behaviour.* Cambridge, MA: MIT Press.

Kenworthy, L., Yerys, B. E., Weinblatt, R., Abrams, D. N., & Wallace, G. L. (2013). Motor demands impact speed of information processing in autism spectrum disorders. *Neuropsychology, 27*, 529–536.

Kermoian, R., & Campos, J. J. (1988). Locomotor experience: A facilitator of spatial cognitive development. *Child Development, 59*, 906–917.

Kosslyn, S. M. (1991). A cognitive neuroscience of visual cognition: Further developments. In R. H. Logie, & M. Denis (Eds.), *Mental images in human cognition* (pp. 351–381). Amsterdam: Elsevier Science.

Koterba, E., Leezenbaum, N. B., & Iverson, J. M. (2012). Object exploration at 6 and 9 months in infants with and without for autism. *Autism, 18*, 97–105.

Kretch, K. S., Franchak, J. M., & Adolph, K. E. (2014). Crawling and walking infants see the world differently. *Child Development, 85*(4), 1503–1518.

Kuschner, E. S., & Bennetto, L. (2007). Looking at the trees, but trying to play in the forest: Visuospatial processing style and play in autism. *Annual Conference of the International Play Association-USA/Canada and the Association for the Study of Play.* Rochester, NY.

Landa, R., & Garret-Mayer, E. (2006). Development in infants with autism spectrum disorders: A prospective study. *Journal of Child Psychology and Psychiatry, 47*, 629–638.

Landau, B. (2002). Spatial cognition. In V. Ramachandran (Ed.), *Encyclopedia of the human brain* (Vol. 4). San Diego, CA: Academic Press.

Lee, V., & Kuhlmeier, V. A. (2013). Young children show a dissociation in looking and pointing behavior in falling events. *Cognitive Development, 28*, 21–30. Available from http://dx.doi.org/10.1016/j.cogdev.2014.04.001.

Lind, S. E., Williams, D. M., Raber, J., Peel, A., & Bowler, D. M. (2013). Spatial navigation impairments among intellectually high-functioning adults with autism spectrum disorder: Exploring relations with theory of mind, episodic memory, and episodic future thinking. *Journal of Abnormal Psychology, 122*, 1189–1199.

López, B. (2015). Beyond modularisation: The need of a socio-neuro-constructionist model of autism. *Journal of Autism and Developmental Disorders, 45*, 31–41. Available from http://dx.doi.org/10.1007/s10803-013-1966-9.10.1007/s10803-013-1966-9.

Mammarella, I. C., & Cornoldi, C. (2014). An analysis of the criteria used to diagnose children with Nonverbal Learning Disability (NLD). *Child Neuropsychology, 20*, 255–280. Available from http://dx.doi.org/10.1080/09297049.2013.796920.

Mammarella, I. C., Lucangeli, D., & Cornoldi, C. (2010). Spatial working memory and arithmetic deficits in children with nonverbal learning difficulties (NLD). *Journal of Learning Disabilities, 43*, 455–468. Available from http://dx.doi.org/10.1177/0022219409355482.

Mash, C., Novak, E., Berthier, N. E., & Keen, R. (2006). What do two-year-olds understand about hidden-object events? *Developmental Psychology, 42*(2), 263–271.

Möhring, W., & Frick, A. (2013). Touching up mental rotation: Effects of manual experience on 6-month-old infants' mental object rotation. *Child Development, 84*, 1554–1565. Available from http://dx.doi.org/10.1111/cdev.12065.

Moreau, D., Mansy-Dannay, A., Clerc, J., & Guerrién, A. (2011). Spatial ability and motor performance: Assessing mental rotation processes in elite and novice athletes. *International Journal of Sport Psychology, 42*, 525–547.

Mottron, L., Dawson, M., Soulières, I., Hubert, B., & Burack, J. (2006). Enhanced perceptual functioning in autism: An update, and eight principles of autistic perception. *Journal of Autism and Developmental Disorders, 36*, 27–43.

Mùth, A., Hönekopp, J., & Falter, C. M. (2014). Visuo-spatial performance in autism: A meta-analysis. *Journal of Autism and Developmental Disorders, 44*, 3245–3263.

Nadel, L., & Hardt, O. (2004). The spatial brain. *Neuropsychology, 18*, 473–476.

Nardini, M., Burgess, N., Breckenridge, K., & Atkinson, J. (2006). Differential developmental trajectories for egocentric, environmental and intrinsic frames of reference in spatial memory. *Cognition, 101*(1), 153–172.

Narimoto, T., Matsuura, N., Takezawa, T., Mitsuhashi, Y., & Hiratani, M. (2013). Spatial short-term memory in children with Nonverbal Learning Disabilities: Impairment in encoding spatial configuration. *The Journal of Genetic Psychology, 174*, 73–87. Available from http://dx.doi.org/10.1080/00221325.2011.641040.

Needham, A., & Libertus, K. (2011). Embodiment in early development. *Wiley Interdisplinary Reviews—Cognitive Science, 2*(1), 117–123.

Newcombe, N., Huttenlocher, J., Drummey, A. B., & Wiley, J. G. (1998). The development of spatial location coding: Place learning and dead reckoning in the second and third years. *Cognitive Development, 13*, 185–200.

Newcombe, N. S., & Huttenlocher, J. (2003). *Making space: The development of spatial representation and reasoning*. Cambridge, MA: MIT Press.

Newcombe, N. S., Uttal, D. H., & Sauter, M. (2013). Spatial development. In P. Zelazo (Ed.), *Oxford handbook of developmental psychology* (Vol. 1, pp. 564–590). New York: Oxford University Press.

Örnkloo, H., & von Hofsten, C. (2007). Fitting objects into holes: On the development of spatial cognition. *Developmental Psychology, 43*, 404–416.

Oudgenoeg-Paz (2014). Walk this way, talk this way: Motor skills, spatial exploration, and the development of spatial cognition and language. *Doctoral dissertation*. The Netherlands: Utrecht University.

Oudgenoeg-Paz, O., Leseman, P. P. M., & Volman, M. J. M. (2014). Can infant self-locomotion and spatial exploration predict spatial memory at school age? *European Journal of Developmental Psychology, 11*(1), 36–48

Oudgenoeg-Paz, O., Leseman, P. P. M., & Volman, M. J. M. (2015). Exploration as a mediator of the relation between the attainment of motor milestones and the development of spatial cognition and language. *Developmental Psychology, 51*, 1241–1253. Available from http://dx.doi.org/10.1037/a0039572.

Ozonoff, S., Macari, S., Young, G. S., Goldring, S., Thompson, M., & Rogers, S. J. (2008). Atypical object exploration at 12 months of age is associated with autism in a prospective sample. *Autism, 12*, 457–472.

Ozonoff, S., Pennington, B. F., & Rogers, S. J. (1991). Executive function deficits in high functioning autistic individuals: Relationship to theory of mind. *Journal of Child Psychology and Psychiatry, 32*, 1081–1105.

Paterson, S. J., Brown, J. H., Gsödl, M. K., Johnson, M. H., & Karmiloff-Smith, A. (1999). Cognitive modularity and genetic disorders. *Science, 268*, 2355–2358. Available from http://dx.doi.org/10.1126/science.286.5448.2355.

Pavlova, M., Sokolov, A., & Krägeloh-Mann, I. (2007). Visual navigation in adolescents with early periventricular lesions: Knowing where, but not getting there. *Cerebral Cortex*, *17*, 363–369. Available from http://dx.doi.org/10.1093/cercor/bhj153.

Pearson, A., Marsh, L., Hamilton, A., & Ropar, D. (2014). Spatial transformations of bodies and objects in adults with autism spectrum disorder. *Journal of Autism and Developmental Disorders*, *44*, 2277–2289.

Pearson, A., Ropar, D., & Hamilton, A. F. D. C. (2013). A review of visual perspective taking in autism spectrum disorder. *Frontiers in Human Neuroscience*, 7, 652. Available from http://dx.doi.org/10.3389/fnhum.2013.00652.

Pellicano, E., Maybery, M., Durkin, K., & Maley, A. (2006). Multiple cognitive capabilities/deficits in children with an autism spectrum disorder: "Weak" central coherence and its relationship to theory of mind and executive control. *Development and Psychopathology*, *18*, 77–98.

Pelphrey, K. A., Reznick, J. S., Goldman, B. D., Sasson, N., Morrow, J., Donahoe, A., et al. (2004). Development of visuospatial short-term memory in the second half of the 1st year. *Developmental Psychology*, *40*(5), 836–851. Available from http://dx.doi.org/10.1037/0012-1649.40.5.836.

Piaget, J. (1954). *The construction of reality in the child*. New York, NY: Basic Books.

Pierce, K., & Courchesne, E. (2001). Evidence for a cerebellar role in reduced exploration and stereotyped behavior in autism. *Biological Psychiatry*, *49*, 655–664.

Postma, A., Sterken, Y., de Vries, L., & de Haan, E. H. F. (2000). Spatial localization in patients with unilateral posterior left or right hemisphere lesions. *Experimental Brain Research*, *134*, 220–227. Available from http://dx.doi.org/10.1007/s002210000430.

Price, T. F., & Harmon-Jones, E. (2010). The effect of embodied emotive states on cognitive categorization. *Emotion*, *10*, 934–938.

Richardson, D. C., Spivey, M. J., Barsalou, L. W., & McRae, K. (2003). Spatial representations activated during real-time comprehension of verbs. *Cognitive Science*, *27*, 767–780. Available from http://dx.doi.org/10.1016/S0364-0213(03)00064-8.

Rogers, S. J. (2004). Developmental regression in autism spectrum disorders. *Mental Retardation and Developmental Disabilities Research Review*, *10*, 139–143. Available from http://dx.doi.org/10.1002/mrdd.20027.

Rosenbaum, P., Paneth, N., Leviton, A., Goldstein, M., Bax, M., Damiano, D., et al. (2007). A report: The definition and classification of cerebral palsy. *Developmental Medicine & Child Neurology (Supplement)*, *109*, 8–14. Available from http://dx.doi.org/10.1111/j.1469-8749.2007.tb12610.x.

Salowitz, N. M. G., Eccarius, P., Karst, J., Carson, A., Schohl, K., Stevens, S., ... Scheidt, R. A. (2013). Brief report: Visuo-spatial guidance of movement during gesture imitation and mirror drawing in children with autism spectrum disorders. *Journal of Autism Spectrum Disorders*, *43*, 985–995.

Savelsbergh, G. J. P., Douwes Dekker, L., Vermeer, A., & Hopkins, B. (1998). Locomoting through apertures of different width: A study of children with cerebral palsy. *Pediatric Rehabilitation*, *2*, 5–13. Available from http://dx.doi.org/10.3109/17518429809078610.

Schutte, A. R., Spencer, J. P., & Schöner, G. (2003). Testing the dynamic field theory: Working memory for locations becomes increasingly precise over development. *Child Development*, *74*(5), 1393–1417.

Schwarzer, G., Freitag, C., Buckel, R., & Lofruthe, A. (2013). Crawling is associated with mental rotation ability by 9-month-old infants. *Infancy*, *18*, 432–441. Available from http://dx.doi.org/10.1111/j.1532-7078.2012.00132.x.

Semrud-Clikeman, M., Goldenring Fine, J., & Bledsoe, J. (2014). Comparison among children with autism spectrum disorder, nonverbal learning disorder and typically developing children on measures of executive functioning. *Journal of Autism and Developmental Disorders*, *44*, 331–342. Available from http://dx.doi.org/10.1007/s10803-013-1871-2.

Shapiro, L. (2007). The embodied cognition research programme. *Philosophy Compass*, *2*(2), 338–346.

Siegler, R. S. (1996). *Emerging minds: The process of change in children's thinking*. New York, NY: Oxford University Press.

Smith, L. B., & Thelen, E. (2003). Development as a dynamic system. *Trends in Cognitive Sciences*, 7(8), 343–348.

Smith, L. B., Thelen, E., Titzer, R., & McLin, D. (1999). Knowing in the context of acting: The task dynamics of the A-not-B error. *Psychological Review*, *106*, 235–260.

Spreen, O. (2011). Nonverbal learning disabilities: A critical review. *Child Neuropsychology*, *17*, 17–33. Available from http://dx.doi.org/10.1080/09297049.2010.546778.

Steele, S. D., Minshew, N. J., Luna, B., & Sweeney, J. A. (2007). Spatial working memory deficits in autism. *Journal of Autism and Developmental Disorders*, *37*, 605–612.

Sutton, J. E. (2006). The development of landmark and beacon use in young children: Evidence from a touchscreen search task. *Developmental Science*, *9*(1), 108–123.

Tamis-Lemonda, C. S., Adolph, K. E., Lobo, S. A., Karasik, L. B., Ishak, S., & Dimitropoulou, K. A. (2008). When infants take mothers' advice: 18-month-olds integrate perceptual and social information to guide motor action. *Developmental Psychology*, *44*(3), 734–746.

Te Velde, A., Savelsbergh, G., Barela, J., & van der Kamp, J. (2003). Safety in road crossing of children with cerebral palsy. *Acta Paediatrica*, *92*, 1197–1204. Available from http://dx.doi.org/10.1111/j.1651-2227.2003.tb02484.x.

Thelen, E. (2000). Grounded in the world: Developmental origins of the embodied mind. *Infancy*, *1*(1), 3–28.

Thelen, E., Schöner, G., Scheier, C., & Smith, L. B. (2001). The dynamics of embodiment: A field theory of infant preservative reaching. *Behavioral and Brain Sciences*, *24*, 1–86.

Thelen, E., & Smith, L. B. (1996). *A dynamic systems approach to the development of cognition and action*. Cambridge, MA: Bradford Books/MIT Press.

Topál, J., Gergely, G., Miklósi, A., Erdőheyi, E., & Csibra, G. (2008). Infants' perseverative search errors are induced by pragmatic misinterpretation. *Science*, *321*, 1831–1833. Available from http://dx.doi.org/10.1126/science.1161437.

Trafton, J. G., & Harrison, A. M. (2011). Embodied spatial cognition. *Topics in Cognitive Science*, *3*, 686–706.

van den Brink, D., & Janzen, G. (2013). Visual spatial cue use for guiding orientation in two-to-three-year-old children. *Frontiers in Psychology*, *4*, 904. Available from http://dx.doi.org/10.3389/fpsyg.2013.00904.

Van Hoogmoed, A. H., van den Brink, D., & Janzen, G. (under review). Toddlers' cue use in navigation.

Volkmar, F. R., Lord, C., Bailey, A., Schultz, R. T., & Klin (2004). Autism and other pervasive developmental disorders. *Journal of Child Psychology and Psychiatry*, *45*, 135–170.

Von Hofsten, C. (2004). An action perspective on motor development. *Trends in Cognitive Sciences*, *8*(6), 266–272.

Von Hofsten, C. (2007). Action in development. *Developmental Science*, *10*(1), 54–60.

Wang, R. F., & Spelke, E. S. (2002). Human spatial representation: Insight from animals. *Trends in Cognitive Sciences*, *6*(9), 376–382.

Wellman, H. M., Cross, D., & Bartsch, K. (1986). Infant search and object permanence: A meta-analysis of the A-not-B error. *Monographs of the Society for Research in Child Development, 51*(3), R5–67.

Wetherby, A. M., Woods, J., Allen, L., Cleary, J., Dickinson, H., & Lord, C. (2004). Early indicators of autism spectrum disorders in the second year of life. *Journal of Autism and Developmental Disorders, 34*, 473–493.

Wexler, M., Kosslyn, S. M., & Berthoz, A. (1998). Motor processes in mental rotation. *Cognition, 68*, 77–94.

Williams, E., Costall, A., & Reddy, V. (1999). Children with autism experience problems with both objects and people. *Journal of Autism and Developmental Disorders, 29*, 367–378.

Wilson, M. (2002). Six views on embodied cognition. *Psychonomic Bulletin & Review, 9*(4), 625–636.

Yerys, B. E., Hepburn, S. L., Pennington, B. F., & Rogers, S. J. (2007). Executive function in preschoolers with autism: Evidence consistent with a secondary deficit. *Journal of Autism Developmental Disorders, 37*, 1068–1079.

Yirmiya, N., & Charman, T. (2010). The prodrome of autism: Early behavioral and biological signs, regression, peri- and post-natal developmental and genetics. *Journal of Child Psychology and Psychiatry, 51*, 432–458.

Zimmer, T., & Volkermar, M. (1987). *MOT—Motoriktest für 4-6jährige Kinder.* Bern: Huber.

CHAPTER 10

Space in Neuropsychological Assessment

Esther van den Berg[1,2] and Carla Ruis[1,3]
[1]Experimental Psychology, Helmholtz Institute, Utrecht University, Utrecht, The Netherlands
[2]Department of Neurology, Erasmus MC University Medical Center, Rotterdam, The Netherlands
[3]Department of Neurology, University Medical Center, Utrecht, The Netherlands

Box 10.1

BOX 10.1 Case Description

XX is a 39-year-old, highly educated man. After acquired brain injury (hippocampus atrophy after incidental ecstasy use) he complained about memory and navigation problems. He tended to forget things people told him and he could not remember appointments adequately. He had great difficulty finding his way in new surroundings, but also in more familiar places. XX got lost several times while riding his bicycle in his hometown. Simply studying a map before leaving did not help him. When he parked his car or bike somewhere, he was not able to find them again.

Extensive neuropsychological assessment revealed a memory disorder (impaired scores on both verbal and nonverbal tests). Because the navigation problems could not properly be assessed by standard neuropsychological tests, a virtual navigation test was administered. Compared to matched control subjects XX had profound difficulties navigating in this virtual surrounding. (Full case report, see Ruis, Postma, Bouvy, & van der Ham, 2015)

10.1 INTRODUCTION

Brain injury may cause disorders in the spatial domain. In the previous chapters a wide range of possible disorders of space have been discussed. When patients experience complaints about their cognitive functioning a neuropsychological assessment is considered to examine the nature and extent of deficits in cognition. Such an assessment typically involves multiple psychometric tests to be administered along with a thorough

Neuropsychology of Space.
DOI: http://dx.doi.org/10.1016/B978-0-12-801638-1.00010-0

investigation of cognitive complaints, medical history, personality characteristics and mood (Lezak, Howieson, Bigler, & Tranel, 2012) (see Box 10.2). Various tests that are administered involve the spatial domain in one way or another, for example, in the assessment of visuospatial

BOX 10.2 Principles of Neuropsychological Assessment

Neuropsychological assessment follows a structured diagnostic cycle. It starts with assessment of a person's complaints, medical history, and aspects of mood and personality. Based on this information, hypotheses are developed as to what the underlying cause of these complaints may be. These hypotheses guide the choice of assessment tools, such as psychometric tests and questionnaires. Following the results of these tests one or more hypotheses may be affirmed or rejected. In complex cases, the results of the assessment may lead to new hypotheses that can be tested. In the final stage a clinical diagnosis is made, including guidance for treatment or rehabilitation.

Assessment of the problem
|
Hypothesis
|
Testing hypothesis
|
Interpretation of the results
|
Evaluation

A typical neuropsychological assessment involves psychometric evaluation of all major cognitive functions, such as memory, language, concentration, perception, and constructive abilities, by performing an extensive test battery. Even when a patient has very specific complaints, for example, complaints that seem to be linked to spatial cognition, it is important to test other cognitive domains to ensure the exact nature of these complaints. One has to be sure that a patient's complaints are not the result of, for example, impaired visual functions or severe general memory problems.

In the case of XX an extensive neuropsychological assessment was administered. He reported memory and navigation problems, and those cognitive domains were studied thoroughly. Other cognitive domains were tested as well, to be sure that they did not interact with the problems reported by XX. Furthermore, extensive testing makes it easier to say something about a patient's strengths and weaknesses, which in turn guides rehabilitation of the complaints. The neuropsychological assessment of XX revealed disorders in

(*Continued*)

BOX 10.2 Principles of Neuropsychological Assessment—cont'd

navigation and memory. The problems in navigation could not be fully explained by the memory disorders. Test scores on other cognitive domains were unimpaired, and executive functions were even above average (Table 10.1).

Table 10.1 Neuropsychological assessment of XX (the tests that assess the spatial domain are in bold and will be described in more detail in this chapter)

Intelligence/overall cognitive functioning	National Adult Reading Test Raven progressive matrices Mini Mental Status Examination
Language	Boston Naming Test Verbal and semantic fluency test
Working memory	Digit Span WAIS-IV **Corsi Block-tapping Test**
Long-term memory	Rey Auditory Verbal Learning Test Stories Rivermead Behavioral Memory Test Doors test **Location Learning Test** **Rey Complex Figure Test—delay** Benton Visual Retention Test **Continuous Visual Memory Test** Visual Association Test
Attention/executive functions/speed of information processing	Trail Making Test Stroop Color Word Test Brixton Test Behavioral Assessment of the Dysexecutive Syndrome
Visuoperception/visuoconstruction	**Judgment of Line Orientation test** **Rey Complex Figure Test—copy**
Navigation	**Virtual Tübingen task**
Symptom validity and questionnaires	Test of Memory Malingering Beck Depression Inventory Symptom Checklist-90

memory or perception. However, questions about spatial cognition are often not routinely asked and complaints in this domain may therefore be underreported. This is surprising since complaints such as failing to find your way around is thought to greatly hamper everyday functioning. The prevalence of complaints in the spatial domain after brain damage is unknown, but complaints of, for example, forgetfulness, mental slowness, and poor concentration are reported by over 50% of patients 6–12 months after cerebral stroke (Hochstenbach, Prigatano, & Mulder, 2005), indicating that a substantial proportion of patients may indeed experience complaints in the spatial domain.

In this chapter we give an overview of the standardized tests and procedures that can be used to assess spatial cognition. Furthermore, we intend to give practical examples of questions that can be asked during neuropsychological assessment to aid clinicians. The final part of this chapter entails ways in which (cognitive) rehabilitation can be used to help patients cope with their deficits in spatial cognition.

10.2 PSYCHOMETRIC TESTS AND PROCEDURES USED TO ASSESS SPACE

Many tests involve the spatial domain. Below we discuss published or frequently used tests and procedures. While one can argue that any test involves space simply because it is administered in the personal space of the patient, we chose only those tests that are explicitly focused on one or more aspects of spatial cognition.

10.2.1 Visual Space Perception

Spatial orientation refers to the ability to identify the position or direction of objects or points in space (Benton & Tranel, 1993). It can be assessed by asking patients to perform spatial transformations such as rotations or inversions of stimuli. Different paper-and-pencil tasks exist which require patients to indicate whether a rotated figure matches the stimulus figure or to mark a test figure to match a stimulus figure (Vandenberg & Kruse, 1978; Fig. 10.1). Computerized versions are also available (Monahan, Harke, & Shelley, 2008), allowing examination of different strategies that can be used to perform mental rotations (Moè, Meneghetti, & Cadinu, 2009).

Visual perception can be assessed by the Visual Object and Space Perception Battery (Warrington & James, 1991). This battery of tests was developed to incorporate different aspects of object and space perception. Tests 1–4 are designed to measure different forms of visual agnosia. The tests are shown to discriminate between patients with left and right hemisphere damage: about 30% of patient with right hemisphere damage fail one or more of the subtests. Tests 5–9 focus on space perception, namely: dot counting, position discrimination, number location (Fig. 10.2), and cube analysis. Again, 30% of patients with right hemisphere damage fail one or

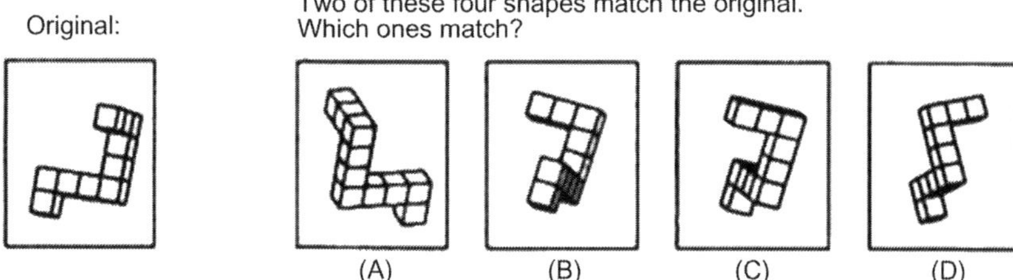

Figure 10.1 Mental rotation. Example of a mental rotation task, based on Shepard and Metzler (1971). Subjects are asked to compare two 3D objects that are rotated. Shepard, R. N., & Metzler, J. T. (1971). Mental rotation of three dimensional objects. Science, 171, 701–703.

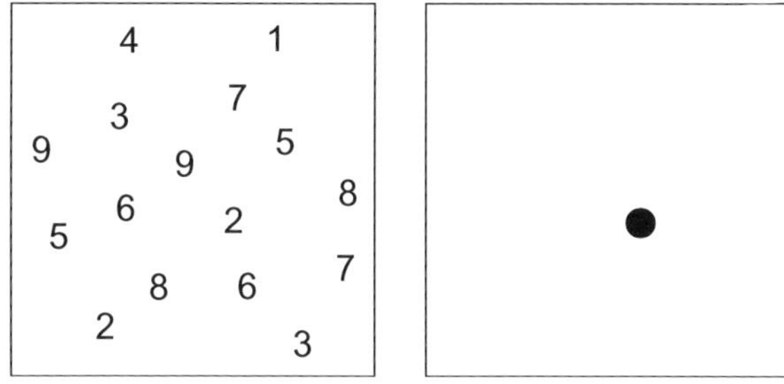

Figure 10.2 VOSP number location. Number location is a subtest of the VOSP measuring object location binding. A person is presented with two panels. The top panel shows different numbers, the lower panel shows a black dot that matches the location of one of the numbers of the top panel. Warrington, E. K., & James, M. (1991). The visual object and space perception battery (VOSP). Bury St. Edmunds, England: Thames Valley Test Co.

more tests, but compared to control subjects 10–15% of patients with left hemisphere damage also fail, indicating involvement of both hemispheres in different aspects of space perception. More recently, the Birmingham Object Recognition Battery (BORB; Riddoch & Humphreys, 1993) was developed as a theory-driven measure of visual perception, similar to the PALPA test in the assessment of language disorders. Whereas many measures of visual perception focus at either low-level processing of features or high-level visual processing such as object recognition, the BORB also allows for assessment of "mid-level" visual processing, including figure–ground segregation, perceptual grouping and global–local processing. The BORB uses a same–different matching paradigm of basic perceptual features, such as orientation, length, position and object size), intermediate visual processes (eg, matching objects different in viewpoint), access to stored perceptual knowledge about objects (object decision), access to semantic knowledge (function and associative matches), and access to names from object (picture naming). Based on the type of errors someone makes on specific subtests of the BORB the nature of the impairment in visual perception can be pinpointed for each individual patient.

Angular relationships are assessed by the Judgment of Line Orientation test (JLO; Benton, Hannay & Varney, 1975), which examines the ability to estimate angular relationships between line segments by visual matching. It was developed as a clinical version of an experimental paradigm using a tachitoscopic stimulus presentation. Patients with right hemisphere damage, particularly those with posterior lesions, show worse performance compared to controls and patients with left hemisphere damage. The items of the JLO allow for different matching strategies, as some of the items can be discriminated based on judgment of shape or configuration of the stimuli whereas others are more strictly spatial in nature. Indeed, Hannay et al. (1987) already showed mainly temporal–occipital blood flow changes rather than temporal–parietal blood flow changes associated with JLO performance. A more recent study in 181 patients used a lesion–symptom mapping approach and showed that impaired JLO performance was associated with lesions in the right posterior parietal region (Tranel, Vianna, Manzel, Damasio, & Grabowski, 2009). In a similar vein, Biesbroek et al. (2014) also performed a lesion–symptom mapping analysis in 111 stroke patients for the JLO and compared this to performance on the Rey Complex Figure Test copy trial. Both tests assess visuospatial perception, but the latter also measures visuospatial construction, and to some extent attention, planning, and executive functioning. Performance on both the JLO and the perceptual part of the Rey Complex Figure Test was affected by lesions in the right frontal, superior temporal, and supramarginal areas. The visuospatial constructive part of the Rey appeared to depend more on right superior and inferior parietal and on occipital areas. Notice Collaer and Nelson (2002) pointed out that the original JLO might be too easy to detect more subtle deficits. Using an adapted format with more line orientations, they observed relatively large sex differences in healthy participants. Trecanni and colleagues (Treccani & Cubelli, 2011; Treccani, Torri, & Cubelli, 2005) used a version in which besides the original JLO items also the mirrored items were included, testing left and right hemisphere damaged patients. On basis of their results they argued for the need to control for attentional factors in the line orientation perception test.

10.2.2 Spatial Attention

Right hemisphere lesions frequently involve absence of awareness (or "inattention") of stimuli in the left visual field. Patients may fail to eat food on the left side of their plate or may consistently bump into objects to their left (see chapter 5). A common way of investigating such hemispatial neglect is by asking a patient to either draw or copy an object or by means of cancelation tasks that require patients to cross out (either timed or untimed) certain targets in an array of stimuli (eg, lines, letters, digits). The nature and severity of hemispatial neglect differs between patients and it is therefore common practice to present patients with more than one test. The Schenkenberg Line Bisection Test (Schenkenberg, Bradford, & Ajax, 1980), for example, consists of 20 lines of different sizes that are centered to either the left, right, or middle of a page. The mean percentage of deviation from the middle is then calculated and compared with normative data. Patients with right hemisphere damage tend to miss shorter lines on the left and center of the page. When using their right hand a clear rightward deviation of the marks is generally observed. The Bells Test (Gauthier, Dehaut, & Joanette, 1989) and the Star cancelation test (Halligan, Cockburn, & Wilson, 1991) are two of the most well-known cancelation tests. The Bells test involves 315 silhouettes of objects distributed on a page. Patients have to circle 35 bells that are scattered among them. These bells are arranged in seven columns of five bells, which allows for documentation of a patient's scanning strategy. The Star cancelation test was designed as a more difficult version of a cancelation task by including stars of different sizes, letters, and words. Targets to be crossed out in this array are 56 small stars (Fig. 10.3). The Behavioral Inattention Test (BIT) is a comprehensive battery that provides a naturalistic set of tests for hemispatial neglect (Wilson, Cockburn, & Halligan, 1988). It consists of different cancelation tests, such as the Star cancelation test, a line bisection test, and several drawing and copying tests. More naturalistic tests in this battery include, for example, reading a menu, copying an address, and navigating a simple map. The BIT thus not only allows for assessment of the presence of hemispatial neglect, but also measures the extent of the neglect on several everyday activities.

All of these tests and procedures also involve other cognitive processes such as visual perception, semantic information or even language comprehension to some degree besides the core spatial functions. Two of the more "spatial" ways of investigating the neglect phenomenon are asking patients to describe a symmetrically organized picture where events on the right and left side of the picture have to be connected to fully understand what is happening in the scene (eg, Cookie theft picture from the

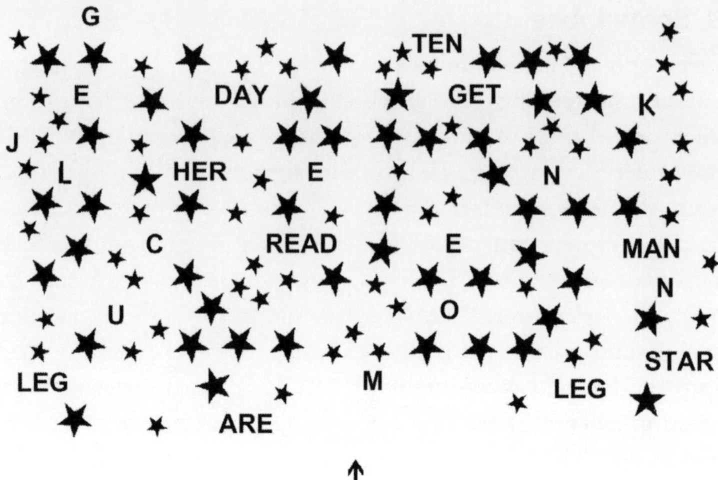

Figure 10.3 Star cancelation. Wilson, B., Cockburn, J., & Baddeley, A. (1991). The Rivermead behavioural memory test manual. Bury St. Edmunds, Suffolk: Thames Valley Test Corporation.

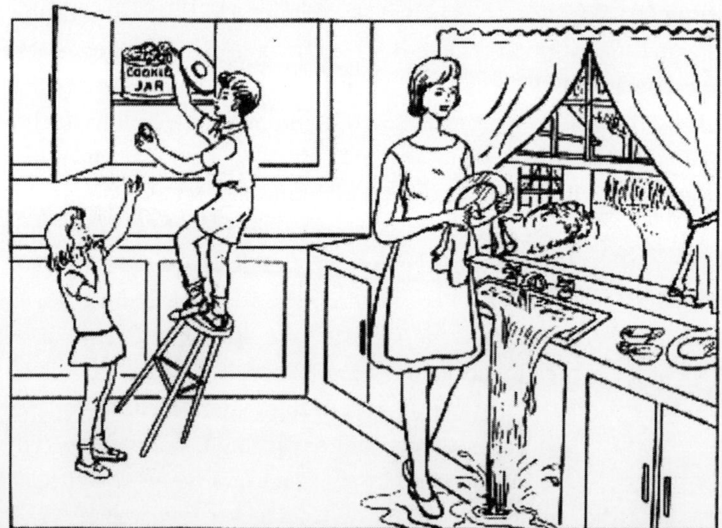

Figure 10.4 Cookie theft. Goodglass, H., Kaplan, E., & Barresi, B. (2001). Boston diagnostic aphasia examination (3rd ed.). Philadelphia: Lippincott Williams & Wilkins.

Boston Diagnostic Aphasia Examination; Fig. 10.4). One may also ask patients to imagine and describe a familiar scene from two viewpoints directly opposite one another. Hemispatial neglect may then be noticed in the form of absence or scarce mentioning of features on the left as opposed to detailed description of details on the right.

10.2.3 Body Space

There are a few psychometric tests available to assess impairments in body space. *Orientation* of body parts can be informally examined by asking patients to name certain body parts indicated by the examiner or to point to body parts on command. *Proprioception* can be assessed by moving the distal parts of fingers or toes up or down without the patient looking. Specific disturbance of *right–left discrimination* can be examined with the Bergen Right–Left Discrimination task (BRLD; Grewe, Ohmann, Markowitsch, & Piefke, 2010) (Fig. 10.5). It consists of sequences of stickmen stimuli of which either the front or the backside is shown. These stimuli have three different arm positions, with two, one, or no arms crossing the midline of the body. Patients are asked to mark either the left or the right hand of each stickman by pencil. Evidently, impaired performance on this task may indicate different deficits. Grewe et al. (2010) argue that right–left discrimination involves (1) sensory integration, (2) application of expressive and receptive language, (3) understanding of the "right–left" concept, and (4) a visual–spatial element (including the ability to mentally manipulate

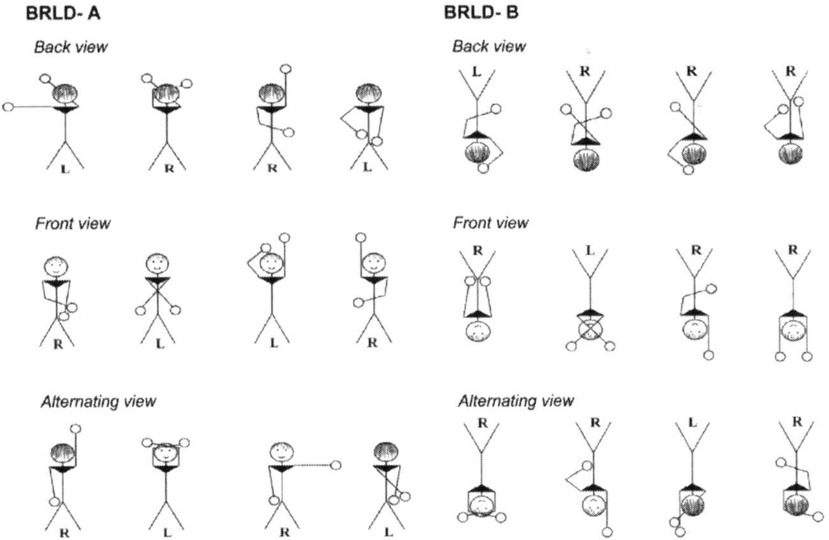
BRLD- A
Back view
Front view
Alternating view
BRLD- B
Back view
Front view
Alternating view
Exemplary items of each of the three subtests with upright stimuli of the BRLD-A (*left*) and inverted stimuli of the BRLD-B (*right*). The letters "R" and "L" indicate that the stickmen's *right* ("R") or *left* ("L") hand has to be marked. Note that each subtest consists of 48 stimuli

Figure 10.5 BRLD. Grewe, P., Ohmann, H. A., Markowitsch, H. J., & Piefke, M. (2010). The Bergen left–right discrimination test: Practice effects, reliable change indices, and strategic performance in the standard and alternate form with inverted stimuli. Cognitive Processing, 15, 159–172.

and rotate). Although the BRLD was not constructed for separate measurement of mental rotation and right–left discrimination, demands on mental rotation abilities is expected to be highest in stimuli that are presented invertedly, as is shown by slower response times on these items compared to noninverted, upright stimuli.

A common disorder of body space is *finger agnosia*, a higher order impairment in naming, orientation, or identification of fingers of oneself or another person. Finger agnosia is viewed as a specific form of autotopagnosia and is generally most evident on examination of the middle three fingers. It is associated with damage to the left angular gyrus. Different assessment procedures exist, most commonly involving patients to identify one (or two) fingers when touched (with and without visual feedback).

10.2.4 Space and Language

Disorders of the spatial domain may involve also language processing (see chapter 6). In categorical spatial representations a person processes the relative spatial location between objects. This is thought to rely in part on language processing: "the chair is to the right of the table"; "the cup is on top of the table." Dedicated testing of spatial language processing is not regularly done in the clinical setting. However, language tests requiring syntactic processing often also include limited testing of spatial language functions. Testing spatial language generally involves a visual scene with two objects and a relational term. Many general tests of language ability or aphasia include items that assess spatial language, such as the Test of Reception of Grammar (Bishop, 1989) or the Token Test subtest of the Aachen Aphasia Test (Huber, Poeck, Weniger, & Willmes, 1983).

10.2.5 Spatial (Working) Memory

Spatial working memory can be assessed with the Corsi Block tapping Test (Kessels, van Zandvoort, Postma, Kappelle, & de Haan, 2000) or similar variants (Berch, Krikorian, & Huha, 1998; Wechsler, 2009) which involves a series of blocks of increasing span length to be tapped by the patient in forward or backward manner (see also chapter 7). Conceptually, the task is highly similar to verbal digit span tasks, but because of the visual presentation the distinction between forward (attention span) and backward (working memory span) conditions is not as clear-cut (Kessels, van den Berg, Ruis, & Brands, 2008). With regard to *spatial long-term memory* a wide range of nonverbal tests is available. One of the most well-known procedures is the immediate and delayed recall of the Rey Complex Figure (Rey, 1964). Patients have to copy the figure and afterward have to draw it from memory. As stated above the copy part of the test measures several functions, including visuospatial perception, visuospatial construction, attention, planning, and executive functioning. A major drawback of the memory part of the Rey Complex Figure Test is that it is heavily confounded by how well a person was able to copy the figure in the first place. It is highly conceivable that a fragmented copy is less well recalled, and this could be unrelated to memory functioning. A more recent and well-validated test involving object location memory is the Location Learning Test (Bucks, Willison, & Byrne, 2000) that consists of a learning phase of 10 pictures of objects placed in a 6 by 6 array. After a 15- or 30-second learning phase, patients are presented with a blank array and 10 cards that each depict an object that was present in the learning phase. Patients have to put all cards on the blank array and a displacement score is calculated. This procedure is repeated five times in total and also consists of a delay trial after 20–30 minutes. A learning index can be calculated as a measure of the steepness of the slope while encoding. The delayed recall procedure indicates the level of retention. While this test is a valid visuospatial alternative for the commonly used Rey Auditory Verbal Learning Test, one has to keep in mind that it is not a nonverbal test per se. Patients can use verbal strategies in the learning phase to remember to location of the object ("the envelope is placed above the keys"). To address these verbal learning strategies in visuospatial memory tasks the Continuous Visual Memory Test (CVMT) was developed (Trahan & Larrabee, 1988). In this test 112 abstract designs are shown with 7 target designs that are repeated 6 times. Patients are asked to discriminate the new stimuli from the repeated stimuli. The task reduces the confounding influence of verbal encoding strategies by using complex, ambiguous designs that restrict verbal labeling. Despite the intuitive design of this task, evidence for involvement of the (nondominant) temporal lobe in performance of the CVMT is limited (Snitz, Roman, & Beniak, 1996). Because of the recognition paradigm, the CVMT is currently recognized as a valuable addition to measuring symptom validity (Henry & Enders, 2007).

10.2.6 Navigation

Tasks to investigate a person's ability to find their way in the world are scarce in standard neuropsychological assessments, but deficits in navigational skills can be readily apparent by asking a person to go from point A to point B. In the Rivermead Behavioral Memory test a specific item has the examiner tracing a short route within the test room (six sections) (Wilson, Cockburn, & Baddeley, 1991). The examinee is next required to retrace the route immediately. Another standardized assessment can be performed by administering a maze test. The Porteus Maze test (Porteus, 1950), for example, consists of multiple mazes in which a person needs to trace the maze printed on paper without entering blind alleys. It requires planning and thinking ahead and thus places a heavy burden on executive functioning. Performance on the Porteus Maze test indeed correlates with other measures of planning, such as the Tower of London and the Wisconsin Card Sorting Test. One of the shortcomings of maze tests is that they may invoke verbal coding strategies. Moreover, performing these mazes takes place in peripersonal space without body updating (see however the use of locomotor mazes, Howard & Templeton, 1966). Most importantly, landmark-based, more allocentric navigation is not assessed. As such, a more promising manner to test navigation and examine its different cognitive elements involves navigation in virtual reality environments. One example discussed in more length in chapter 8 is aspects of navigation is the Virtual Tübingen task (see also chapter 8), where a person watches a movie of a route through the (virtual) German city of Tübingen and is asked a variety of questions concerning scene recognition, route knowledge, and other aspects of navigation ability afterward. This task illustrates the use of virtual reality-based procedures to examine the underlying cause of navigational problems for different patients. Important advantages are control of pretest familiarity, resemblance to natural environments (ecological validity), and the fact that also patients with limited physical mobility can participate. At the same time a disadvantage of virtual reality navigation is that the locomotion components are excluded.

10.3 COMPLAINTS IN SPATIAL COGNITION: SUGGESTIONS FOR HISTORY TAKING

An important part of the neuropsychological assessment is history taking. Questions about cognitive complaints but also about daily functioning lead to more specific neuropsychological hypotheses and guides the choice of the type of tests that will be administrated. Clinicians are used to ask detailed questions about memory performance, attention, and executive functioning in daily life. Questions regarding spatial cognition are less frequently asked, which may lead to underreporting of complaints. The following questions may aid clinical assessment of spatial cognition (see Box 10.3, based on the clinical experience of the authors). Clinicians are advised to adjust the questions according to patient-specific circumstances.

BOX 10.3 Suggestions for History Taking

1. Do you experience problems in finding your way...
   ... to familiar places, such as the grocery store or going to work?
   ... to unfamiliar places, for example, when you are on holiday?
   ... back to the starting point when hiking a trail?
2. Can you find your way back to your car when you leave this building?
3. Can you visualize your surroundings to determine where you are?
4. When you ask directions, do you prefer a verbal description ("go left at the next street") or a drawn map?
5. Do you use/recognize landmarks such as churches, bridges, or crossroads when you visit a city?
6. Can you point toward the main exit in the building where you currently are?
7. Do you experience problems in reading a map?
8. Do you play games? Can you think ahead when playing chess or checkers?
9. Can you imagine to turn small objects to see the back or the bottom?
10. Can you estimate how much luggage fits in a suitcase or how much wrapping paper is needed to wrap a gift?
11. Do you experience difficulty in estimating distance or size, for example, in traffic of while putting your cup on a table?
12. Do your body parts feel like they below to your body?
13. Do you experience difficulty in distinguishing left or right?
14. Can you describe what is behind you when standing in your living room facing the window?

10.4 REHABILITATION

Cognitive rehabilitation has rapidly expanded in the last decades. Patients who experience brain damage, such as stroke or traumatic brain injury, are currently provided detailed guidance to optimize their recovery and, most importantly, to aid that person in obtaining or maintaining

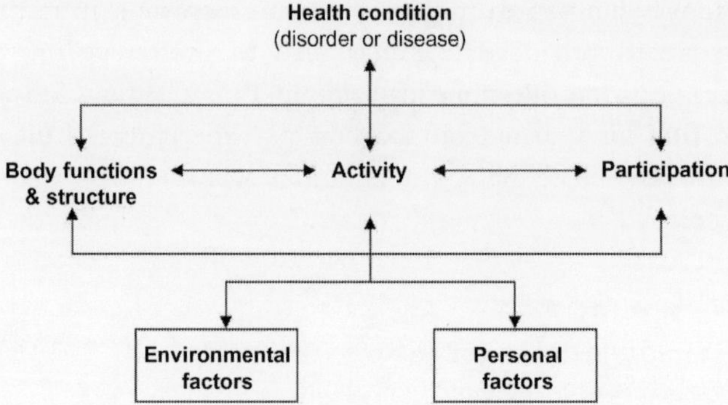

Figure 10.6 ICF model. World Health Organization (2001). International Classification of Functioning, Disability and Health (ICF), resolution WHA 54.21.

physical, psychological, social, and vocational well-being. The International Classification of Functioning, Disability and Health (ICF) Model (World Health Organization, 2001) provides a conceptual framework to classify the consequences of brain damage into different levels of functioning (Fig. 10.6): impairment in body functions/structure, activity, and participation. With regard to the case description at the start of this chapter, the hippocampal atrophy and the navigational impairments observed in neuropsychological assessment would be considered impairment at the level of body function/structure. His inability to find his way while using his car or bicycle can be classified as impairment at the activity level. Should this impairment lead to inability to successfully manage his job or social activities, then this would be considered impairment at the level of participation.

This distinction in levels of functioning already shows that cognitive rehabilitation as a whole is not one clear-cut treatment and that measuring effectiveness of any such rehabilitation method can be challenging. Three different types of cognitive rehabilitation methods are generally distinguished (for an overview see eg, Wilson, 1997). Classic cognitive rehabilitation comprises of "drill and practise" exercises. The assumption behind this approach is to remediate or retrain deficits in cognitive functioning. With regard to spatial cognition this would, for example, imply a person to be trained in finding the solution in a computerized maze-task. Retraining exercises appear intuitive and are thought to stimulate dendritic sprouting of neurons in associated areas in the brain, but evidence for its effectiveness at this level is very limited. Moreover, at the level of functioning there is a clear problem of generalization of these types of procedures. While a person may develop considerable skill in the trained task, there is no convincing evidence that the cognitive processes that underlie this skill improve and, furthermore, one may question whether a person can find his way better in day-to-day life. This line of reasoning has led to the development of rehabilitation methods focused on strategy training. This view of cognitive rehabilitation is focused on teaching patients alternative behaviors to compensate for impaired functions. Patients can learn to optimally use remaining spatial functions or use other cognitive functions, such as verbal memory, to counter spatial deficits. In case of severe deficits external compensatory strategies can be used. With regard to spatial cognition deficits some compensatory strategies are easily applied. Patients may learn to use computerized navigation in their car or on their smartphones (see Box 10.4). Specific routes can be

BOX 10.4 Dealing With Navigation Problems (Case XX)

Ten years after the onset of the navigation complaints and 3 years after the neuropsychological assessment that revealed a significant navigation disorder, XX still has to cope with his cognitive deficits every day. His complaints did not diminish over time; he still gets lost sometimes in his hometown, even on routes that he has successfully used several times before. The complaints make XX uncertain, especially when he is among other people. In the past 10 years, XX has learned to cope with his deficits in a way that they are hampering his daily life less. He makes use of several compensatory strategies. He uses navigation tools on his cell phone to find his way through the city. Making use of such a tool is helpful for XX to stay calm, instead of feeling anxious of whether he would find his way around. Furthermore, XX taught himself to make very specific notes about the place where he parked his car or bike (how far down the street, on which side, front of the care pointing in which direction), so that he could find back the specific place more easily.

trained in real life to ensure better recovery from memory. Patients can learn to make use of landmarks in their day-to-day surroundings or memorize verbal descriptions of well-known routes ("go left at the third crossing"). With regard to hemispatial neglect promising results are observed following prism adaptation (see chapter X). A relatively new method that is particularly of interest in spatial cognition is the use of virtual reality. Chapter X already showed some applications with regard to navigation problems. Virtual reality allows for complete control over information presented to patients and provides real world-like surroundings available for training.

In *holistic* neuropsychological rehabilitation (Ben-Yishay & Gold, 1990) different methods are combined. It may consist of inventions directed at remediation of cognitive deficits, but explicitly includes interventions focused on emotional mastery, interpersonal communication, and social competencies. All interventions are focused on effective use of residual cognitive abilities, rather than restoration of cognitive impairments per se. In this approach rehabilitation of deficits in spatial cognition can also be focused on fear of losing one's way or the impact of dependence on others or external aid on a person's feeling of self-worth.

10.5 SUMMARY AND CONCLUSION

Complaints in spatial cognition are common following brain damage. Despite hampering everyday functioning, these complaints are underreported and rarely assessed in clinical practice. However, different measures of spatial memory, perception, and attention are available. Fewer published tests focus on body space and spatial language. Detailed questions about spatial cognition and administration of specific space tests can be a valuable addition to the neuropsychological assessment. In our view, investigating cognitive complaints and assessment of the spatial domain should be part of routine neuropsychological assessment. This is relevant for all persons who suffer from brain damage, but may be particularly evident for patients suffering from relatively mild brain damage, who are expected to return to their professional lives and may be greatly hampered by a diminished ability to find their way around. Neuropsychological assessment should at a minimum include measures of spatial memory and perception, for which several validated measures are currently available.

REFERENCES

Benton, A., & Tranel, D. (1993). Visuoperceptual, visuospatial, and visuoconstructive disorders. In K. M. Heilman, & E. Valenstein (Eds.), *Clinical Neuropsychology* (3rd editon, pp. 165–214). New York: Oxford University Press.

Benton, A. L., Hannay, H. J., & Varney, N. R. (1975). Visual perception of line direction in patients with unilateral brain disease. *Neurology, 25*, 907–910.

Ben-Yishay, Y., & Gold, I. (1990). Therapeutic mileau approach to neuropsychological rehabilitation. In R. L. Wood (Ed.), *Neurobehavioral Sequelae of Traumatic Brain Injury* (pp. 194–218). New York: Taylor & Francis.

Berch, D. B., Krikorian, R., & Huha, E. M. (1998). The Corsi block-tapping task: Methodological and theoretical considerations. *Brain and Cognition*, *38*, 317–338.

Biesbroek, J. M., van Zandvoort, M. J., Kuijf, H. J., Weaver, N. A., Kappelle, L. J., Vos, P. C., & Utrecht, V. C. I. Study Group (2014). The anatomy of visuospatial construction revealed by lesion–symptom mapping. *Neuropsychologia*, *62*, 68–76.

Bishop, D. V. (1989). *Test of reception of grammar* (2nd ed.) Manchester: Age & Cognitive Performance Research Center, University of Manchester.

Bucks, R. S., Willison, J. R., & Byrne, L. M. T. (2000). *Location Learning Test*. Burry St. Edmunds, UK: Thames Valley Test Company.

Collaer, M. L., & Nelson, J. D. (2002). Large visuospatial sex difference in line judgment: Possible role of attentional factors. *Brain and Cognition*, *49*(1), 1–12.

Gauthier, L., Dehaut, F., & Joanette, Y. (1989). The Bells Test: A quantitative and qualitative test for visual neglect. *International Journal of Clinical Neuropsychology*, *11*, 49–54.

Goodglass, H., Kaplan, E., & Barresi, B. (2001). *Boston diagnostic aphasia examination* (3rd ed.). Philadelphia: Lippincott Williams & Wilkins.

Grewe, P., Ohmann, H. A., Markowitsch, H. J., & Piefke, M. (2010). The Bergen left–right discrimination test: Practice effects, reliable change indices, and strategic performance in the standard and alternate form with inverted stimuli. *Cognitive Processing*, *15*, 159–172.

Halligan, P. W., Cockburn, J., & Wilson, B. A. (1991). The behavioural assessment of visual neglect. *Neuropsychological Rehabilitation*, *1*, 5–32.

Hannay, H. J., Falgout, J. C., Leli, D. A., Katholl, C. A., Halsey, J. H., & Wills, E. L. (1987). Focal right temporo-occipital blood flow changes associated with judgment of line orientation. *Neuropsychologia*, *25*, 755–763.

Henry, G. K., & Enders, C. (2007). Probable malingering and performance on the Continuous Visual Memory Test. *Applied Neuropsychology.*, *14*(4), 267–274.

Hochstenbach, J., Prigatano, G., & Mulder, T. (2005). Patients' and relatives' reports of disturbances 9 months after stroke: Subjective changes in physical functioning, cognition, emotion, and behavior. *Archives of Physical Medicine and Rehabiliation*, *86*, 1587–1593.

Howard, I. P., & Templeton, W. B. (1966). *Human spatial orientation*. London: Wiley.

Huber, W., Poeck, K., Weniger, D., & Willmes, K. (1983). *Der Aachener Aphasie Test (AAT)*. Göttingen: Hogrefe.

Kessels, R. P., van den Berg, E., Ruis, C., & Brands, A. M. (2008). The backward span of the Corsi Block-Tapping Task and its association with the WAIS-III Digit Span. *Assessment*, *15*, 426–434.

Kessels, R. P., van Zandvoort, M. J., Postma, A., Kappelle, L. J., & de Haan, E. H. (2000). The Corsi Block-Tapping Task: Standardization and normative data. *Applied Neuropsychology*, *7*, 252–258.

Lezak, M. D., Howieson, D. B., Bigler, E. D., & Tranel, D. (2012). *Neuropsychological assessment* (5th ed.) New York: Oxford University Press.

Moè, A., Meneghetti, C., & Cadinu, M. (2009). Women and mental rotation: Incremental theory and spatial strategy use enhance performance. *Personality and Individual Differences*, *46*, 187–191.

Monahan, J. S., Harke, M. A., & Shelley, J. R. (2008). Computerizing the mental rotations test: Are gender differences maintained? *Behavior Research Methods*, *40*, 422–427.

Porteus, S. (1950). *The Porteus maze test and intelligence*. Palo Alto: Pacific Books.

Rey, A. (1964). *L'examen clinique en psychologie [Clinical assessment in psychology]*. Paris, France: Presses Universitaires de France.

Riddoch, M. J., & Humphreys, G. W. (1993). *The Birmingham Object Recognition Battery*. London: Erlbaum.

Ruis, C., Postma, A., Bouvy, W., & van der Ham, I. (2015). Cognitive disorders after sporadic ecstasy use? A case report. *Neurocase*, *21*, 351–357.

Schenkenberg, T., Bradford, D. C., & Ajax, E. T. (1980). Line bisection and unilateral visual neglect in patients with neurologic impairment. *Neurology*, *30*, 509–517.

Shepard, R. N., & Metzler, J. T. (1971). Mental rotation of three dimensional objects. *Science*, *171*, 701–703.

Snitz, B. E., Roman, D. D., & Beniak, T. E. (1996). Efficacy of the Continuous Visual Memory Test in lateralizing temporal lobe dysfunction in chronic complex-partial epilepsy. *Journal of Clinical and Experimental Neuropsychology.*, *18*(5), 747–754.

Trahan, D. E., & Larrabee, G. J. (1988). *Continuous Visual Memory Test: Professional manual.* Odessa, FL: Psychological Assessment Resources.

Tranel, D., Vianna, E., Manzel, K., Damasio, H., & Grabowski, T. (2009). Neuroanatomical correlated of the Benton Facial Recognition Test and Judgment of Line Orientation Test. *Journal of Clinical and Experimental Neuropsychology*, *31*, 219–233.

Treccani, B., & Cubelli, R. (2011). The need for a revised version of the Benton judgment of line orientation test. *Journal of Clinical and Experimental Neuropsychology*, *33*(2), 249–256.

Treccani, B., Torri, T., & Cubelli, R. (2005). Is judgement of line orientation selectively impaired in right brain damaged patients? *Neuropsychologia*, *43*(4), 598–608.

Vandenberg, S. G., & Kruse, A. R. (1978). Mental rotations, a group test of three dimensional spatial visualization. *Perceptual and Motor Skills*, *47*, 599–604.

Warrington, E. K., & James, M. (1991). *The visual object and space perception battery (VOSP).* Bury St. Edmunds, England: Thames Valley Test Co.

Wechsler, D. (2009). *Wechsler Memory Scale (WMS-IV).* New York: The Psychological Corporation.

Wilson, B., Cockburn, J., & Baddeley, A. (1991). *The Rivermead behavioural memory test manual.* Bury St. Edmunds, Suffolk: Thames Valley Test Corporation.

Wilson, B. A., Cockburn, J., & Halligan, P. (1988). *Behavioural Inattention Test.* Flempton: Thamse Valley Test Company.

Wilson, B. A. (1997). Cognitive rehabilitation: How it is and how it might be. *Journal of International Neuropsychological Society*, *3*, 487–496.

World Health Organization. (2001). International Classification of Functioning, Disability and Health (ICF), resolution WHA 54.21.

INDEX

Note: Page numbers followed by "*b*," "*f*," and "*t*" refer to boxes, figures, and tables, respectively.

N

O

T

U

V

W

Printed and bound by CPI Group (UK) Ltd, Croydon, CR0 4YY

11/06/2025

01899189-0003